Recurrent Pregnancy Loss

SERIES IN MATERNAL-FETAL MEDICINE

Forthcoming

Vincenzo Berghella, *Obstetric Evidence Based Guidelines*
ISBN 9780415701884

Vincenzo Berghella, *Maternal-Fetal Evidence Based Guidelines*
ISBN 9780415432818

Of related interest

Joseph J Apuzzio, Anthony M Vintzelos, Leslie Iffy, *Operative Obstetrics*
ISBN 9781842142844

Isaac Blickstein, Louis G Keith, *Prenatal Assessment of Multiple Pregnancy*
ISBN 9780415384247

Tom Bourne, George Condous, *Handbook of Early Pregnancy Care*
ISBN 9781842143230

Gian Carlo Di Renzo, Umberto Simeoni, *The Prenate and Neonate: The transition to extrauterine life*
ISBN 9781842140444

Asim Kurjak, Guillermo Azumendi, *The Fetus in Three Dimensions: Imaging, Embryology and Fetoscopy*
ISBN 9780415375238

Asim Kurjak, Frank A Chervenak, *Textbook of Perinatal Medicine,* second edition
ISBN 9781842143339

Catherine Nelson-Piercy, *Handbook of Obstetric Medicine,* third edition
ISBN 9781841845807

Dario Paladini, Paolo Volpe, *Ultrasound of Congenital Fetal Anomalies*
ISBN 9780415414449

Donald M Peebles, Leslie Myatt, *Inflammation and Pregnancy*
ISBN 9781842142721

Felice Petraglia, Jerome F Strauss, Gerson Weiss, Steven G Gabbe, *Preterm Birth: Mechanisms, Mediators, Prediction, Prevention and Interventions*
ISBN 9780415392273

Ruben A Quintero, *Twin-Twin Transfusion Syndrome*
ISBN 9781842142981

Baskaran Thilaganathan, Shanthi Sairam, Aris T Papageorghiou, Amor Bhide, *Problem Based Obstetric Ultrasound*
ISBN 9780415407281

Recurrent Pregnancy Loss Causes, Controversies and Treatment

Edited by

Howard JA Carp MB BS FRCOG

Professor, Department of Obstetrics and Gynecology
Sheba Medical Center
Tel Hashomer
and
Sackler School of Medicine
Tel Aviv University
Tel Aviv
Israel

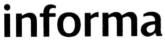
healthcare

© 2007 Informa UK Ltd

First published in the United Kingdom in 2007 by Informa Healthcare, Telephone House, 69–77 Paul Street, London, EC2A 4LQ. Informa Healthcare is a trading division of Informa UK Ltd. Registered office, 37/41 Mortimer Street, London W1T 3JH. Registered in England and Wales number 1072954.

Tel: +44 (0)20 7017 5000
Fax: +44 (0)20 7017 6336
Website: www.informahealthcare.com

Although every effort has been made to ensure that all owners of copyright material have been acknowledged in this publication, we would be glad to acknowledge in subsequent reprints or editions any omissions brought to our attention.

Although every effort has been made to ensure that drug doses and other information are presented accurately in this publication, the ultimate responsibility rests with the prescribing physician. Neither the publishers nor the authors can be held responsible for errors or for any consequences arising from the use of information contained herein. For detailed prescribing information or instructions on the use of any product or procedure discussed herein, please consult the prescribing information or instructional material issued by the manufacturer.

A CIP record for this book is available from the British Library.

Library of Congress Cataloging-in-Publication Data

Data available on application

ISBN-10: 0 415 42130 6
ISBN-13: 978 0 415 42130 0

Distributed in North and South America by
Taylor & Francis
6000 Broken Sound Parkway, NW (Suite 300)
Boca Raton, FL 33487, USA

Within Continental USA
Tel: 1 (800) 272 7737; Fax: 1 (800) 374 3401
Outside Continental USA
Tel: (561) 994 0555; Fax: (561) 361 6018
Email: orders@crcpress.com

Distributed in the rest of the world by
Thomson Publishing Services
Cheriton House
North Way
Andover, Hampshire SP10 5BE, UK
Tel: +44 (0)1264 332424
Email: tps.tandfsalesorder@thomson.com

Composition by CEPHA IMAGING PVT LTD, Bangalore, India.

Printed and bound in India by Replika Press Pvt. Ltd.

Contents

Contributors

Eytan R Barnea MD FACOG
Chairman, The Society for the Investigation of
    Early Pregnancy
Clinical Associate Professor of Obstetrics,
    Gynecology and Reproductive Sciences
UMDNJ/Robert Wood Johnson Medical School
Cherry Hill, NJ
USA

Miri Blank PhD
Associate Professor of Immunology
Sackler Faculty of Medicine
Tel-Aviv University
and
Center for Autoimmune Diseases
Sheba Medical Center
Tel-Hashomer
Israel

Zvi Borochowitz MD
Professor of Pediatrics and Medical Genetics,
Director, Simon Winter Institute for Human
    Genetics
and
Institute for Human Genetics
Technion-Rappaport Faculty of Medicine
Haifa
Israel

Benjamin Brenner MD
Professor of Hematology, Technion Israel Institute
    of Technology
Director, Thrombosis and Hemostasis Unit
Rambam Medical Center
Haifa
Israel

Howard JA Carp MB BS FRCOG
Professor, Department of Obstetrics and
    Gynecology
Sheba Medical Center
Tel Hashomer
and
Sackler School of Medicine
Tel Aviv University
Tel Aviv
Israel

Jerome H Check MD PhD
Robert Wood Johnson Medical School at Camden
Melrose Park, PA
and
University of Medicine and Dentistry of
New Jersey
Newark, NJ
USA

Ole B Christiansen MD DMSC
Fertility Clinic
Rigshospitalet
Copenhagen
Denmark

David Clark MD PhD DiplABIM FRCPC FRCPED
Emeritus Professor of Medicine
McMaster University
Hamilton
Ontario
Canada

Carolyn Coulam MD
Director, Millennova Immunology Laboratories;
Director, Pregnancy Loss Center
and
Director of Research, Rinehart Center for
    Reproductive Medicine
Chicago, IL
USA

Howard Cuckle MA MSc DPhil
Adjunct Professor of Obstetrics and Gynecology
Columbia University
New York, NY
USA
and
Emeritus Professor
University of Leeds
Leeds
UK

Salim Daya MBChB MSc FRCSC
Hamilton
Ontario
Canada

Paul Devroey MD PhD
Professor, Centre for Reproductive Medicine
University Hospital
Dutch-speaking Brussels Free University
Belgium

Patricio Donoso MD
Centre for Reproductive Medicine
University Hospital
Dutch-speaking Brussels Free University
Belgium

Roy G Farquharson MD FRCOG
Clinical Director, Liverpool Women's Hospital
Liverpool
UK

Andrea Riccardo Genazzani MD PhD
Director of Obstetrics and Gynecology
Hospital S Chiara
University of Pisa
Pisa
Italy

Mordechai Goldenberg MD
Professor, Chaim Sheba Medical Center
Tel-Hashomer
and
The Sackler School of Medicine
Tel Aviv University
Tel Aviv
Israel

Mindy Gross
Ra'anana
Israel

JG Grudzinskas MD
The London Bridge Fertility
Gynaecology and Genetics Centre
London
UK

Nigel Harris MD DM
Vice Chancellor, University of West Indies
Kingston
Jamaica

Israel Hendler MD
Assistant Professor, Wayne State University
Detroit, MI
USA
and
Sheba Medical Center
Tel Hashomer
Israel

Aida Inbal MD
Associate Professor of Hematology
Sackler Faculty of Medicine
Tel Aviv University
and
Director of Thrombosis and Hemostasis Unit
Rabin Medical Center
Petah Tikva
Israel

Lucia Lazzeri MD
Section of Obstetrics and Gynecology
Policlinics Le Scotte
University of Siena
Siena
Italy

Pelle G Lindqvist MD PhD
Associate Professor and Senior Consultant
Malmö University Hospital
Malmö
Sweden

Stefano Luisi MD PhD
Section of Obstetrics and Gynecology
Policlinics Le Scotte
University of Siena
Siena
Italy

Shazia Malik MBChB (hon), MRCOG
St Mary's Hospital NHS Trust
London
UK

Thomas Philipp MD
Assistant Professor
Ludwig Boltzman Institute of Gynecology and
    Obstetrics
Danube Hospital
Vienna
Austria

Siobhan M Quenby MD MRCOG
Senior Lecturer, University Department of
    Obstetrics and Gynaecology
Liverpool Women's Hospital
Liverpool
UK

Raj Rai BSc MD MRCOG
Senior Lecturer and Consultant Gynaecologist
Imperial College London
St Mary's Hospital
London
UK

Lesley Regan MD FRCOG
Professor of Obstetrics and Gynaecology
Imperial College London
St Mary's Hospital
London
UK

Daniel S Seidman MD MMSc
Professor, Chaim Sheba Medical Center
Tel-Hashomer
and
Sackler School of Medicine
Tel Aviv University
Tel Aviv
Israel

Keren Shakhar PhD
Department of Oncological Sciences
Mount Sinai School of Medicine
New York, NY
USA

Yaniv Sherer MD
Instructor in Internal Medicine
Sackler Faculty of Medicine
Tel Aviv University
Tel Aviv
and
Center for Autoimmune Diseases
Sheba Medical Center
Tel-Hashomer
Israel

Yehuda Shoenfeld MD
Professor of Internal Medicine
Sackler Faculty of Medicine,
Incumbent of the Laura Schwartz Kipp Chair for
    Research of Autoimmune Diseases
Tel-Aviv University
Tel Aviv
and
Director, Department of Medicine 'B' and Center
    for Autoimmune Diseases
Sheba Medical Center
Tel-Hashomer
Israel

Joe Leigh Simpson MD
Professor of Obstetrics and Gynecology
Professor of Molecular and Human Genetics
Baylor College of Medicine
Houston, TX
USA

Vladimir Toder MD PhD
Professor in Embryology
Sackler School of Medicine
Tel-Aviv University
Ramat-Aviv
Israel

Arkady Torchinsky MD PhD DSc
Principal Research Associate
Sackler School of Medicine
Tel-Aviv University
Ramat-Aviv
Israel

Gilad Twig MD PhD
Center for Autoimmune Diseases
Sheba Medical Center
Tel-Hashomer
and
Sackler Faculty of Medicine
Tel-Aviv University
Tel Aviv
Israel

Andre Van Steirteghem MD PhD
Professor Emeritus
Centre for Reproductive Medicine
University Hospital
Dutch-Speaking Brussels Free University
Belgium

Marighoula Varla-Leftherioti MD PhD
Head of the Immunobiology Department
'Helena Venizelou' Maternity Hospital
Athens
Greece

David Alan Viniker MD FRCOG
Consultant Obstetrician and Gynaecologist
Whipps Cross University Hospital
Loughton
UK

James Walker MD FRCOG FRCP Edin FRCPS Glas
Professor of Obstetrics and Gynaecology
St James's University Hospital
Leeds
UK

Wendell A Wilson MD FRCP
Professor of Medicine, Arthritis and
    Rheumatology
Center of Excellence
Louisiana State University Medical Center
New Orleans, LA
USA

Victor YH Yu MD MSc FRACP FRCP FRCP Ed FRCP Glas
Professor of Neonatology
Clinical Director of Ritchie Centre for Baby
    Health Research
Monash University
Melbourne
Australia

Foreword

'Children are the anchors that hold a mother to life'

Sophocles, *Phaedra*

In almost all traditions, the importance of procreation is inherent in man's very creation; both Old and New Testaments of the Bible refer to the tragic plight of barren women, eloquently describing the pain and agony of childlessness. However, records dated far earlier than the Bible confirm that fertility has been a constant fundamental priority and preoccupation, in all societies, throughout the ages of man. Fertility symbols are clearly identified in the relics of prehistoric times, of ancient civilizations in all parts of the world, a recognition of the concept that man's existence depends upon the renewal of fertility. The above quotation was written by Sophocles 2500 years ago. The ancient Canaanites and Greeks had gods of fertility – Ashtarte and Hermes. Today, infertility is recognized as a disease by the World Health Organization and by numerous healthcare providers throughout the world. Recurrent pregnancy loss represents one aspect of disordered fertility. Recurrent pregnancy loss has been described as the 'orphan' of infertility, as this condition is often overlooked in the larger process of research and management of fertility. Recurrent pregnancy loss is a heterogeneous condition, with numerous causes and numerous treatment options. It is multidisciplinary, involving gynecology, genetics, endocrinology, immunology, pediatrics, and internal medicine. Whatever the cause and possible treatment, the psychological implications are enormous. Both partners may feel that they have failed in their parenting role. Couples have divorced with mutual recriminations, each blaming the other. Even when pregnancy does succeed, it may be fraught with the fear of another loss. This anxiety is multipled when the diagnosis remains unexplained.

This book will be welcomed by many investigators and clinicians working in the field of recurrent pregnancy loss. There are chapters governing basic scientific topics such as cytokines, mechanisms of action of antiphospholipid antibodies, and signaling between mother and fetus. The major advances in genetics, including pregestational diagnosis, immunology, endocrinology, and thrombotic mechanisms, have been described in depth. The methodology of clinical research and the application of evidence-based medicine to clinical practice have been explained comprehensively. The problems of midtrimester loss and late obstetric complications are aired, including the problems associated with extreme prematurity and possible resulting handicaps, and recent views on the role of cerclage in prevention. However, as is inevitable in clinical practice, there are many controversies, leaving the clinician in a quandary, as how to help the patient. Hence, there are six debates, and one opinion article, that try to bring the relevant points before the clinician, to aid in deciding the most appropriate management. However, we must never forget that at the end of the line is a patient. Therefore, the chapter on psychological mechanisms and the connection between psychological mechanisms and the immune and other systems is welcome. The story told by the patient in Chapter 22 is most touching, and reminds us of the real problem at hand.

It is hoped that this book will be read by specialists working in recurrent pregnancy loss clinics and associated disciplines who wish to keep up to date, and generalists who wish to gain a comprehensive view of developments in the field. The 'half-life' of scientific knowledge has been said to be ten years. However, many advances are occurring so quickly that a 'half-life' of ten years seems to be out of date. It is to be hoped that the advances in scientific and clinical knowledge will continue at this pace, in order to improve the management of the patients and to allow those still unable to have children to fulfil this most basic of human desires.

Professor Bruno Lunenfeld MD PhD FRCOG FACOG (Hon) P.O.G.S. (Hon)

Professor Emeritus at Faculty of Life Sciences
Bar-Ilan University
President of the International Society for the Study
of the Aging Male (ISSAM)
General Secretary of The Asian–Pacific Initiative
on Reproductive Endocrinology (ASPIRE)
Member of the Israel Government National
Council for Obstetrics, Genetics and Neonatology

Preface

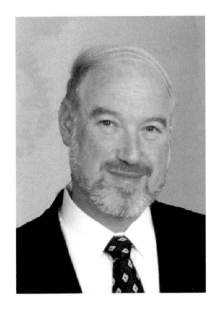

Prof Howard JA Carp MB BS FRCOG
Professor, Department of Obstetrics and Gynecology,
Sheba Medical Center, Tel Hashomer, and
Sackler School of Medicine, Tel Aviv University,
Tel Aviv, Israel

Recurrent pregnancy loss is a vexing clinical problem as the cause often remains unexplained despite the major advances in genetics and immunology. Treatment is often controversial and ranges from "masterly inactivity", to an approach which could be considered as "over aggressive". The problem is distressing to couples, who understandably expect answers and solutions, and frustrating for the physician who often does not have these answers, particularly in the face of ever-changing and conflicting recommendations. This book tries to summarize those controversies, and discuss the scientific basis for various causes of pregnancy loss in depth, and to debate the various treatment modalities which have been used in recent years. Hence, it is hoped that this book describes the accumulating data in a way which is both scientifically sound and also clinically useful, and which may improve the care of these couples.

The book is planned for general gynecologists, and specialists working in the field. Each contributing author is an authority on a specific area of recurrent pregnancy loss. I would like to thank each author for the time and effort taken in preparing the manuscripts to make publication of this book possible. I would also like to thank those responsible in a more indirect way for the publication of this book; my teachers over the years, particularly Prof. Shlomo Mashiach for his constant help and encouragement in my work in recurrent pregnancy loss. Thanks go to my collaborators, Prof's Yehuda Shoenfeld, Aida Inbal, Ephraim Gazit, and Vladimir Toder, and special recognition goes to the greatest teachers of all, the patients.

1. Epidemiology of recurrent pregnancy loss

Ole B Christiansen

INTRODUCTION

Epidemiology can be defined as 'the scientific study of disease frequency, determinants of disease, and the distribution of disease in a population'. The determinants of disease considered in epidemiological studies are normally demographic parameters (age, sex, occupation, and economic status), in addition to some clinical parameters relevant for the specific disease (e.g., tobacco and alcohol consumption, and reproductive and family history) – all information that can be obtained through registers and questionnaires, whereas parameters requiring special interventions such as blood samples are normally not included in purely epidemiological studies.

DEFINITION OF MISCARRIAGE AND RECURRENT PREGNANCY LOSS

The term 'miscarriage' (or 'abortion') is used to describe a pregnancy that fails to progress, resulting in death and expulsion of the embryo or fetus. The generally accepted definition stipulates that the fetus or embryo should weigh 500 g or less – a stage that corresponds to a gestational age of up to 20 weeks, according to the World Health Organization (WHO).[1] Unfortunately, this definition is not used consistently, and pregnancy losses at higher gestational ages are also classified as miscarriage in some studies instead of as stillbirth or preterm neonatal death. Thus, from a definitional perspective, it is important to characterize the population being studied so that comparisons across therapeutic trials can be made more appropriately and reliably.

Recurrent miscarriage should be defined, according to the above definition of miscarriage, as at least three consecutive miscarriages, whereas recurrent pregnancy loss (RPL) could also include pregnancy losses up to gestational week 28. However, there is no consensus regarding the definition of recurrent miscarriage or RPL.[2] Pregnancy losses after week 20 are rare, so defining recurrent miscarriage and RPL as above will result in almost identical populations.

Unfortunately, many studies include women with only two previous miscarriages in studies of recurrent miscarriage/RPL, which, from an epidemiological point of view, is very problematic. This issue will be discussed later.

EPIDEMIOLOGICAL PARAMETERS RELEVANT FOR RPL

OCCURRENCE

The incidence of RPL is the number of new women each year (or in some other defined period) suffering their third consecutive pregnancy loss, while the prevalence of RPL is the number of women in a population who, at a specific timepoint, have had three or more consecutive pregnancy losses. The incidence or prevalence is often expressed as a rate of those individuals being at risk for the disorder. The number in the denominator could be all women in the population, women of fertile age, or women who had attempted pregnancy at least two or three times. Indeed, the estimate of the incidence or prevalence of RPL is very uncertain, since in most countries there is no nationwide registration of miscarriages or RPL, and many early miscarriages are not treated in hospitals and thus are not registered. There is no valid estimate of the incidence of RPL, whereas there are a few estimates of its prevalence. One of the most informative studies of the prevalence of RPL was performed by Alberman,[3] who asked female doctors to report retrospectively about the outcome of their previous pregnancies. Seven hundred and forty-two women had had three previous pregnancies, and 355 women had had four previous pregnancies. Nine women (0.8%) had had three or more consecutive pregnancy losses. This study is probably the best estimate of the prevalence of RPL, since the cohort was restricted to women who had attempted pregnancy at least three times. As the study consisted of physicians, delayed menstruation, induced abortions, ectopic pregnancies, and miscarriages were unlikely to be misclassified. However, since the study was carried out before 1980, many early miscarriages may not have been registered due to a lack of highly sensitive human chorionic gonadotropin (hCG) tests and ultrasound examinations at that time. Furthermore, female doctors may not reflect the background population: they may be healthier than other women, which may lower the miscarriage risk, but (due to their long education) they may be older than other women when attempting pregnancy, which increases the miscarriage risk.

Other estimates of the prevalence of RPL are generally in accordance with that of Alberman. A RPL prevalence of 2.3% was found in 432 randomly identified women in a multicenter study.[4] In a group of 5901 Norwegian women with at least two pregnancies screened for *Toxoplasma* antibodies, 1.4% had experienced RPL.[5] Data from a Danish questionnaire-based study[6] found, in a random sample of 493 women with at least two intrauterine pregnancies, that 0.6% had had at least three consecutive miscarriages, 0.8% at least three consecutive pregnancy losses during all trimesters, and 1.8% at least three, not necessarily consecutive, losses at some time during pregnancy. Overall, these studies thus find the prevalence of RPL to be between 0.6% and 2.3%.

NUMBER OF PREVIOUS MISCARRIAGES

Almost all prospective studies of RPL patients show remarkable consistency in finding an increasing risk of miscarriage as the number of previous miscarriages increases. The chance of subsequent live birth in untreated RPL patients with 3, 4, and 5 or more miscarriages has been found to be 42–86%, 41–72%, and 23–51%, respectively[7–10] (Figure 1.1). The significant variability in the estimate of the subsequent risk of miscarriage in RPL patients can probably be attributed to the time of ascertainment of the pregnancies (Figure 1.2), since the average age of the patients and the duration of follow-up in the various studies were not different. The information in Figure 1.2 is based on the data given in the literature[8,10,11] or data that can unequivocally be deduced from the literature. In studies where the patients are urged to contact the department for inclusion in a treatment trial as soon as menstruation is delayed by 2–3 days, and a highly sensitive pregnancy test is positive,[10] almost all preclinical losses (including biochemical pregnancies) are identified, and the patients will be registered as having a high fetal loss rate (47.1%) but a low non-pregnancy rate (14.7%) during the observation period. In studies where the patients are told to call the department in gestational week 6–7 to be included in treatment trials,[11] or patients are

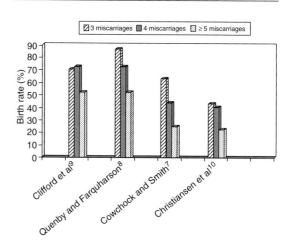

Figure 1.1 Subsequent birth rate according to the number of previous miscarriages in patients with recurrent pregnancy loss reported in four studies of untreated or placebo-treated patients.

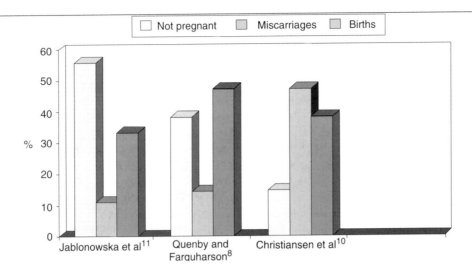

Figure 1.2 Incidence of subsequent live births and miscarriages. Christiansen et al[10] indicated the proportion of miscarriages as preclinical and clinical (56.3% were clinical and 43.7% were preclinical). All miscarriages, except one in the series by Jablonowska et al[11] series and all in the series by Quenby and Farquharson,[8] were clinical. $p = 0.001$ for the differences between the not-pregnant rates and $p < 0.0001$ for differences between the miscarriage rates in the three studies.

enrolled only after ultrasonographic demonstration of fetal heart activity,[8] most preclinical miscarriages are not ascertained, and therefore significantly higher non-pregnancy rates (38.3–55.6%) and significantly lower miscarriage rates (11.1–14.4%) are registered (Figure 1.2). The subsequent probability of a live birth in RPL can best be estimated from the placebo arm of studies of RPL (Figure 1.2), because in placebo-controlled trials the ascertainment of pregnancies is generally better than in non-randomized studies since the patients are included according to a strict protocol and are more closely monitored in early pregnancy. Hence, more very early pregnancy losses are included in placebo-controlled trials and the live birth rate in the placebo-arm is expected to be lower than in non-randomized studies. In accordance with this, Carp et al[12] have shown that the live birth rate in untreated patients in randomized studies was 15–20% lower than that of non-randomized patients independent of the number of previous miscarriages.

The prognostical negative effect of the number of previous miscarriages could, in theory, be attributed to the fact that maternal age and the presence of age-related risk factors for miscarriages are positively correlated to gravidity. However, in multivariate analyses of clinical and paraclinical parameters of potentially prognostic importance in RPL, the number of previous miscarriages has without exception remained the strongest prognostic parameter, even after adjustment for other risk factors.[7,13,14]

MATERNAL AGE

In a register-based study of 634 272 Danish women achieving pregnancy between 1978 and 1992 and who attended a hospital during the pregnancy,[15] the miscarriage rates were almost identical in women of age 30–34 years with RPL and those of age 35–39 (38–40%), but increased to 70% in women aged 40–44 (Figure 1.3). It seems that the impact of age on the miscarriage rate in RPL is quite modest until age 40, but beyond this age it is the strongest prognostic factor. In concordance with this, several multivariate analyses[7,13,14] of prognostic variables for live births in RPL patients (almost all of whom were

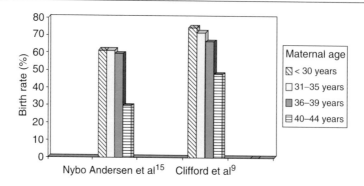

Figure 1.3 Subsequent birth rate according to maternal age in patients with recurrent pregnancy loss.

younger than 40) found that maternal age was not a significant predictor of miscarriage after adjustment for other relevant independent variables, the adjusted odds ratios (OR) for live birth being very similar in two studies: 0.93 (95% confidence interval (CI) 0.8–1.1)[7] and 0.94 (95% CI 0.9–1.0).[13]

SUBGROUPS OF RPL

The pregnancy history in women with RPL may include pregnancies that have ended in live births. Three different groups can be identified that should be assessed separately:

- The primary RPL group consists of women with three or more consecutive pregnancy losses with no pregnancy progressing beyond 20 weeks gestation.
- The secondary RPL group consists of women who have had three or more pregnancy losses following a pregnancy that progressed beyond 20 weeks' gestation (which may have ended in live birth, or less commonly a stillbirth or neonatal death).
- The tertiary RPL group (which is a group that has not been well characterized or studied) consists of women who have had several pregnancy losses before a pregnancy that progressed beyond 20 weeks' gestation followed by at least three more pregnancy losses.[12]

In some studies, secondary RPL is defined as RPL after a live birth or a pregnancy that progressed beyond gestational week 28;[12,16] however, in this survey, 20 weeks is taken as the cut-off point.

Unfortunately, few studies separate the patients into primary or secondary RPL, which may indicate that the authors consider the two disorders as identical entities. It is indeed possible that secondary RPL is not a particular entity but just the clinical appearance of the RPL syndrome among patients who, by chance, instead of delivering a child after three or four miscarriages deliver an infant in the first pregnancy and subsequently experience a series of miscarriages. However, if the chance of delivering a child is equal in all consecutive pregnancies of women destined to experience RPL, we would expect the prevalence of patients with secondary RPL and at least four miscarriages who delivered a child in the first pregnancy to be equal to that of those who had delivered a child in the second pregnancy. We studied a cohort of patients with secondary RPL and four miscarriages[17,18] and found that four times as many had had a successful outcome in the first pregnancy compared with the second pregnancy (Table 1.1). Since it is unlikely that patients in the latter group have a lower likelihood of being admitted to our clinic than patients in the former group, we conclude that the risk of suffering RPL is much higher after a birth in the first pregnancy than in the second pregnancy. This observation supports the theory that some risk

Table 1.1 Distribution of patients with secondary recurrent pregnancy loss (RPL) and at at least four miscarriages according to the order of the birth in the pregnancy sequence

Pregnancy outcomes[a]	Type of RPL	Observed prevalence	Expected prevalence	p-value
B, M, M, M, M,...	Secondary RPL	82 (79.6%)	51.5[b] (50.0%)	< 0.00005
M, B, M, M, M,...	Secondary RPL	21 (20.4%)	51.5[b] (50.0%)	

[a]B, birth; M, miscarriage.
[b]Expected distribution of patients with secondary RPL and at least four miscarriages.

factors for RPL have a high chance of developing during the first ongoing pregnancy and that secondary RPL is not a chance phenomenon.

If primary and secondary RPL have different pathophysiological backgrounds, we should expect different prognoses for the two conditions. Summarizing the placebo-treated patients included in our placebo-controlled trials of immunotherapy,[10,19] the live birth rate was 17/35 = 48.6% in the first pregnancy in women with primary RPL, compared with 11/34 = 32.4% in women with secondary RPL (not significantly different) matched for number of previous miscarriages and age. Other studies have reported success rates[8,9] in the two subsets that are not different, which must be considered to be the commonly accepted view.

In the secondary RPL group, however, the sex of the firstborn seems to affect the prognosis. In a prospective study of 182 patients with secondary RPL followed up from 1986 to 2002,[17] the cumulative chance of giving birth to a child after a series of miscarriages was 58% in patients with a male firstborn, compared with 76% in those with a female firstborn ($p = 0.01$). The hazard ratio for a live birth (the relative chance for live birth adjusted for the follow-up period and a series of prognostic factors) in patients with a male firstborn was 0.59 (95% CI 0.41–0.86) compared with those with a female firstborn. The previous birth of a boy is therefore a prognostic negative factor in these patients, which may be attributed to immunization against male-specific minor histocompatibility antigens (HY antigens) in the first ongoing pregnancy.

RPL patients with second-trimester losses also constitute a subset with particular characteristics. Drakeley et al[20] found that 25% of their RPL patients had had at least one second-trimester loss. Among 228 RPL patients admitted to our clinic in 2000–2004, 39 (17.1%) had experienced a mixture of first- and second-trimester miscarriages, but only three had suffered exclusively second-trimester losses. Since almost all patients with second-trimester miscarriages had experienced at least one first-trimester miscarriage, early and late RPL must have pathogenetic factors that partially overlap – but the observation that the overwhelming majority of patients only suffer first-trimester miscarriages suggests that some pathogenetic factors are specific for those with early miscarriages. Several prospective studies indicate that a history of one or more second-trimester pregnancy losses is a strong risk factor for a poor prognosis,[21,22] which also suggests that some pathogenetic factors are specific for patients with late losses.

FAMILIAL AGGREGATION

Few studies have investigated the genetics of RPL in families of RPL couples with normal chromosomes. Results from the published family studies are shown in Table 1.2. Johnson et al[23] and Alexander et al[24] compared the prevalence of three not necessarily consecutive miscarriages among blood relatives of women with RPL with the corresponding prevalence in relatives of fertile controls. Ho et al[25] compared the prevalence of RPL in relatives of couples with RPL with that in relatives of fertile control couples. The data concerning the relatives were those stated by the probands. Christiansen et al[26] obtained information concerning relatives' pregnancy outcomes from questionnaires completed by the relatives themselves, and the stated pregnancy

Table 1.2 Studies of occurrence of recurrent pregnancy loss (RPL) in relatives of women with RPL

Reference and kind of relatives studied	RPL rate in relatives (%)	RPL rate in controls (%)	p-value
Johnson et al[23] Blood relatives	12.2	7.3	
Alexander et al[24] Mothers and sisters	7.0	0.0	0.02
Ho et al[25] First degree relatives	1.4	0.2	0.0001
Christiansen et al[26] Sisters	10.6	1.8	0.00005
Brothers' wives	6.3	1.8	NS

NS, not significant.

loses were confirmed from hospitals' and practitioners' records. The prevalence of at least three, not necessarily consecutive, pregnancy losses in relatives with at least two pregnancies was compared with an external control group.[6] Table 1.2 shows that the risk of RPL in first-degree relatives of RPL patients is 2–7 times higher than in the background population. The relative frequency λ (the frequency of RPL in relatives divided by the frequency in the general population) is a measure of the degree of heritability of a disorder: the higher the value of λ, the higher is the genetic component. For type 1 ('insulin-dependent') diabetes mellitus, λ for sisters is 15, suggesting a high degree of heritability. In the Danish RPL study,[26] λ can be calculated to be 5.9 for sisters and 3.5 for brothers's wives when compared with the prevalence in the general population,[6] indicating a moderate degree of heritability. If a condition is determined by multifactorial or polygenic inheritance, it is expected that λ equals the inverse square root of the population prevalence, i.e., $1/\sqrt{0.018} = 7.5$, which is very close to the observed λ in sisters, and this emphasizes the hypothesis that RPL is a disorder following a polygenic mode of inheritance.[27]

PARTNER SPECIFICITY

It is commonly assumed that unexplained RPL is a partner-specific condition, and a criterion that all pregnancies should be with the same partner has been included in the definition of primary and secondary RPL by some authors.[28] However, no study has really addressed the question of partner specificity. Out of 228 RPL patients admitted to our clinic in 2000–2004, 38 (16.7%) had experienced miscarriages with two or more partners, and with regard to pregnancy prognosis they do not behave differently from those who had all pregnancies with the same partner. In a multivariate analysis (Nielsen et al, unpublished work), we have found that, after adjustment for all relevant prognostic factors, the chance of a subsequent live birth was not different in patients with secondary RPL who have had all pregnancies with the same partner compared with those who have had two different partners. The observation that there is a clear familial predisposition to RPL, at least in the female partner (Table 1.2), also argues against RPL as being partner-specific.

CLINICAL ASSOCIATIONS

An association has been found between RPL and various late obstetric complications. These are fully described in Chapter 16.

LIFESTYLE FACTORS

Lifestyle factors are rarely, if ever, major causes of RPL; however, epidemiological studies have indicated that a series of lifestyle factors can increase the risk of miscarriage. There is good evidence that obesity,[29,30] high daily caffeine intake,[31–34] alcohol consumption,[34] and use of non-steroidal anti-inflammatory drugs[35,36] increase the risk of miscarriage significantly. Social class and occupation also increase the chance of miscarriage, with the greatest risk ocurring in women exposed to high physical or psychological stress during work.[37,38] Several studies now also indicate that previous subfertility or infertility treatment may increase the risk of miscarriage.[14,39]

INTEGRATION OF EPIDEMIOLOGICAL FACTORS IN THE RESEARCH AND MANAGEMENT OF RPL

OCCURRENCE

Estimation of the prevalence of RPL has several applications: it can be used for comparing risks of RPL between different populations or in subgroups within the same population, and it can be used for comparing change in risk over time – which is necessary for identifying risk factors. Furthermore, the observation that the prevalence of RPL is greater than 1% indicates that RPL is not a random event but rather a disorder affecting women who have an increased risk of pregnancy loss. In theory, a woman could have RPL, and each of the three consecutive pregnancy losses may be caused by the same factors as those causing 'sporadic' miscarriages, especially fetal chromosome abnormalities. However, if all RPL cases were caused by a random accumulation of 'sporadic' miscarriages, the prevalence of RPL should be $0.14^3 = 0.27\%$ (based on a prevalence of 14% for single pregnancy loss[6]) rather than 1%. The prevalence of 1% indicates that at least three out of four RPL cases are caused by non-random factors that increase the risk of miscarriage in each pregnancy.

NUMBER OF MISCARRIAGES

It is clear from the evidence showing that the number of previous miscarriages is the most important prognostic factor in RPL that this parameter has to be taken into account when planning therapeutic trials. The ideal trial should stratify for the number of previous miscarriages, with randomization between control and experimental treatments within each stratum. To date, such a study has not been undertaken. It is quite likely that by stratifying the sample by number of previous miscarriages, the effect of the experimental intervention will become easier to demonstrate in those women with higher numbers of previous miscarriages than in those with fewer previous miscarriages, because the spontaneous success rate is so much lower in the former group.[12,40]

Unfortunately, in many studies, patients with only two previous miscarriages are included. The occurrence of two miscarriages may in many cases be a chance phenomenon caused by de novo fetal chromosome abnormalities (in particular, autosomal trisomies) rather than a recurrent maternal factor. Cytogenetic evaluations of specimens of sporadic abortions have revealed an overall incidence of chromosomal abnormalities of 43%.[41] Thus, in theory, in $0.43 \times 0.43 = 18.5\%$ of all women with two consecutive miscarriages, the cause is the occurrence of two chromosomally abnormal conceptions. The inclusion of women with only two early miscarriages in a study of RPL will 'dilute' the estimate of the risk factor (in case–control and cohort studies) or the treatment effect in controlled clinical trials. The proportion of RPL patients in whom the disorder can be explained by a random accumulation of 'sporadic' miscarriages declines with the number of previous miscarriages.[42] Conversely, the proportion of cases that can be explained by a factor increasing the risk of miscarriage of euploid embryos may increase with the number of previous miscarriages. Hence, the frequency of many immunological risk factors[43–45] and the possible effect of immunotherapy,[12,40] increase and the frequency of chromosomally abnormal abortions decreases,[46] with the number of previous pregnancy losses.

MATERNAL AGE

Because increased maternal age increases the subsequent miscarriage rate, stratification for age should be taken into account in therapeutic trials. However, in RPL, age seems to display a significant impact on pregnancy outome only after age 40[15] (Figure 1.3). Consequently, it may be sufficient to stratify according to two age groups: below and above 40. Advanced age is associated with several disorders such as uterine fibroids and endocrine and autoimmune abnormalities, so age is a confounding factor that should be adjusted for when the real impact of these disorders on subsequent reproductive performance is assessed.

SUBGROUPS OF RPL

If secondary and primary RPL and RPL with first- and second-trimester losses have different pathogenetic backgrounds, the frequency of recognized risk factors for RPL and the efficacy of treatments may differ between the groups. Indeed, a series of studies have provided data suggesting that such differences exist (Table 1.3).

The factor V Leiden mutation is the commonest cause of activated protein C (APC) resistance, which is a risk factor for thrombosis and is probably also associated with RPL.[47] Wramsby et al[48] found factor V Leiden to be significantly associated with primary but not secondary RPL, and Rai et al[49] found that APC resistance was significantly associated with the absence of a previous live birth among patients with RPL. In a study of three congenital thrombophilic factors (including the factor V Leiden mutation), 25.5% with primary RPL compared with 15.1% of those with secondary RPL were positive for at least one factor.[50] The literature thus points towards a lower prevalence of factor V Leiden/APC resistance in secondary rather than primary RPL patients. Most studies also point towards a higher prevalence of thrombophilic factors, especially the factor V Leiden mutation in patients with second-trimester miscarriages compared with those with only early losses.[47,51]

It is unclear whether parental chromosome abnormalities (e.g., balanced translocations) have a different prevalence in primary or secondary RPL. In a review[52] of 79 relevant studies on the prevalence of parental chromosome abnormalities in couples with RPL, a higher frequency of aberrations (3.7%) was found in couples with multiple pregnancy losses and one or more live births compared with couples with exclusively repeated pregnancy losses, among whom it was 2.9%. Franssen et al[53] found that the frequency of parental chromosome abnormalities was not different between couples with RPL including a live birth and RPL couples without a previous birth. The frequency of parental chromosome anomalies thus seems to be almost similar in primary and secondary RPL, and the consequence is that screening of parental chromosomes should be a part of the routine workup in both types of RPL.

A series of immunological parameters have been described as being important for RPL and would be expected to show a different distribution between the subgroups of RPL patients if the pathogenetic backgrounds were different. Research in immunological factors in RPL has concentrated on alloantibodies, autoantibodies, natural killer (NK) cells, and HLA (human leukocyte antigen) molecules of the major histocompatibility complex (MHC).

Table 1.3 The prevalence of risk factors or effect of treatments in patients with primary and secondary recurrent pregnancy loss (RPL) and RPL with second-trimester losses (late RPL)

Risk factor or treatment	Prevalence/effect in secondary vs primary RPL	Prevalence/effect in late vs early primary RPL
Parental chromosome abnormality	Equal	NA
Antipaternal antibodies	Higher	Higher
Antiphospholipid antibodies	Lower or equal	Higher
Thrombophilia factors	Lower	Higher
Natural killer cell activity	Lower	NA
HLA-DR3	Higher	NA
Allogeneic lymphocyte immunization	Lower	NA
Treatment with intravenous immunoglobulin	Higher	NA

NA, cannot be estimated.

There is much evidence that the maternal immune system recognizes and reacts to the trophoblast and fetus in an ongoing pregnancy: alloantibodies directed against paternal/fetal HLA antigens are produced with increased gestation[54] due to traffic of fetal cells into the mother's circulation in the third trimester and at delivery. Anti-HLA antibodies often persist for years and can therefore be found more often in women with secondary compared with primary RPL,[55] but seem not to exhibit any pathological action.[19,56]

Most autoantibodies can be found with increased prevalence in patients with RPL, and their presence is associated with a poor pregnancy prognosis;[13] however, few studies of autoantibodies in RPL have differentiated between primary and secondary RPL. In patients with primary RPL, the prevalence of positive anticardiolipin or antinuclear antibody concentrations has been reported to be higher than in those with secondary RPL.[13,57,58] None of the individual differences were statistically significant, but the clear trend emphasizes the importance that future studies of autoantibodies in RPL clearly distinguish between primary and secondary RPL. There is, however, a consensus that antiphospholipid antibodies (aPL) display a stronger association with late miscarriages than with early RPL[51] – a fact that is integrated into the definition of the antiphospholipid (APS) syndrome.[59] APS is considered to be present in an aPL-positive patient with a history of only one death of a normal fetus beyond week 10, whereas at least three miscarriages are needed for the diagnosis in an APL-positive patient with miscarriages before 10 weeks.

NK-cell cytotoxicity, an important factor in innate immune defence, has been reported to be predictive for a poor prognosis in patients with RPL.[60] Only one study has differentiated between primary and secondary RPL.[16] NK-cell activity in peripheral blood has been reported to be significantly increased in women with primary but not secondary RPL when compared with controls.[16]

Class II HLA alleles are associated with most immunological disorders. In the largest published case–control study of HLA-DR alleles in patients with RPL,[45] the immunological high-responder allele HLA-DR3 was found significantly more often in the total patient group than in controls (OR 1.4, $p < 0.02$). However, among the 250 patients with secondary RPL, the frequency of the HLA-DR3 phenotype was 32.4%, compared with 21.0% in controls ($p < 0.006$). In patients with primary RPL, the frequency of the HLA-DR3 phenotype was 21.8%, which was clearly similar to that of controls. It is thus clear that HLA-DR3 is only associated with secondary RPL but not with primary RPL.

The finding that increased NK cytotoxicity is associated with primary RPL indicates that excessive innate immunity may be associated with primary RPL. However, the association between particular HLA-DR alleles and secondary RPL, and the epidemiological evidence that immunization against the male-specific HY antigen plays a role in secondary RPL,[17] indicate that adaptive immunity may have a role in secondary RPL, since recognition of alloantigens by T lymphocytes and subsequent sensitization requires involvement of HLA-DR antigens.

There is evidence that immunotherapy such as allogeneic lymphocyte injections/infusions or intravenous immunoglobulin (IVIG) exhibit different effects in primary and secondary RPL, respectively (Table 1.3).

FAMILIAL AGGREGATION

As discussed above, family studies (Table 1.2) have shown that the RPL prevalence in siblings of RPL probands is in accordance with a multifactorial model for the inheritance of RPL. In internal medicine and other disciplines, the development of many common diseases (e.g., arterial hypertension, diabetes mellitus, and schizophrenia) is thought to be determined by a multifactorial threshold model. One risk factor is not sufficient to cause disease, but when several intrinsic and extrinsic factors come together in the same individual (or couple), the risk exceeds a threshold level and disease develops. In recent years, research has identified a series of predisposing factors for RPL. So many risk factors have now been identified that it is very common to find several in the same patient. Both thrombophilic[61] and immunogenetic[62] risk factors seem to aggregate significantly more frequently than expected in RPL patients and the presence of several risk factors in the same couples affects the pregnancy prognosis negatively,[63,64] indicating that they may exhibit an additive or multiplicative effect on the RPL risk. Traditionally, the causes of RPL have been divided into single sufficient factors as slices of a pie: uterine malformations 10%, endocrine factors 10%, APL 15%, etc., which, together with the unexplained group, comprise 100%. This model is probably not adequate due to the above arguments. We therefore encourage scientists and clinicians working in the area of RPL to think in a threshold rather than a pie model.[65] The clinical implication is that, in principle, an RPL patient should be screened for all potential risk factors and the investigation should not stop as soon as the first risk factor has been identified. The recognition that RPL exhibits a high degree of heritability paves the way for the identification of susceptibility genes for RPL through the performance of genetic linkage analyses in families with several siblings experiencing miscarriage or RPL. Such linkage analyses have already documented that genes in the HLA region are important pathogenetic factors in RPL.[66]

PARTNER SPECIFICITY

Early studies on HLA in RPL were based on the hypothesis that increased HLA similarity between partners would lead to inadequate maternal protective immune responses and fetal loss. Although a considerable number of studies on HLA sharing in couples with RPL have been performed, the evidence did not support this hypothesis.[67,68] If good-quality epidemiological studies showing little evidence of partner specificity in RPL had been performed (Nielsen et al, unpublished work) prior to the HLA-sharing studies, the theories of increased HLA-sharing between RPL spouses might not have developed.

CLINICAL ASSOCIATIONS

Women with a history of RPL exhibit a significantly increased risk of late pregnancy complications. Hence, all RPL patients should be offered increased surveillance in late pregnancy (e.g., repeated ultrasound examinations) to decrease perinatal mortality and morbidity. A series of factors associated with RPL – aPL, hereditary thrombophilias, and mannose-binding lectin deficiency – have also been associated with low birthweight.[44,51] Since RPL per se seems to be associated with low birthweight, prospective studies of the effect of the mentioned factors on perinatal complications should be adjusted for the confounding effect of the number and type (midtrimester losses) of previous miscarriages.

LIFESTYLE FACTORS

As mentioned above, a number of lifestyle factors, including obesity, occupation, alcohol and caffeine consumption, and subfertility, are important risk factors for miscarriage. RPL is a complex disorder where lifestyle factors are expected to modify the effect of the non-lifestyle (intrinsic) factors discussed previously. The prevalence of the most important lifestyle factors should be described in research publications for both patients and controls, in order to document that studies assessing non-lifestyle risk factors or pregnancy outcome are matched for lifestyle factors. Since it is likely that smoking aggravates the effect of thrombophilic risk factors on pregnancy loss, details about smoking habits should be reported in all studies of RPL and thrombophilia. Another example of the importance of adjusting for lifestyle factors is that of the relationship between polycystic ovary syndrome (PCOS) and RPL. It is generally recognized that women with PCOS exhibit an increased rate of miscarriage and RPL. However, when adjustment for obesity is undertaken in multivariate analyses, the miscarriage rate in PCOS is not dependent on polycystic ovarian pathology or PCOS-associated endocrine abnormalities.[30]

CONCLUSIONS

Throughout medical science, epidemiological studies can provide indispensable knowledge when basic laboratory research, case–control studies, or controlled treatment trials are planned and carried out. This is also true in RPL. However, it seems that epidemiological knowledge has only been integrated to a very limited degree into the current clinical research and management of RPL.

The population prevalence of RPL is much higher than would be expected if RPL were merely a random accumulation of 'sporadic' miscarriages, and this indicates that most RPL cases are caused by factors increasing an individual couple's miscarriage risk.

Estimates of the future miscarriage risk in RPL patients vary significantly between studies, mainly due to different methods of ascertainment and monitoring. Some studies have estimated the prognosis too optimistically, as preclinical pregnancy losses have been classified as non-pregnancies. To overcome this potential source of error, in future treatment trials the take-home baby rate per time unit may be a better outcome measure than the miscarriage rate per registered pregnancy

Not only is the number of previous miscarriages the strongest prognostic factor, but with an increased number of previous miscarriages, fetal aneuploidy seems to play a decreasing role and maternal factors an increasing pathogenic role. Therefore, stratification by the number of previous miscarriages is important both in association studies and in treatment trials. Primary and seconday RPL, from an epidemiological point of view, also seem to be distinct entities, and in many case–control and treatment studies these two subgroups have indeed been found to behave quite differently (Table 1.3).

There are almost no studies addressing the issue of partner specificity in RPL, and such studies are urgently needed. However, a series of family studies have unanimously found a familial aggregation of miscarriage and RPL among first-degree relatives of RPL patients – especially sisters – which indicates a significant degree of heritability. The pattern of inheritance is multifactorial, and this is also in accordance with clinical evidence: several risk factors for RPL can very often be found in a single patient, and an aggregation of risk factors aggravates the pregnancy prognosis.

A series of studies have unanimously reported that RPL is associated with a series of complications in late pregnancy: reduced birthweight caused by increased risk for preterm birth and intrauterine growth retardation. It remains to be clarified from multivariate analyses which clinical and paraclinical factors among RPL patients determine the risks in late pregnancy.

Lifestyle factors are unfortunately rarely mentioned or are only reported very superficially in clinical studies in RPL. Since lifestyle factors can cause miscarriage by themselves, or through interaction with intrinsic factors, they should be reported in more detail in future studies, and appropriate stratification should be performed.

In conclusion, the multifactorial and polygenic background of RPL should be included in the models used for the pathogenesis of RPL. Additionally, the recognition of the different natures and pathogenic background of primary and secondary RPL, and the different nature of RPL with few miscarriages as opposed to RPL with many miscarriages, should help eliminate the practice of combining data from too heterogeneous studies for meta-analysis.

REFERENCES

1. World Health Organization. Recommended definitions; terminology and format for statistical tables related to the perinatal period. Acta Obstet Gynecol Scand 1977; 56:247–53.

2. Farquharson R, Jauniaux E, Exalto N, on behalf of the ESHRE Special Interest Group for Early Pregnancy (SIGEP). Updated and revised nomenclature for the description of early pregnancy events. Hum Reprod 2005; 20:3008–11.

3. Alberman E. The epidemiology of repeated abortion. In: Beard RW, Sharp F, eds. Early Pregnancy Loss: Mechanisms and Treatment. London: Springer-Verlag; 1988:9–17.

4. Warburton D, Strobino B. Recurrent spontaneous abortion. In: Bennet MJ, Edmonds DK, eds. Spontaneous and Recurrent Abortion. Oxford: Blackwell Scientific, 1987:193.

5. Stray-Pedersen B, Lorentzen-Styr AM. The prevalence of *Toxoplasma* antibodies among 11,736 pregnant women in Norway. Scand J Infect Dis 1979; 11:159–65.

6. Fertility and Employment 1979. The Danish Data Archives No. 0363, Odense University.

7. Cowchock FS, Smith JB. Predictors for live birth after unexplained spontaneous abortions: correlations between immunological test results, obstetric histories, and outcome of the next pregnancy without treatment. Am J Obstet Gynecol 1992; 167:1208–12.

8. Quenby SM, Farquharson RG. Predicting recurring miscarriage: What is important? Obstet Gynecol 1993; 82:132–8.

9. Clifford K, Rai R, Regan L. Future pregnancy outcome in unexplained recurrent first trimester miscarriage. Hum Reprod 1997; 12:387–9.

10. Christiansen OB, Pedersen B, Rosgaard A, et al. A randomized, double-blind, placebo-controlled trial of intravenous immunoglobulin

in the prevention of recurrent miscarriage: evidence for a therapeutic effect in women with secondary recurrent miscarriage. Hum Reprod 2002; 17:809–16.

11. Jablonowska B, Selbing A, Palfi M, et al. Prevention of recurrent spontaneous abortion by intravenous immunoglobulin: a double-blind placebo-controlled study. Hum Reprod 1999; 14:838–41.

12. Carp HJ, Toder V, Torchinsky A, et al. Allogenic leukocyte immunization after five or more miscarriages. Recurrent Miscarriage Immunotherapy Trialists Group. Hum Reprod 1997; 12:250–5.

13. Nielsen HS, Christiansen OB. Prognostic impact of anticardiolipin antibodies in women with recurrent miscarriages negative for the lupus anticoagulant. Hum Reprod 2005; 20:1720–8.

14. Cauchi MN, Coulam CB, Cowchock S, et al. Predictive factors in recurrent spontaneous abortion – a multicenter study. Am J Reprod Immunol 1995; 33:165–70.

15. Nybo Andersen AM, Wohlfahrt J, Christens P, et al. Maternal age and fetal loss: population based register study. BMJ 2000; 320:1708–12.

16. Shakhar K, Ben-Eliyahu S, Loewenthal R, et al. Differences in number and activity of peripheral natural killer cells in primary versus secondary recurrent miscarriage. Fertil Steril 2003; 80:368–75.

17. Christiansen OB, Pedersen B, Nielsen HS, et al. Impact of the sex of first child on the prognosis in secondary recurrent miscarriage. Hum Reprod 2004; 19:2946–51.

18. Christiansen OB, Kolte AM, Nielsen HS. Secondary recurrent miscarriage – unique entity with repect to etiology and treatment. Curr Women's Health Rev 2006; 2:119–24.

19. Christiansen OB, Mathiesen O, Husth M, et al. Placebo-controlled trial of active immunization with third party leukocytes in recurrent miscarriage. Acta Obstet Gynecol Scand 1994; 73:261–8.

20. Drakeley AJ, Quenby S, Farquharson RG. Mid-trimester loss; appraisal of a screening protocol. Hum Reprod 1998; 13:1471–9.

21. Cowchock FS, Smith JB, David S, et al. Paternal mononuclear cell immunization therapy for repeated miscarriage: predictive variables for pregnancy success. Am J Reprod Immunol 1990; 22:12–17.

22. Goldenberg RL, Mayberry SK, Copper RL, et al. Pregnancy outcome following a second-trimester loss. Obstet Gynecol 1993; 81:444–6.

23. Johnson PM, Chia KV, Risk JM, et al. Immunological and immuno-genetic investigation of recurrent spontaneous abortion. Dis Mark 1988; 6:163–171.

24. Alexander SA, Latinne D, Debruyere M, et al. Belgian experience with repeat immunization in recurrent spontaneous abortion. In: Beard RW, Sharp F, eds. Early Pregnancy Loss: Mechanisms and Treatment. London: Springer-Verlag, 1988:355–63.

25. Ho H, Gill TJ, Hsieh C, et al. The prevalence of recurrent spontaneous abortion, cancer, and congenital anomalies in the families of couples with recurrent spontaneous abortions or gestational trophoblastic tumors. Am J Obstet Gynecol 1991; 165:461–6.

26. Christiansen OB, Mathiesen O, Lauritsen JG, et al. Idiopathic recurrent spontaneous abortion. Evidence of a familial predisposition. Acta Obstet Gynecol Scand 1990; 69:597–601.

27. Emery AEH. Methodology in Medical Genetics. 2nd rev edn. Edinburgh; Churchill Livingstone, 1986.

28. Stephenson MD. Frequency of factors associated with habitual abortion in 197 couples. Fertil Steril 1996; 66:124–9.

29. Fedorcsak P, Storeng R, Dale PO, et al. Obesity is a risk factor for early pregnancy loss after IVF or ICSI. Acta Obstet Gynecol Scand 2000; 79:43–8.

30. Wang JX, Davies MJ, Norman RJ. Polycystic ovarian syndrome and the risk of spontaneous abortion following assisted reproductive technology treatment. Hum Reprod 2001; 16:2606–9.

31. Infante-Rivard C, Fernandez A, Gauthier R et al. Fetal loss associated with caffeine intake before and during pregnancy. JAMA 1993; 270:2940–3.

32. Fenster L, Hubbard AE, Swan SH, et al. Caffeinated beverages, decaffeinated coffee, and spontaneous abortion. Epidemiology 1997; 8:515–23.

33. Giannelli M, Doyle P, Roman E, et al. The effect of caffeine consumption and nausea on the risk of miscarriage. Paediatr Perinat Epidemiol 2003; 17:316–23.

34. Rasch V. Cigarette, alcohol, and caffeine consumption: risk factors for spontaneous abortion. Acta Obstet Gynecol Scand 2003; 82:182–8.

35. Nielsen GL, Sorensen HT, Larsen H, et al. Risk of adverse outcome and miscarriage in pregnant users of non-steroidal anti-inflammatory drugs: population based observational study and case-control study. BMJ 2001; 322:266–70.

36. Li DK, Liu L, Odouli R. Exposure to nonsteroidal anti-inflammarory drugs during pregnancy and risk of miscarriage: population based cohort study. BMJ 2003; 327:368–72.

37. Brandt LP, Nielsen CV. Job stress and adverse outcome of pregnancy: a causal link or recall bias? Am J Epidemiol 1992; 35:302–11.

38. Florack EI, Zielhuis GA, Pellegrino JE, et al. Occupational physical activity and the occurence of spontaneous abortion. Int J Epidemiol 1993; 22:878–84.

39. Wang JX, Norman RJ, Wilcox AJ. Incidence of spontaneous abortion among pregnancies produced by assisted reproductive technology. Hum Reprod 2004; 19:272–7.

40. Daya S, Gunby J, and The Recurrent Miscarriage Trialists Group. The effectiveness of allogeneic leukocyte immunization in unexplained primary recurrent abortion. Am J Reprod Immunol 1994; 32:294–302.

41. Creasy R. The cytogenetics of spontaneous abortion in humans. In: Beard RW, Sharp F, eds. Early Pregnancy Loss: Mechanisms and Treatment. London: Springer-Verlag, 1988:293–304.

42. Christiansen OB. A fresh look at the causes and treatment of recurrent miscarriage, especially its immunological aspects. Hum Reprod Update 1996; 2:271–93.

43. Pfeiffer KA, Fimmers R, Engels G, et al. The HLA-G genotype is potentially assoiated with idiopathic recurrent spontaneous abortion. Mol Hum Reprod 2001; 7:373–8.

44. Kruse C, Rosgaard A, Steffensen R, et al. Low serum level of mannan-binding lectin is a determinant for pregnancy outcome in women with recurrent spontaneous abortion. Am J Obstet Gynecol 2002; 187:1313–20.

45. Kruse C, Steffensen R, Varming K, et al. A study of HLA-DR and -DQ alleles in 588 patients and 562 controls confirms that HLA-DRB1*03 is associated with recurrent miscarriage. Hum Reprod 2004; 19:1215–21.

46. Ogasawara M, Aoki K, Okada S, et al. Embryonic karyotype of abortuses in relation to the number of previous miscarriages. Fertil Steril 2000; 73:300.

47. Rey E, Kahn SR, David M, Shrier I. Thrombophilic disorders and fetal loss: a meta-analysis. Lancet 2003; 361:901–8.

48. Wramsby ML, Sten-Linder M, Bremme K. Primary habitual abortions are associated with high frequency of factor V Leiden mutation. Fertil Steril 2000; 74:987–91.

49. Rai R, Shlebak A, Cohen H, et al. Factor V Leiden and acquired activated protein C resistance among 1000 women with recurrent miscarriage. Hum Reprod 2001; 16:961–5.

50. Carp H, Salomon O, Seidman D, et al. Prevalence of genetic markers for thrombophilia in recurrent pregnancy loss. Hum Reprod 2002; 17:1633–7.

51. Roque H, Paidas MJ, Funai EF, et al. Maternal thrombophilias are not associated with early pregnancy loss. Thromb Haemost 2004; 91: 290–5.

52. Tharapel AT, Tharapel SA, Bannerman RM. Recurrent pregnancy losses and chromosome abnormalities: a review. Br J Obstet Gynaecol 1985; 92:899–914.

53. Franssen MTM, Korevaar JC, Leschot NJ, et al. Selective chromosome analysis in couples with two or more miscarriages: case-control study. BMJ 2005; 331:137–41.

54. Regan L. A prospective study of spontaneous abortion. In: Beard RW, Sharp F, eds. Early Pregnancy Loss. Mechanisms and Treatment. London: Springer-Verlag, 1988:23–37.

55. Coulam CB. Immunological tests in the evaluation of reproductive disorders: a critical review. Am J Obstet Gynecol 1992; 167:1844–51.

56. Sargent IL, Wilkins T, Redman CWG. Maternal immune responses to the fetus in early pregnancy and recurrent miscarriage. Lancet 1988; ii:1099–104.

57. Cowchock S, Bruce Smith J, Gocial B. Antibodies to phospholipids and nuclear antigens in patients with repeated abortions. Am J Obstet Gynecol 1986; 155:1002–10.

58. Rai R, Regan L, Clifford K, et al. Antiphospholipid antibodies and β_2-glycoprotein-I in 500 women with recurrent miscarriage: results of a comprehensive screening approach. Hum Reprod 1995:10:2001–5.

59. Wilson WA, Gharavi AE, Koike T, et al. International concensus statement on preliminary classification criteria for definite antiphospholipid syndrome: report of an international workshop. Arthritis Rheum 1999; 42:309–11.

60. Aoki K, Kajiura S, Matsumoto Y, et al. Preconceptional natural-killer activity as a predictor of miscarriage. Lancet 1995; 345:1340–2.

61. Coulam CB, Jeyendran RS, Fishel LA, Roussev R. Multiple thromobophilic gene mutations rather than specific gene mutations are risk factors for recurrent miscarriage. Am J Reprod Immunol 2006; 55:360–8.

62. Hviid TV, Christiansen OB. Linkage disequilibrium between human leukocyte antigen (HLA) class II and HLA-G – possible implications for human reproduction and autoimmune disease. Hum Immunol 2005; 66:688–99.

63. Jivraj S, Rai R, Underwood J, et al. Genetic thrombophilic mutations among couples with recurrent miscarriage. Hum Reprod 2006; 21: 1161–5.

64. Christiansen OB, Kruse C, Steffenson R, Varming K. HLA Class II, mannan-binding lectin (MBL) and recurrent miscarriage. Presented at the European Congress of Reproductive Immunology, Plzen, 2004, Abstract I30 in special issue of Am J Reprod Immunol.

65. Christiansen OB, Nybo-Andersen AM, Bosch E, et al. Evidence-based investigations and treatments of recurrent pregnancy loss. Fertil Steril 2005; 83:821–39.

66. Christiansen OB, Andersen HH, Hojbjerre M, et al. Maternal HLA Class II allogenotypes are markers for the predisposition to fetal losses in families of women with unexplained recurrent fetal loss. Eur J Immunogenetics 1995; 22:323–34.

67. Christiansen OB, Riisom K, Lauritsen JG, et al. No increased histocompatibility antigen sharing in couples with idiopathic habitual abortions. Hum Reprod 1989; 4:160–2.

68. Ober C, van der Ven K. HLA and fertility. In: Hunt JB, ed. HLA and the Maternal–Fetal Relationship. Austin, TX:. RG Landers, 1996:133–56.

2. Signaling between embryo and mother in early pregnancy: Basis for development of tolerance

Eytan R Barnea

THE HYPOTHESIS

In 1978, Beer and Billingham,[1] while working on immunological recognition mechanisms in mammalian pregnancy, published their view that the maternal system is aware of the presence of the early embryo, and actively responds to it. This was surprising, considering the differences in genetic make-up of the mother and fetus (semi or total), and was contrary to the prevailing opinion at that time, which considered that the trophoblast was hypoantigenic, as a protection from cellular immunity. Beer and Billingham[1] suggested that unique HLA (human leukocyte antigen) molecules are presented to the maternal system, the responses to which play a role in establishing and maintaining pregnancy. A decade later, Billingham and Head[2] suggested that local cell-based immunosuppressive and immunoprotective activity in the placenta was mediated by suppressor and other unknown cells. Billingham and Head[2] further suggested that HLA sharing in the parents leads to lack of maternal recognition and is therefore the basis for rejection, i.e., miscarriage.

Hansel and Hickey[3] examined various compounds that might be involved in the maternal recognition of pregnancy, with an emphasis on domestic animals. They found several proteins, including embryo-derived platelet-activating factor (PAF), a trophoblastic protein with an antiluteolytic effect. Further progress regarding embryo–maternal recognition was provided by Weitlauf,[4] who reported that embryo-conditioned media has a specific effect on the rat uterus compared with control media or that produced by deciduomata (a non-pregnant environment). This strongly suggested communication between embryo and mother before implantation, but specific factors were never identified.

Later studies have recognized that there are multiple types of placenta in mammals. The hemochorial placenta (found in the human and the mouse) is associated with intimate interaction, while in other species there is less invasiveness (an example is the pig placenta, which communicates with the endometrium through the histiotroph). In addition, the secretory products of different types of placentas also differ: human chorionic gonadotropin (hCG) in humans, prolactin in rodents,[5] etc.

Despite such diversity at implantation, there are features that are common to the development of all mammals before implantation: egg and sperm fusion, and progressive development of the fertilized embryo up to the blastocyst stage. In a recent review, Moffet and Loke[6] concluded that pregnancy is not a classical acceptance/rejection phenomenon, and the specific compounds derived from the conceptus and the receptors present on immune cells need to be identified to better understand the unique interaction in pregnancy.

The present review provides the rationale for early pregnancy recognition, with an emphasis on compounds that appear to be present prior to implantation. It discusses previous and recent data strongly suggesting that preimplantation factor (PIF) is a unique, universal compound that initiates pregnancy recognition (and tolerance) in mammalian pregnancy. This recognition starts prior to direct embryo–maternal contact in the uterus.

RESCUE OF THE CORPUS LUTEUM

Following ovulation, the corpus luteum (CL) is formed and secretes progesterone, which has a trophic effect on the endometrium. Studies have shown that a variety of signals can rescue the CL. These include hCG in humans, prolactin in rodents, and estrogen in pigs, indicating that the CL-rescuing signals are species-specific. When cow and mare uteruses are removed, prostaglandin $F_{2\alpha}$ ($PGF_{2\alpha}$) is not released and the CL persists long term; therefore, the presence of the conceptus actually prevents luteolysis.[7] But the presence of an embryo is not necessary, and hCG injections, for example, can prolong the lifespan of the CL to a certain degree. This contrasts with the uterus, in which a viable embryo must be present in order for the endometrium to become receptive. Thus, recognition of pregnancy and successful implantation take place before the stage when rescue of the CL occurs, strongly suggesting that there is no linkage between tolerance and the CL.

DOES THE EMBRYO–MATERNAL DIALOGUE START PRIOR TO IMPLANTATION?

As we have seen, the CL initially does not need the conceptus, and can persist for a few weeks before it undergoes spontaneous regression, at menses. Therefore, the embryo–maternal dialogue required for implantation likely does not involve the CL. In humans, for example, implantation takes place 1 week before the CL would undergo regression. If the CL were involved in embryo recognition, it could take place only when there was intimate embryo–maternal contact. But this is clearly not the case, and the search for the elements involved in the early interaction has been long going. First, here, we give a brief rationale of the need for maternal recognition of the embryo shortly after fertilization.

THE FERTILIZATION PROCESS

The released mature egg reaches the ampular region and survives for only 12–24 hours unless it is fertilized. There is a one-in-three chance of fertilization occurring. Once the sperm penetrates the egg at fertilization, it becomes 'invisible' to the maternal immune system. As expected, following egg/sperm fusion, there is no maternally induced immune rejection, for as long as the egg membrane does not change its characteristics (expressing foreign antigens). Once foreign antigens are expressed, the fertilized egg rapidly becomes surrounded by the zona pellucida, a hard and impenetrable shell that wards off maternal immune cells. Further immune protection is provided by maternal cumulus oophorus cells, which further prevent direct access of maternal immune cells to the embryo. However, the cumulus cells persist only for a few days after fertilization, as their primary role is to facilitate tubal transport of the embryo towards the uterus. The cumulus has immune cells that secrete cytokines, and may serve as a first relay system for propagating embryo-derived signaling.[8] Indeed, it has been shown that within 8 hours after fertilization, there is emargination of platelets from the peripheral blood in mice.[9]

Embryonic cell proliferation up to the 8-cell stage is rather orderly. The blastomeres are totipotential (i.e., each of them could develop into a complete embryo). This process lasts approximately 3 days while the embryo travels within the fallopian tube. The speed of development is a good index to evaluate embryonic health with respect to likelihood for implantation.

Evidence that the embryo may have an active role in immune recognition was suggested by studies showing that embryo-conditioned medium has immune-suppressive properties.[10,11] However, the compounds responsible for this immune effect have not been fully characterized. Further data suggested that a variety of compounds can be identified in the maternal circulation prior to implantation, compared with non-pregnant subjects. However, whether the putative embryo-specific secreted products and the early-stage circulatory compounds are the same remains unclear. If the embryo-secreted products and circulatory compounds are identical, very low concentrations of embryo-secreted compounds could reach the maternal circulation and cause changes in maternal immunity to initiate tolerance. Obviously, this would mean that the embryo plays a role in developing tolerance even prior to implantation. This signaling would also explain pathological pregnancies in which implantation occurs in sites outside the uterus, including the fallopian tube, ovary, or even (rarely) in the abdominal cavity on the bowel. Ectopic pregnancies strongly suggest that maternal recognition of pregnancy must be systemic – not localized to the uterus.

Moreover, experience with transfer of donor (genetically dissimilar) embryos has shown high implantation and pregnancy success rates, further implicating the role of the embryo in the recognition process. There is a 4- to 5-day delay between fertilization and implantation, which is replicated in embryo transfer following in vitro fertilization (IVF). The delay suggests that this time is required to establish tolerance and prime the endometrium, making it both receptive and accommodating for the incoming embryo.

GENOMIC ELEMENTS IN RECOGNITION

Recent data show that the embryo expresses its genome as early as the 2-cell stage. Thus, in the earliest stages of development, the embryo becomes a partial or total 'non-self' from the perspective of the mother. Thus, development of the zona pellucida as a protection against maternal adversity becomes necessary. It has recently been been observed that there is a major downregulation of genes in the preimplantation embryo compared with the unfertilized egg.[12] This downregulation may protect the embryo by minimizing its vulnerability, and in a mostly anerobic environment it may be advantageous to shut down non-essential functions that are not necessary for survival. Additionally, the few genes that are upregulated may have an important physiological role. Novel genes that are expressed very early may lead to early maternal recognition of pregnancy.[13]

UNIQUE PHENOMENA REQUIRE UNIQUE SIGNALS

In order for a semi- or totally foreign embryo (or even a cross-species transfer) to implant and lead to successful progeny, unique embryo-derived signals must be present, due to the absence of a host-versus-graft or graft-versus-host reaction. Moreover, the maternal system must accommodate and nurture the conceptus until delivery, and any immune tolerance is therefore *conditional*, because rejection may take place at any moment until delivery. In addition, such a unique phenomenon would have to be pregnancy-specific; for tolerance to be successful, the embryo must be viable and the maternal system receptive. The signal must be present early in embryo development, must be potent, and must have specific sites of action both on the maternal immune system and on the endometrium. The signal must also be universally mammalian, because the same early phenomenon takes place in all mammals (and any diversity only occurs at the implantation phase).

What properties would such a signal have? It would *modulate* the maternal immune system without suppressing it. This is essential, because during pregnancy the mother is exposed to pathogens and her ability to maintain an effective immune system to combat disease is essential for survival – both for her and for the embryo. Therefore, the signal would have to allow maternal immunity to function unimpeded, allowing it to fight bacteria, viruses, and parasites, while maintaining the tolerance toward the embryo. The tolerance that this signal creates must not be excessive; otherwise the mother's ability to reject a defective embryo or seriously infected fetus would be inhibited. Of course, most defective embryos are rejected early, and, in case of infection, premature labor frequently ensues. An additional role of this signal would be to prime the endometrium, and make the uterine environment hospitable to the embryo. Finally, it is clear that as the embryo–maternal interaction becomes intimate, the dynamics change, and there are complex events that take place that could be labeled as a *maintenance* of tolerance rather than the initiation that is the topic of this chapter.

The following is a discussion of the compounds implicated so far in early pregnancy events prior to implantation. Unfortunately, most knowledge to date about the embryo–maternal immune interaction involves study of uterine milieu during implantation.

Briefly, there is a tolerant (Th2) cytokine balance in pregnancy: increased interleukin-4 (IL-4), IL-5, and IL-10 and reduced Th1-type cytokines, such as IL-2, interferon-γ (IFN-γ) and tumor necrosis factor α (TNF-α).[14] However, excess Th1 cytokines are associated with reproductive failure.[15] The preimplantation embryo may protect itself from maternal immune rejection by promoting a Th2 phenotype.[3] Activated natural killer (NK) cells cause a Th1-type response, while increased peripheral T lymphocytes express progesterone receptors, and protect by releasing IL-10 and transforming growth factor β (TGF-β).[16] NK cells may also inhibit excessive trophoblast invasiveness by recognizing unusual fetal trophoblast major histocompatibility complex (MHC) ligands.[15] Other non-pregnancy-specific compounds may also be involved: sex steroids, integrins and IL-1b have no mRNA for receptors in the embryo. While insulin- like growth factors (IGFs) have receptors, the ligands expressed in the early embryo have trophic effects on the embryo. They are modulated by embryonic IGF-binding protein 3 (IGFBP-3). Leukemia inhibitory factor (LIF) and colony-stimulating factors that stimulate matrix metalloproteinases (MMPs) are also involved, and inhibition of mucin 1 (MUC-1) expression on the endometrial surface facilitates implantation.[17,18] The presence of regulatory T cells (T_{reg}, CD4$^+$CD25$^+$) increases prior to implantation, suggesting early embryo signaling.[19] This cannot be due to semen-induced factors, since implantation after embryo transfer following IVF without contact with semen is also associated with upregulated T cells.

However, none of these compounds are pregnancy-specific, and therefore cannot be the initiating signal for tolerance. In contrast, failure to implant is frequent and may be caused by any disruption of the delicate balance between the uterine epithelial lining, which becomes the decidua, and the embryo. The endometrium can be hostile due to immune disruptors, such as high peripheral levels of NK cells, altered hormonal priming, infection, and deficient integrin expression. The role of antiphospholipid antibodies, for example, in failed implantation is still being debated.[20] The embryo can also fail to implant due to deficient expression of adhesion molecules (MMPs) as well as the lack of secretory and cellular elements that aid in the immune maternal recognition of pregnancy.[21] In addition, some embryos may only partially or temporarily implant, later dislodging into the fallopian tube, leading to chemical or ectopic pregnancy. Recent data show an imbalance toward stimulatory overinhibitory NK-cell receptors: CD158a and CD158b inhibitory receptor expression by CD56^{dim}CD16$^+$ and CD56^{bright}CD16$^-$ NK cells was decreased, while CD161-activating receptor expression by CD56$^+$CD3$^+$ NKT cells was increased, in patients with implantation failures.[22]

WHICH CURRENTLY KNOWN COMPOUND COULD BE THE UNIVERSAL TOLERANCE BIOMARKER?

The main diagnostic marker for human pregnancy is hCG, but it does not reflect pregnancy viability, it cannot be detected early in embryo culture media, and its persistence in the circulation after pregnancy has terminated greatly limits its clinical use. hCG has an important role in the maintenance of the corpus luteum following implantation, and it has been shown to be involved in altering the biochemical behavior and morphology of endometrial cell types, by acting on a specific binding site (CG/LH-R). A local immunological role has also been ascribed to hCG.[23] However, hCG is not pregnancy-specific, is unique to humans, and, significantly, is also found in various cancers. It appears that most of the effect of hCG in supporting pregnancy is at implantation and beyond.

PLATELET-ACTIVATING FACTOR

PAF is an acetylated phosphoglyceride expressed by the embryo in both humans and rodents. Its role is mostly local within the fallopian tube, aiding in the transfer of the embryo into the uterus.[24] However, in other species, other compounds play this role; for example, in horses, prostaglandin E is secreted by the morula. PAF also has a trophic effect on the embryo.[25]

PAF is not pregnancy-specific, and is present in platelets, leukocytes, and endothelial cells. Therefore, it is clear that PAF could not be a unique signal required for pregnancy tolerance.

EARLY PREGNANCY FACTOR

Early pregnancy factor (EPF) has been identified as chaperonin 10, a 12 kDa protein. It can be detected prior to implantation in the maternal circulation.[26] EPF has been shown to influence immune effects mediating the suppressive effect by binding T cells, NK cells, and monocytes. The receptor for EPF is not a functional homologue of chaperonin 10.[27] EPF activity in the serum is determined by decreased rosette formation using a cumbersome bioassay. Similar activity in mare and cow serum is related to a 26 kDa protein that is different from the chaperonin molecule.[28] In addition, EPF is not pregnancy-specific; it is also present is several non-pregnant tissues, including in the serum of patients with ovarian cancer.[29]

HLA-G

The embryo and trophoblast express non-classical forms of HLA-G, which may protect them against NK-mediated lysis, and lead to apoptosis of allo-geneic cytotoxic CD8[+] T cells by Fas ligands.[30] But HLA-G-negative embryos may implant, and therefore HLA-G is not essential for implantation.[31] Recent data have shown that NK cells, which are dominant in the decidua, express a receptor for KIR2DL4, which interacts with HLA-G; however, a multiparous woman who lacked the receptor still had normal pregnancies.[32] Also, HLA-G polymorphism has been investigated in recurrent spontaneous abortion, but no difference has been found between the fertile and abortion-prone populations.[33] HLA-G can be detected in human embryo culture media by specific immunoassays. However, pregnancy can also occur in its absence. When present, there is a higher pregnancy rate, and therefore HLA-G testing has been used to determine which embryos should be transferred after IVF.[34] However, the soluble forms are not secreted by the trophoblast, but are cleaved from membrane-bound HLA-G1.[35] Thus, HLA-G may be necessary, but is certainly not sufficient, for initiating maternal tolerance of pregnancy.

PREIMPLANTATION FACTOR

Over the past several years, our team's studies have focused in identifying and documenting the role of PIF in mammalian pregnancy. PIF is only found in pregnancy, is similar in all mammals, and is found very early, shortly after fertilization – all of which suggest that PIF is the factor initiating maternal recognition of pregnancy.

Earlier work had shown that viable human and rabbit human embryo culture media contain unidentified immune modulatory compounds.[10,11] We developed a novel bioassay and reported that viable human and mouse embryo-conditioned culture media, and human and porcine pregnancy serum, contain immune-modulatory compounds that increase rosette formation between donor lymphocytes and platelets in the presence of CD2MAb due to PIF, a low-molecular-weight peptide(s).[36–42] A bioassay, unlike an immune assay, is a reflection of a biological phenomenon, which led us to study whether the compounds present in embryo culture media are also present in the maternal circulation.

The presence of PIF activity in maternal sera 4 days after embryo transfer was followed in 27/38 (71%) live births, while only 3 pregnancies occurred from 114 embryo transfers (3%) with non-detectable PIF activity, due to delayed implantation. In human pregnancy, detection of PIF activity in maternal sera predicted viable pregnancy after IVF with excellent sensitivity, specificity, and positive and negative predictive values (88%, 95%, 94%, and 90%, respectively) in 65 patients beginning 4 days after embryo transfer. In a retrospective study, the presence of PIF was found to be highly specific (100%) for pregnancy.[36] The accuracy of the PIF assay in predicting successful and non-viable pregnancies has been confirmed in another study.[37] Furthermore, the premature disappearance of PIF activity led to embryonic demise, approximately 3 weeks prior to decline in hCG levels.

Chromosomal analysis of these spontaneous abortuses revealed the presence of an abnormal karyotype in over 60%. Only one woman who lost a euploid conceptus had PIF activity that was positive 4 days after embryo transfer.[38]

The next stage focused on identifying PIF and elucidating its biological role. The biochemical nature of PIF was examined by isolating it from viable mouse embryo-conditioned media using a multistep process including affinity chromatography and high-performance liquid chromatography (HPLC).[42] The peptide responsible for the biological activity generated by the bioassay was isolated. It was found to be a novel 15-amino-acid peptide sharing partial sequence homology with the circumsporozoite protein of the malaria parasite. The peptide that was initially identified in mouse embryo culture media was also found to be present in human embryos. Due to the simple structure of PIF, a synthetic analog was designed that mimics the native peptide's properties. It was now possible to examine the biological effects of PIF in vitro and in vivo and to generate highly specific antibodies (polyclonal and monoclonal) that could detect and measure the presence of PIF in both gestational tissues and peripheral blood.

Synthetic PIF was shown to have a potent dose- and time-dependent effect by mostly affecting mitogen-activated human immune cells. This was shown by blocking peripheral blood mononuclear cell (PBMC) proliferation, modulating the secretion of both Th1 and Th2 cytokines, favoring the latter. These effects were exerted through apparently novel binding sites, and a mechanism of action distinct from that of immunosuppressive agents (Barnea et al, unpublished work). We have demonstrated that PIF indeed has a beneficial effect on various immune disorders including multiple sclerosis, juvenile diabetes, and graft vs host disease (due to transfer of foreign immune cells to a host) using relevant mouse models (Barnea et al, unpublished work). These effects were achieved without toxicity, and low-dose short-term therapy led to either prevention or long-term protection against disease. The work on synthetic PIF concurred with our earlier studies where short-term PIF treatment

of mated mice led to decreased rates of fetal absorption (Barnea et al, unpublished work). PIF is being examined in additional models in preparation for clinical trials. Thus, one aspect of the activity of PIF, namely its immunomodulatory properties, is a necessity in pregnancy. Moreover, the effect is cross-species, since the peptide originally derived from the mouse is effective on human cells.

The second characteristic of PIF, in order for it to be relevant to the very early stages of embryo development, is its ability to interact with the endometrium. Our data show that PIF has a clear effect on human endometrial cells, increasing receptivity molecules. The presence of PIF as determined by bioassay[36] was recently validated in primate blood and was shown to be associated with subsequent endometrial pre-epithelial plaque reaction, angiogenesis, and stromal compaction, as an index of impending implantation.[37]

The next task was to show whether PIF can be detected in the early stages of pregnancy and is capable of exerting its effects in low concentrations at the relevant time. The initial observations using the PIF bioassay in both normal pregnancy serum and viable embryo-conditioned media have been confirmed. Using various enzyme-linked immunosorbent assay (ELISA) formats, we have measured PIF concentrations in maternal blood 8–10 days after embryo transfers that led to successful pregnancies. Very recent data have also shown that a sensitive ELISA (using monoclonal antibodies) can detect pregnancy within 5 days of insemination in cows. In addition, we have measured PIF concentrations in both viable single human (4–8 cells) and mouse embryo culture media (Barnea, Roussev, and Coulam, unpublished work). These data demonstrated the link between the presence of the peptide in peripheral blood in sufficient amounts to explain its observed biological effects.

CONCLUSIONS

In conclusion, three essential elements are required for pregnancy to succeed: a viable embryo, immune tolerance, and a receptive uterus. Based on our data, PIF plays a major role in all three aspects: it is only secreted by viable embryos, it modulates the maternal immune system towards tolerance prior to implantation, and it primes the endometrium for implantation. Thus, PIF is a true biomarker for pregnancy that can be used for both diagnostic and therapeutic purposes in pregnancy and other conditions.

A PIF-ELISA could be used to investigate very early pregnancy events and help to improve various aspects of reproduction. In IVF, PIF-ELISA could be used to detect the viability of fertilized embryos by testing the embryo culture media. Consequently, the current low pregnancy rates (20–25%) associated with morphological analysis for embryo viability might be greatly improved, and the multiple-pregnancy rate associated with current IVF practices might be reduced. In addition, very early events in human pregnancy remain poorly explored, especially those at the peri-implantation period. Measuring PIF levels may help us to better understand the events taking place during this period. Furthermore, PIF assays might be used to monitor high-risk pregnancies, such as recurrent pregnancy loss; immunocytochemistry of premature-labor placentas has documented very low or absent expression of PIF. These potential applications of PIF, and the possible treatment of various immune disorders, remain to be fully explored.

REFERENCES

1. Beer AE, Billingham RE. Maternal immunological recognition mechanisms during pregnancy. Ciba Found Symp 1978; 64:293–322.
2. Billingham RE, Head JR. Recipient treatment to overcome the allograft reaction, with special reference to nature's own solution. Prog Clin Biol Res 1986; 224:159–85.
3. Hansel W, Hickey GJ. Early pregnancy signals in domestic animals. Ann NY Acad Sci 1988; 541:472–84.
4. Weitlauf HM. Embryonic signaling at implantation in the mouse. Prog Clin Biol Res 1989; 294:359–76.
5. Soares JM. The prolactin and growth hormone families: pregnancy-specific hormones/cytokines at the maternal–fetal interface. Reprod Biol Endocrinol 2004; 2:51.
6. Moffett A, Loke YW. The immunological paradox of pregnancy: a reappraisal. Placenta 2004; 25:1–8.
7. Wright JM, Kiracofe JH, Beeman KB. Factors associated with shortened estrous cycles after abortion in beef heifers. J Anim Sci 1988; 66:3185–9.
8. Piccinni MP. Scaletti C, Malvilia C, et al. Production of IL-4 and leukemia inhibitory factor by T cells of the cumulus oophorus: a favorable microenvironment for pre-implantation embryo development. Eur J Immunol 2001; 24:31–7.
9. O'Neill C. Partial characterization of the embryo-derived platelet-activating factor in mice. J Reprod Fertil 1985; 75:285–290.
10. Pinkas H, Fisch B, Tadir Y, et al. Immunesuppressive activity in culture media containing oocytes fertilized in vitro. Arch Androl 1992; 28:53–59.
11. Fortin M, Oulette MJ, Lambert RD. TGF-β and PGE₂ in rabbit blastocoelic fluid can modulate GM-CSF production by human lymphocytes. Am J Reprod Immunol 1997; 38:129–39.
12. Alizadeh Z, Kageyama SI, Aoki F. Degradation of maternal mRNA in mouse embryos: selective degradation of specific mRNAs after fertilization. Mol Reprod Dev 2005; 72:281–90.
13. Sharma, S, Murphy S, Barnea ER. Genes regulating implantation and fetal development: a focus on mouse knockout models. Front Biosci 2006; 20:2123–37.
14. Choudhury SR, Knapp LA. Human reproductive failure I: immunological factors. Hum Reprod Update 2001; 7:113–34.
15. Raghupathy R. Th1-type immunity is incompatible with successful pregnancy. Immunol Today 1997; 18:478–82.
16. Druckman R, Druckman MA. Progesterone and the immunology of pregnancy. J Steroid Biochem Mol Biol 2005; 97:389–96.
17. Kralickova M, Sima P, Rokyta Z. Role of leukemia-inhibitory factor gene mutations in infertile women: the embryo–endometrial cytokine cross talk during implantation – a delicate homeostatic equilibrium. Folia Microbiol (Praha) 2005; 50:179–86.
18. Aplin JD, Kimber SJ. Trophoblast-uterine interactions at implantation. Reprod Biol Endocrinol 2004; 2:48.
19. Somerset DA, Zheng Y, Kilby MD, Sansom DM, Drayson MT. Normal human pregnancy is associated with an elevation in the human suppressive CD25+CD4+ regulatory T-cell subset. Immunology 2004; 112:38–43.
20. Francis J, Rai R, Sebire NJ, et al. Impaired expression of endometrial differentiation markers and complement regulatory proteins in patients with recurrent pregnancy loss associated with antiphospholipid syndrome. Mol Hum Reprod 2006; 12:435–42.
21. Buckingham KL, Stone PR, Smith JF, Chamley LW. Antiphospholipid antibodies in serum and follicular fluid – Is there a correlation with IVF implantation failure? Hum Reprod 2006; 21:728–34.
22. Ntrivalas EI, Bowser CR, Kwak-Kim J, Beaman KD, Gilman-Sachs A. Expression of killer immunoglobulin-like receptors on peripheral blood NK cell subsets of women with recurrent spontaneous abortions or implantation failures. Am J Reprod Immunol 2005; 53:215–21.
23. Cameo P, Srisuparp S, Strakova S, Fazleabas AT. Chorionic gonadotropin and uterine dialogue in the primate. Reprod Biol Endocrinol 2004; 2:50.
24. O'Niell C. The role of PAF in embryo physiology. Hum Reprod Update 2005; 11:215–28.
25. Roudboush WE, Wininger JD, Jones AE, et al. Embryonic platelet-activating factor: an indicator of embryo viability. Hum Reprod 2002; 17:1306–10.
26. Cavanagh AC, Morton H. The purification of early-pregnancy factor to homogeneity from human platelets and identification as chaperonin 10. Eur J Biochem 1994; 222:551–60.
27. Ohnuma K, Ito K, Takahashi J, Nambo Y, Miyake Y. Partial purification of mare early pregnancy factor. Am J Reprod Immunol 2004; 51:95–101.
28. Athanasas-Platsis C, Somodevilla-Torres MJ, Morton H, Cavanagh AC. Investigation of the immunocompetent cells that bind early pregnancy factor and preliminary studies of the early pregnancy factor target molecule. Immunol Cell Biol 2004; 82:361–9.

29. Akyol S, Gercel-Taylor C, Reynolds HS, Taylor DD. HSP-10 in ovarian cancer: expression and suppression of T-cell signaling. Gynecol Oncol 2006; 101:481–6.

30. Fuzzi B, Rizzo R, Criscuoli L, et al. HLA-G expression in early embryos is a fundamental prerequisite for the obtainment of pregnancy. Eur J Immunol 2002; 32:311–15.

31. Bainbridge D, Ellis S, Le Bouteiller P, Sargent I. HLA-G remains a mystery. Trends Immunol 2001; 22:548–52.

32. Gomez-Lozano N, de Pablo R, Puente S, Vilches C. Recognition of HLA-G by the NK receptor KIR2DL4 is not essential for human reproduction. Eur J Immunol 2003; 33:639–44.

33. Yan WH, Fan LA, Yang JQ, et al. HLA-G polymorphism in a Chinese Han population with recurrent spontaneous abortion. Int J Immunogenet 2006; 33:55–8.

34. Criscuoli L, Rizzo R, Fuzzi B, et al. Lack of histocompatibility leukocyte antigen-G expression in early embryos is not related to germinal defects or impairment of interleukin-10 production by embryos. Gynecol Endocrinol 2005; 20:264–9.

35. Sargent IL. Does 'soluble' HLA-G really exist? Another twist to the tale. Mol Human Reprod 2005; 11:695–8.

36. Barnea ER, Lahijani KI, Roussev R, Barnea JD, Coulam CB. Use of lymphocyte platelet binding assay for detecting a preimplantation factor: a quantitative assay. Am J Reprod Immunol 1994; 32:133–8.

37. Rosario GX, Modi ND, Sachdeva G, et al. Morphological events in the primate endometrium in the presence of a preimplantation embryo, detected by the serum preimplantation assay. Hum Reprod 2005; 20:61–71.

38. Coulam CB, Roussev RG, Thomasson EJ, Barnea ER. Preimplantation factor (PIF) predicts subsequent pregnancy loss. Am J Reprod Immunol 1995; 34:88–92.

39. Roussev RG, Coulam CB, Kaider BD, Yarkoni M, et al. Embryonic origin of preimplantation factor (PIF): biological activity and partial characterization. Mol Hum Reprod 1996; 2:883–7.

40. Roussev RG, Barnea ER, Thomason EJ, Coulam CB. A novel bioassay for detection of preimplantation factor (PIF). Am J Reprod Immunol 1995; 33:68–73.

41. Barnea ER, Simon J, Levine SP, et al. Progress in characterization of pre-implantation factor in embryo cultures and in vivo. Am J Reprod Immunol 1999; 42:95–9.

42. Barnea ER. Insight into early pregnancy: emerging role of the embryo. Am J Reprod Immunol 2004; 51:319–22.

3. Genetics of spontaneous abortions

Joe Leigh Simpson

INTRODUCTION

Genetic factors are the most common causes of spontaneous abortions. From 50% to 80% of first-trimester abortions show chromosomal abnormalities. Additionally, there are other genetic causes distinct from chromosomal abnormalities. Single-gene abnormalities are almost unexplored in spontaneous abortions, although single-gene defects are a more common cause of birth defects in liveborns than chromosomal abnormalities. Many causes of repeated abortions that are commonly classified as 'non-genetic' are actually the result of perturbations of gene products such as factor V Leiden, and other genes associated with thromboembolism, and alloimmune pregnancy loss (which may involve shared human leukocyte antigen (HLA) molecules). In this chapter, we shall restrict the discussion to the frequency and most common genetic causes of sporadic and recurrent abortions.

CHROMOSOMAL ABNORMALITIES IN PREIMPLANTATION EMBRYOS

The frequency of losses in human preimplantation embryos is very high.[1,2] This is reflected by pregnancy rates being no more than 25–35% per embryo transfer in assisted reproductive technology (ART), even in experienced hands. Of morphologically normal embryos, no less than 25% show chromosomal abnormalities (aneuploidy or polyploidy).[3] This is based on studies using fluorescence in situ hybridization (FISH) with chromosome-specific probes for only seven to nine chromosomes; rates would doubtless be higher if it were possible to routinely perform a complete karyotype or microarray analysis on a blastomere. The 25% aneuploidy rate in morphologically normal embryos is consistent with

6% aneuploidy in sperm from ostensibly normal males[4,5] and in 20% in oocytes.[6,7] Aneuploidy rates in embryos and oocytes increase as maternal age increases.

Chromosomal abnormalities are even more frequent in morphologically abnormal embryos. Using FISH with chromosome-specific probes, abnormality rates of 50–75% can be observed, even when not all chromosomes are tested.[3]

CHROMOSOMAL ABNORMALITIES: THE MOST FREQUENT EXPLANATION FOR CLINICALLY RECOGNIZED SPONTANEOUS ABORTIONS

FREQUENCY

No less than 50% of clinically recognized pregnancy losses show a chromosomal abnormality.[8–10] This figure is based on analysis of spontaneously expelled products. If chorionic villus sampling (CVS) is performed after ultrasound diagnosis of fetal demise, the frequency is 75–90%.[11,12] Comparative genomic hybridization (CGH; microarray analysis) also reveals abnormalities in abortuses that are not evident by karyotype.[13] Using chromosomal microarrays, additional abnormalities can be detected. Schaeffer et al[14] performed CGH using microarrays on 41 abortuses that had previously been analyzed by karyotype. Array analysis revealed heretofore unrecognized abnormalities in 4 of the 41 cases.

In the second trimester, chromosomal abnormalities are less frequent. The actual frequency is not certain, because many abortuses recognized in the second trimester are really missed abortions that were retained in utero after a first-trimester demise. It has long been recognized that fetal demise may precede spontaneous expulsion of the products of conception by several weeks.[15] The anomalies seen in second-trimester abortions are similar to those observed in liveborn infants: trisomies 13, 18, and 21; monosomy X; and sex chromosomal polysomies. The frequency of these anomalies is estimated to be approximately 15%.

In third-trimester losses (stillborn infants), the frequency of chromosomal abnormalities is 5%.[16] This incidence is less than that observed in earlier abortuses, but greater than the 0.6% found in live-borns. A major problem in assessing the frequency of chromosomal abnormalities is that maceration ensues soon after fetal death – usually days in advance of delivery. Hefler et al[17] found that 63% of 139 third-trimester losses were macerated, impeding accurate morphological assessment and cytogenetic studies. Again, a large series of stillbirths studied by microarray analysis would be informative.

SPECTRUM OF CHROMOSOMAL ABNORMALITIES

AUTOSOMAL TRISOMY

Autosomal trisomies comprise approximately 50% of cytogenetically abnormal spontaneous abortions. Trisomy for every chromosome has now been observed. Table 3.1 shows frequencies in one series. The most common trisomies are 16, 22, 21, 15, 13, and 14 (in descending order). Trisomy 16 is rarely, if ever, observed in liveborns in non-mosaic form, but is the most common aberration in the abortus. These six chromosomes in aggregate account for 70% of trisomies – an important consideration in selecting probes to exclude aneuploidy in preimplantation genetic diagnosis (PGD).

Correlations between placental morphological abnormalities and specific trisomies have been attempted, but remain imprecise. Attempts are complicated by non-specific villous changes following fetal demise in utero. Thus, low predictive value exists when placental histology is used to distinguish aneuploid from euploid abortuses. A few correlations are valid. Fetuses with trisomies incompatible with life grow more slowly than those with trisomies compatible with life (e.g., trisomies 13, 18, and 21). The mean crown–rump length (CRL) for the latter is 20.65 mm, compared with only 10.66 mm for the former.[18] Either fetuses with non-lethal trisomies live longer than those with lethal

Table 3.1 Chromosomal completion in spontaneous abortions; recognized clinically in the first trimester[a]

Completion	Frequency	Percentage
Normal: 46,XX or 46,XY		54.1
Triploidy:		7.7
69,XXX	2.7	
69,XYX	0.2	
69,XXY	4.0	
Other	0.8	
Tetraploidy:		2.6
92,XXX	1.5	
92,XXYY	0.55	
Not stated	0.55	
Monosomy X		18.6
Structural abnormalities		1.5
Sex-chromosomal polysomy:		0.2
47,XXX	0.05	
47,XXY	0.15	
Autosomal monosomy (G)		0.1
Autosomal trisomy for chromosomes:		22.3
1	0	
2	1.11	
3	0.25	
4	0.64	
5	0.04	
6	0.14	
7	0.89	
8	0.79	
9	0.72	
10	0.36	
11	0.04	
12	0.18	
13	1.07	
14	0.82	
15	1.68	
16	7.27	
17	0.18	
18	1.15	
19	0.01	
20	0.61	
21	2.11	
22	2.26	
Double trisomy		0.7
Mosaic trisomy		1.3
Other abnormalities or not specified		0.9
		100.0

[a] Pooled data from several series, as referenced by Simpson and Bombard.[10]

trisomies, or the fetuses with lethal trisomies also exhibit greater intrauterine growth retardation (IUGR), or both. Abortuses from non-lethal trisomies (13, 18, and 21) tend to show anomalies consistent with those found in full-term liveborn trisomic infants.[18,19] Malformations observed may be more severe than those found in induced abortuses detected after prenatal diagnosis.

Most trisomies show a maternal age effect, but the effect varies among chromosomes. The maternal age correlates positively with errors at meiosis I, the most common cytological explanation for trisomies. The proportion of trisomies that arise at meiosis I versus meiosis II varies among aneuploidies. Virtually all trisomy 16 cases are maternal in origin, and arise in meiosis I.[20] In trisomies 13 and 21, 90% are maternal, usually arising at meiosis I. In trisomy 18, however, two-thirds of the 90% of the maternal origin cases arise at meiosis II.[21,22] Maternal meiosis errors correlate not only with advanced maternal age, but also with decreased or absent meiotic recombination.[21–23] The mechanism invoked to explain this relationship is the product-line hypothesis. Oocytes ovulated earlier in life are believed to be more likely to have undergone genetic recombination and hence are less predisposed to non-disjunction.[24] The location of the recombinant event on the chromosome and the exact nature of recombination are pivotal, as discussed elsewhere.[25]

Errors in paternal meiosis account for 10% of acrocentric (13, 14, 15, 21, and 22) trisomies.[26] In non-acrocentric trisomies paternal meiotic errors are equally likely to arise at meiosis I or II.[27] Paternal meiotic errors account for 10% of trisomy 21 cases, and for some cases of trisomy 2 abortuses. A paternal contribution is uncommon in other abortus trisomies.

The ability to analyze polar bodies (1st and 2nd) for PGD has generated a new body of information on maternal meiosis.[28] This topic is beyond the scope of this chapter, and it remains unclear whether the abnormalities detected in polar bodies are as directly applicable to clinically recognized abortuses as they clear are to preimplantation embryos. Polar body studies have revealed that rates of meiosis I errors are only marginally higher (41.7% versus 35.2) than meiosis II errors; errors in both meiosis I and II are not uncommon.[28] The relative distribution of errors thus differs from that observed in trisomies recovered later in pregnancy.

DOUBLE TRISOMY

The frequency of double trisomy in abortuses is more common than expected by chance. The frequency varies more than for other chromosomal abnormalities, which may reflect vicissitudes of culture (failure) or differences in sample characteristics (maternal or gestational age). Table 3.1 (based on series collected up to 1987) shows that double trisomies accounted for 0.7% of abortuses. A similar prevalence was observed in pooled data tabulated in 1997 by Reddy.[29] However, a more recent report of 517 abortuses found double trisomies in 2.2% of 321 successfully karyotyped abortuses.[30] Double trisomies most often involve the X chromosome, but may involve the Y chromosme, or autosomes 21, 18, 16, 22, 13, 8, 2, and 15 in descending order (Table 3.2). Diego-Alvarez et al[30] have described the exact combinations of the 178 reported double trisomies. In liveborns, approximately 50 double trisomies have been reported.[31] In liveborns, usually one of the additional chromosomes is an X and the other is 13, 18, or 21.

The gestational age was 8.7 ± 2.2 weeks at abortion in double trisomies in Reddy's[29] series, compared with 10.1 ± 2.9 weeks for a single trisomy. In the series of Diego-Alvarez et al,[30] the gestational age was 8.2 ± 1.7 for double trisomies. The sex ratio was approximately 1 in both series.

Morphological examination usually reveals an empty sac[29,30] and only occasionally an embryo.

Table 3.2 Chromosomes involved in double-trisomy abortuses[30]

Chromosome	1	2	3	4	5	6	7	8	9	10	11	12	13	14	15	16	17	18	19	20	21	22	X/Y	Total
No. of cases	0	15	0	5	4	3	7	18	5	2	1	2	18	7	13	37	2	44	0	8	66	20	79	360

In one study, 5 of 7 double trisomies showed no morphological detail;[30] one was anembryonic and the other (48,XXX,+18) showed hydrops fetalis.

Advanced maternal age is a striking feature.[29–31] In the series of Diego-Alvarez et al,[30] the mean maternal age was 39.7 ± 3.4 years. Almost all analyzed cases originated at maternal meiosis. As expected, the stage of meiotic error is consistent with that expected for single trisomies. Thus, double trisomy involving chromosome 18 is more likely to show meiosis II errors than 48,XX,+16,+21.

POLYPLOIDY

In polyploidy, more than two haploid chromosomal complements exist. Non-mosaic triploidy ($3n = 69$) and tetraploidy ($4n = 92$) are not common in abortuses (Table 3.1). Diploid/triploid mosaicism is found in approximately 30% of blastocysts. However, placental mosaicism of this type is thought to involve trophoectoderm rather than the embryo per se (inner cell mass), and will therefore not be discussed here.[32] Of general interest, however, is the association between diandric (paternally inherited) triploidy and hydatidiform mole. A 'partial mole' exists if molar tissue and fetal parts coexist. Partial (triploid) moles must be distinguished from the more common 'complete' hydatidiform moles. Complete moles are 46,XX, exclusively of androgenetic origin, and exclusively villous tissue.[33]

Placental findings in diandric triploid placentas include a disproportionately large gestational sac, focal (partial) hydropic degeneration of placental villi, and trophoblast hyperplasia.[34] Placental hydropic changes are progressive, and hence difficult to identify early in early pregnancy. Irrespective of chromosomal status, placental villi also undergo non-specific hydropic degeneration following fetal demise. This makes histological and cytogenetic corrections difficult. Embryonic/fetal malformations associated with triploid abortuses include neural tube defects and omphaloceles – anomalies reminiscent of those in triploid conceptuses surviving to term. Facial dysmorphia and limb abnormalities have also been reported.[35] There is no correlation between embryonic morphology and parental origin (diandry or digyny).[35]

Triploid abortuses are usually 69,XXY or 69,XXX. The origin has long been presumed to be due to dispermy, and this has been verified.[33,36,37] Triploidy may follow either fertilization by two haploid sperm or fertilization by single diploid sperm.[37,38]

TETRAPLOIDY

Tetraploidy ($4n = 92$) is uncommon, rarely progressing beyond 2–3 weeks of embryonic life. This chromosomal abnormality can be associated with persistent trophoblastic disease, and thus needs to be identified in order to provide appropriate follow-up. Tetraploidy in embryonic tissue should be distinguished from the not uncommon, and clinically insignificant, tetraploid cells found in amniotic fluid. Although uncommon, true fetal tetraploidy does exist,[39] and probably arises from failure of cytokinesis.[40] Failure of cytokinesis has been deduced on the basis of chromosomal complement (92,XXXX or 92,XXYY), and more recently confirmed by molecular studies.[41]

MONOSOMY X

Monosomy X accounts for 15–20% of chromosomally abnormal specimens. Autosomal monosomy appears to be lethal prior to or just beyond implantation, and thus seems not to persist to clinical recognition. Early monosomy X abortuses usually consist of only an umbilical cord stump. If survival persists until later in gestation, anomalies characteristic of Turner syndrome may be seen. These include cystic hygromas, generalized edema, and cardiac defects. Unlike liveborn 45,X individuals, 45,X abortuses show germ cells; however, germ cells rarely develop beyond the primordial stage. The pathogenesis of 45,X germ cell failure seems to be rapid attrition of germ cells, rather than failure of germ cell development.[42,43] Rapid attrition of germ cells explains the rare but well-documented pregnancies occurring in 45,X individuals. Mosaicism (45,X/46,XX) need not necessarily be invoked as the mechanism explaining pregnancies.[44]

Approximately 80% of monosomy X occurs as a result of paternal sex chromosome loss.[45]

Consequently, there is a lack of a maternal age effect in 45,X. An inverse age effect has been reported.

SEX CHROMOSOMAL POLYSOMY (X OR Y)

The complements 47,XXY and 47,XYY each occur in about 1 per 800 liveborn male births; 47,XXX occurs in 1 per 800 female births. X or Y polysomies are slightly (10%) more common in abortuses than in liveborns.

RECURRENT ANEUPLOIDY

DOES RECURRENT ANEUPLOIDY EXIST?

In first-trimester abortions, recurrent aneuploidy occurs more often than expected by chance. However, a lack of consensus exists on the extent to which numerical chromosomal abnormalities (aneuploidy) explain recurrent losses. In my view, recurrent aneuploidy is a frequent explanation – at least until the number of losses exceeds 4. This reasoning is based on observations that the chromosomal complements of abortuses in a given family are more likely to be either recurrently normal or recurrently abnormal (Table 3.3). That is, if the complement of the first abortus is abnormal, the likelihood is increased that the complement of the second abortus will also be abnormal.[46] Recurrence usually involves trisomy. The ramifications become significant with respect to therapeutic management (or lack thereof).

Some of the non-random distributions reflect an increasing incidence of aneuploidy as maternal age increases. Adjustments for maternal age account for some of the ostensibly non-random distribution, and, in the opinion of Warburton et al,[46] precluded a relationship. The study by Warburton et al[46] pooled cases from a New York City sample and a Hawaii sample.[47] However, a confounder is that in the New York City cases, the inclusion criteria extended to 28 weeks' gestation; these cases predictably had a lower overall aneuploidy rate than the earlier-gestation sample from Hawaii. Hence, recurrent aneuploidy that had previously seemed to clearly exist in the Hawaii sample of Hassold et al,[47] but was not statistically confirmed by Warburton et al.[46] Studying recurrent aneuploidy in preimplantation embryos has since seemingly convinced Warburton of the concept of recurrent aneuploidy.[48]

A different approach that also supports the concept of recurrent aneuploidy is calculation of aneuploidy rates in prenatal diagnosis samples, in comparison with prior pregnancy outcome. Bianco et al[48] studied 46 939 women undergoing prenatal genetic diagnosis (CVS or amniocentesis). The prevalence of aneuploidy increased progressively as the number of prior spontaneous abortuses increased (Table 3.4): 1.39% with no prior abortuses, 1.67% after one, 1.84% after two, and 2.18% after three abortions. After adjustments for

---

Table 3.3 Recurrent aneuploidy: relationship between karyotypes of successive abortuses[46]

Complement of first abortus	Complement of second abortus					
	Normal	Trisomy	Monosomy	Triploidy	Tetraploidy	De novo rearrangement
Normal	142	18	5	7	3	2
Trisomy	31	30	1	4	3	1
Monosomy X	7	5	3	3	0	0
Triploidy	7	4	1	4	0	0
Tetraploidy	3	1	0	2	0	0
De novo Rearrangement	1	3	0	0	0	0

Table 3.4 Risk of aneuploidy by number of prior miscarriage; stratified by maternal age. Comparison is with women with no spontaneous abortions, controlling for parity and indications for prenatal diagnosis[49]

No. of prior spontaneous abortions	Maternal age < 35 years	
	Adjusted OR for trisomy 13, 18, or 21[a]	Adjusted OR for all aneuploidies[a]
0	1.00	1.00
1	1.27 (0.74–2.08)	1.19 (0.78–1.84)
2	1.31 (0.80–2.13)	1.21 (0.94–1.58)
≥3	1.36 (0.46–2.73)	1.41 (0.56–3.19)

No. of prior spontaneous abortions	Maternal age > 35 years	
	Adjusted OR for trisomy 13, 18, or 21[a]	Adjusted OR for all aneuploidies[a]
0	1.00	1.00
1	1.23 (1.04–1.52)	1.23 (1.00–1.52)
2	1.34 (1.01–1.82)	1.30 (0.99–1.74)
≥3	1.56 (1.03–2.31)	1.68 (1.12–2.52)

[a] OR, odds ratio. 95% confidence interval in parenthesis.

maternal age, ethnicity, and type of invasive procedure (a surrogate indicator of gestational age), the odds ratios were 1.21 (95% confidence interval (CI) 1.01–1.47), 1.26, and 1.51, respectively. These findings thus confirmed an earlier study by Drugan et al.[50]

Further supporting recurrent aneuploidy as a genuine phenomenon is the occurrence of trisomic preimplantation embryos in successive ART cycles. Rubio et al[51] showed increased aneuploid embryos in couples with repeated abortions, compared with couples undergoing PGD for mendelian indications. Frequencies of chromosomal abnormalities were 71% versus 45%, respectively. In a similar study, Munne et al[48] found rates to be 37% versus 21% in women under age 35 years, and 34% versus 31.5% in women over 35 years.

CONSEQUENCES FOR GENETIC COUNSELING

If couples are predisposed to recurrent aneuploidy, they might logically be at increased risk not only for aneuploid abortuses but also for aneuploid liveborns. The trisomic autosome in a subsequent pregnancy might not always confer lethality, but might be compatible with life (e.g., trisomy 21). Indeed, the risk of liveborn trisomy 21 following an aneuploid abortus has long been considered to be

about 1%.[52] Based on first-trimester trisomies, which may or may not survive, Snijders and Nicholaides[53] reported a recurrence rate of 0.7% following trisomy 21 and 0.7% following trisomy 18. Bianco et al[49] describe the consequences of a prior abortion of unknown karyotype. If abortions are recurrent but no information is available on the chromosomal status, the odds ratios provided by Bianco et al[49] can be applied to give a patient specific risk (Table 3.4). For example, if the a priori Down syndrome risk is 1 in 300, a woman's calculated risk after 3 abortions would be 1/300 × 1.5, or 1/200.

EXPECTATIONS OF THE KARYOTYPE IN RECURRENT ABORTION

The concept of recurrent aneuploidy has certain corollaries, one of which has been the subject of controversy. Given the existence of recurrent aneuploidy, and that 50% of all abortuses are abnormal cytogenetically, aneuploidy should be as likely to be detected in a recurrent abortus as in a sporadic abortus. This has proved to be true in most series. Stern et al[54] found a 57% prevalence of chromosomal abnormalities among abortuses of repetitively aborting women – a frequency coincidentally identical among abortuses of sporadically aborting women. Among 420 abortuses obtained from women with repeated losses, Stephenson et al[55] found 46% chromosomal abnormalities; 31% of the original sample was trisomic. Their comparison was unselected pooled data, which showed 48% of abortuses to be abnormal; 27% of the original sample was trisomic.

Other authors have concluded that a recurrent abortus is likely to be cytogenetically normal whereas a sporadic abortuses will be cytogenetically abnormal. Carp et al[56] found that among women having three or more abortuses, the likelihood that the abortus would have an abnormal karyotype was 29%. After an aneuploid abortus, the likelihood of a subsequent live birth was 68% (13 of 19). If the abortus was euploid, the subsequent live birth rate was 41% (16 of 39). One explanation for the difference between this study and those cited above might be a different referral pattern, for example biased toward autoimmune causes. A second possibility is simply the small numbers in each subgroup. A third and more likely possibility is the increased gestational age in this sample. That only 29% of abortuses in the series of Carp et al[56] were chromosomally abnormal is consistent with inclusion criteria extending to 20 weeks' gestation. There is less reason to expect recurrent aneuploidy in the second trimester, given the low (15%) frequency of chromosomal abnormalities in the second trimester. A fourth possibility is the higher mean number of previous pregnancy losses (4.7) in the series of Carp et al.[56]

RELATIONSHIP OF RECURRENT ANEUPLOIDY TO NUMBER OF LOSSES

Although recurrent aneuploidy appears to exist with two or three losses, this does not necessarily hold for higher-order losses. These seem more likely to be cytogenetically normal.[57] Maternal factors thus become plausible explanations when numbers of losses exceed four. Consecutive losses of high number also favor non-aneuploid explanations, because one would not necessarily expect every single abortus to be aneuploid.

CONSEQUENCES FOR CLINICAL MANAGEMENT

That recurrent aneuploidy exists dictates that neither a genetic nor a non-genetic etiology should be assumed on the basis of number of losses. Often, there is no information concerning the chromosomal status of prior abortuses. However, paraffin blocks of products of conception are suitable for FISH analysis of chromosomes most likely to be trisomic (13, 14, 16, 18, 21, and 22). Chromosomal microarrays may also yield information on paraffin block specimens.[58] If no information can be obtained, it is less clear whether prenatal genetic diagnosis is appropriate. However, the risk of an aneuploid offspring is still increased, and indeed can be calculated as discussed above.[49] The small but finite risk of amniocentesis or CVS is especially troublesome to couples who have had difficulty maintaining a pregnancy. Non-invasive approaches may be the preferable initial option, but the sensitivity for detecting aneuploidy does not exceed 85–95%.[59] PGD is another option. The selective transfer of euploid embryos clearly decreases clinical abortions in couples with RPL.[60,61] Studies are underway to verify the expected increase in liveborns.

STRUCTURAL CHROMOSOMAL REARRANGEMENTS: TRANSLOCATIONS

Structural chromosomal rearrangements are an important cause of recurrent abortions, but account for only 1.5% of all abortuses. The presence of a balanced rearrangement in one parent can result in an unbalanced translocation in the offspring.[62] Phenotypic consequences depend on the specific duplicated or deficient chromosomal segments.

FREQUENCY

A balanced translocation is found in 4–5% of couples experiencing repeated losses.[63–65] These individuals are themselves phenotypically normal, but their offspring (abortuses or abnormal liveborns) may show chromosomal duplications or deficiencies as a result of normal meiotic segregation. The frequency of balanced translocations is higher in females than males,[63] and if there is a family history of a stillborn or abnormal liveborn.[65]

The likelihood of detecting a translocation heterozygote does not necessarily reflect maternal age,[66] nor does the likelihood of detecting a balanced translocation substantially differ after 1, 2, or 3 miscarriages. In the tabulation by Simpson et al,[63] detection rates in females after 2, 3, 4, and 5 losses were 0.8%, 1.7%, 2.3%, and 2.9%, respectively. For males, the respective rates were 1.2%, 1.9%, 2.4%, and 0 (0/39). In the study by Goddijn et al,[66] the odds ratios for finding a balanced translocation after 2, 3, and 4 or more losses were 1.4 (95% CI 0.4–4.8), 2.2 (0.4–12.5), and 2.1 (0.3–15.4), respectively.

LIKELIHOOD OF ABNORMAL LIVEBORNS

There are two general types of translocations: Robertsonian and reciprocal. Robertsonian translocations involve centric fusion of an acrocentric (13, 14, 15, 21, 22) chromosome. The theoretical risk of a parent with t(14q;21q) having a liveborn child with Down syndrome is 33%. However, the empirical risks are considerably less, given the lethality of certain complements. The risks are 2% if the father carries a translocation involving chromosome 21 and 10% if the mother carries such a translocation.[67,68] Robertsonian (centric fusion) translocations involving chromosomes other than chromosome 21 show lower empirical risks. In t(13q;14q), the risk for liveborn trisomy 13 is 1% or less. This low risk presumably reflects the lethality of many segregant products (trisomies and monosomies).

In reciprocal translocations, interchanges occur between two or more metacentric chromosomes. Empirical data for specific translocations are usually not available, and generalizations are typically made on the basis of pooled data derived from many different translocations. As in Robertsonian translocations, the theoretical risks for abnormal offspring (unbalanced reciprocal translocations) are much greater than the empirical risks. The sex differences are less apparent. The risks are 12% for

offspring of either female heterozygotes or male heterozygotes.[67,68]

The mode of ascertainment is important in counseling. The frequency of unbalanced fetuses is lower if a parental balanced translocation was ascertained through repetitive abortions (3%) than through anomalous liveborns (nearly 20%).[67] Presumably, the likelihood of severely unbalanced products (e.g., 3:1 segregation) is greater in the former. Detecting a chromosomal rearrangement in a parent obviously dictates that prenatal cytogenetic studies should be offered. Even if there is normal transmission of chromosomes involved in the translocation, a different chromosome could be aneuploid (interchromosomal effect).

LIKELIHOOD OF SUBSEQUENT ABORTIONS

Distinct from the likelihood of unbalanced segregants is the quantitative likelihood of subsequent abortion. Does this differ from the expected 65–70% live birth rate observed in the general population with recurrent pregnancy loss (RPL)? A less favorable prognosis has been reported. In the study by Sugiura-Ogasawara et al,[69] the loss rates were 61% (11/18) for couples in which the male partner had a translocation and 72.4% (21/29) if the female partner had the translocation. Of 1184 couples with two or more miscarriages who had normal karyotypes, the miscarriage rate, by contrast, was only 28.3% (335/1184).[69] In 2004, Carp et al[70] reported that 45.2% (33/73) pregnancies of couples with a translocation heterozygote resulted in a live birth, compared with 55.3% (325/588) without a translocation. The same group later found a similar percentage of normal and balanced karyotypes (74%) in embryos of translocation heterozygotes as well as embryos of couples without a translocation (77%).[71] Carp et al[71] concluded that any decrease in the live birth rate was due to factors unrelated to the chromosomal imbalance. Different results have been reported by others. Goddijn et al[66] reported only 26% miscarriages among 43 pregnancies in 25 carrier couples. However, almost half of the patients in the series of Goddijn et al[66] (55/115) had only two miscarriages, which may account for the different results. Stephenson and Sierra[72] studied 1893 couples, 40 of whom had a balanced translocation (28 reciprocal and 12 Robertsonian). Among 35 monitored pregnancies in the reciprocal translocation group, the live birth rate was 63% (22/35); in the Robertsonian translocation group, it was 69% (9/13). These data are comparable to those in the general RPL population. However, the proportion of structurally unbalanced abortuses was increased. Among abortuses of the translocation heterozygote couples, 13 of 36 (36%) were unbalanced, 11 of 36 (30%) aneuploid for another chromosome (interchromosomal effect), and only 12 of 36 (33%) normal. Among recurrent miscarriage couples not having a translocation, the rates were 2%, 44%, and 54%, respectively. These findings are at odds with those of Carp et al.[71] However, the series of Stephenson and Sierra[72] included 7 patients (14%) with two previous losses, whereas that of Carp et al[71] was restricted to patients with three or more losses (mean 4.27). The different number of previous losses may partially explain the different results.

Rarely, a translocation precludes a normal liveborn infant. This occurs when a translocation involves homologous acrocentric chromosomes (e.g., t(13q;13q) or t(21q;21q)). The only possibility of normalcy is if trisomic rescue occurs; i.e., the 'additional' chromosome is 'expelled' from the nucleus to yield the normal chromosomal number with one homologous chromosome. If the father carries a homologous structural rearrangement, artificial insemination may be appropriate. If the mother carries the rearrangement, donor oocytes or donor embryos should be considered.

In conclusion, when a balanced translocation is detected in a couple experiencing recurrent abortions, the prognosis for a live birth remains uncertain compared with the situation if a translocation had not been detected.[70] In my opinion, the increased frequency of loss dictates offering the option of PGD, given that 80–100% of embryos can be non-viable.[28,73] The strategy is to identify and transfer only the (few) balanced embryos. Indeed, this decreases the likelihood of abortion.[28,60]

INVERSIONS

In an inversion, the order of genes is reversed. The clinical consequence is analogous to that of a translocation, in that individuals heterozygous for an inversion are normal but their genes are rearranged. Likewise, these individuals suffer untoward reproductive consequences as result of normal meiotic phenomena. However, crossing-over involving the inverted segment may produce unbalanced gametes. Duplication exists for some regions and deficiency for others. There are two types of inversions. In pericentric inversions, breaks occur in both arms. In paracentric inversions, breaks occur on the same arm. The frequency of inversions in couples having repetitive abortions is less than 1%.

LIKELIHOOD OF ABNORMAL LIVEBORNS

Females with a pericentric inversion have a 7% risk of abnormal liveborns; males carry about a 5% risk.[74] Pericentric inversions ascertained through phenotypically normal probands are less likely to result in abnormal live infants. The extent of origin of the crossing within the inverted segment influences the likelihood of a fetal anomaly. The clinical outcome is paradoxical. Inversions involving only a small portion of the total chromosomal length are usually lethal because, when recombinants arise, they yield large duplications or deficiencies. By contrast, products of larger inversions, involving 30–60% of the total chromosomal length, are relatively more likely to survive.[74] On a molecular level, inversions less than 100 Mbp appear not to exert undue untoward outcomes.[75] There were no recombinants in a tabulation when inversion was less than 50 Mbp (40% of chromosome) length and only a few around 50 Mbp (40–50%) length; a higher number occurred if the inversion was greater than100 Mbp.[75]

Data are limited on recurrence risks involving paracentric inversions. Theoretically, there should be a lower risk of unbalanced products of clinical consequence than with pericentric inversions, because nearly all paracentric recombinants should be lethal. However, both abortions and abnormal liveborns have been observed within the same kindred. The risk for unbalanced viable offspring has been tabulated to be 4%.[76]

LIKELIHOOD OF SUBSEQUENT ABORTIONS

Few data exist on the likelihood of abortion following the detection of an inversion in one of the parents. In the series of Stephenson and Sierra,[72] there were 7 inversion carriers with 35 pregnancies; 31% were livebirths and 69% miscarriages (24/35). In the series of Carp et al,[70] 8 of 15 pregnancies (53%) were live births. These outcomes are less favorable than in the general population, but data are sparse.

DEVELOPMENTAL GENES: MENDELIAN
AND POLYGENIC/MULTIFACTORIAL

From 50% to 80% of first-trimester abortuses show chromosomal abnormalities. Casual deductions might lead one to conclude that the other 20–50% might not have a genetic etiology. However, this would not be correct, because mendelian and polygenic/multifactorial disorders show chromosomal abnormalities. Indeed, these conditions far more commonly explain congenital anomalies in liveborns than do chromosomal abnormalities. Thus, it would be naive to assume that mendelian and polygenic/multifactorial factors do not play pivotal roles in embryonic mortality. The difficulty is that few of the many genes required for differentiation have been identified, despite there being a myriad of potential candidate genes. As one example, Baek[77] enumerated over 30 highly plausible candidate genes. Many genes in animals are known to produce lethality, as demonstrated by null mutants (knockouts) in mice. In embryonic humans, lethality is recognized for certain genes (e.g., *OCT4*), but studies in embryos that survive until the first trimester are limited.

Embryos that abort because of mendelian or polygenic factors may or may not show structural anomalies. However, a structural anomaly found in an abortion having a normal chromosomal complement may still point to a genetic etiology. The lack of cytogenetic data on dissected specimens has made it difficult to determine the exact role that non-cytogenetic mechanisms play in early embryonic maldevelopment. Philipp and Kalousek[78] sought to address this by correlating the cytogenetic status of missed abortions with morphological abnormalities observed at embryoscopy. Embryos with chromosomal abnormalities usually showed one or more external anomalies, but some euploid embryos also showed anatomical anomalies.

Indirect evidence further points to a mendelian etiology in human abortuses. Mosaicism may be restricted to the placenta, the embryo per se being normal. Termed 'confined placental mosaicism,' this phenomenon has as a corollary uniparental disomy (UPD). In UPD, both homologues for a given chromosome are derived from a single parent. UPD is thought to occur as result of expulsion of a chromosome from a trisomic zygote ('trisomic rescue'). Although the karyotype would be euploid (46,XX or 46,XY), genes on the involved chromosome have a 1 in 3 likelihood of having the genetic contribution of only one single parent. Indeed, uniparental disomy for chromosome 21 has been detected in an embryonic abortus.[79] Lethality would occur if that chromosome contains an imprinted gene that needed to be inherited from the parent whose chromosome was excluded. (The same problems can occur in trisomic rescue involving a robertsonian translocation.) Another mechanism involves a heterozygous mutant that became homozygous (actually doubly hemizygous) through trisomic rescue.

Another mechanism indirectly pointing to the existence of mutant genes is skewed X-inactivation. Among 48 women having two prior losses with no obvious explanation, 7 (14.6%) had skewed X-inactivation as defined by 90% of their X chromosomes originating from one parent (expected 50%); only 1 of 67 controls (1.5%) showed skewed X-inactivation.[80] The non-random distribution could be explained by lethality for an X-linked gene on the X chromosome of a single parent. Thus, male offspring of a woman with skewed X-inactivation might preferentially be aborted. The loss could be the specific result of UPD per se, or it could reflect the sole contribution by the single parent having a lethal gene (heterozygosity). Pedigrees consistent with this hypothesis have been reported.[81]

REFERENCES

1. Plachot M, Junca AM, Mandelbaum J, et al. Chromosome investigations in early life. II. Human preimplantation embryos. Hum Reprod 1987; 2:29–35.
2. Papadopoulos G, Templeton AA, Fisk N, et al. The frequency of chromosome anomalies in human preimplantation embryos after in-vitro fertilization. Hum Reprod 1989; 4:91–8.
3. Munné S, Alikani M, Tomkin G, et al. Embryo morphology, developmental rates, and maternal age are correlated with chromosome abnormalities. Fertil Steril 1995; 64:382–91.
4. Egozcue J, Blanco J, Vidal F. Chromosome studies in human sperm nuclei using fluorescence in-situ hybridization (FISH). Hum Reprod Update 1997; 3:441–52.
5. Pellestor F, Anahory T, Hamamah S. The chromosomal analysis of human oocytes. An overview of established procedures. Hum Reprod Update 2005; 11:15–32.
6. Plachot M. Genetics in human oocytes. In: Boutaleb Y, ed. New Concepts in Reproduction. Lancater, UK: Parthenon, 1992:367.
7. Martin R. Chromosomal analysis of human spermatozoa. In: Verlinsky Y, Kuliev A, eds. Preimplantation Genetics. New York: Plenum Press, 1991:91–102.
8. Boue J, Boue A, Lazar P. Retrospective and prospective epidemiological studies of 1500 karyotyped spontaneous human abortions. Teratology 1975; 12:11–26.
9. Hassold TJ. A cytogenetic study of repeated spontaneous abortions. Am J Hum Genet 1980; 32:723–30.
10. Simpson JL, Bombard AT. Chromosomal abnormalities in spontaneous abortion: frequency, pathology and genetic counseling. In: Edmonds KB, ed. Spontaneous Abortion. Oxford: Blackwell, 1987: 51–76.
11. Sorokin Y, Johnson MP, Uhlmann WR, et al. Postmortem chorionic villus sampling: correlation of cytogenetic and ultrasound findings. Am J Med Genet 1991; 39:314–16.
12. Strom CM, Ginsberg N, Applebaum M, et al. Analyses of 95 first-trimester spontaneous abortions by chorionic villus sampling and karyotype. J Assist Reprod Genet 1992; 9:458–61.
13. Ellett K, Buxton EJ, Luesley DM. The effect of ethnic origin on the rate of spontaneous late mid-trimester abortion. Ethn Dis 1992; 2:84–6.
14. Schaeffer AJ, Chung J, Heretis K, et al. Comparative genomic hybridization-array analysis enhances the detection of aneuploidies and submicroscopic imbalances in spontaneous miscarriages. Am J Hum Genet 2004; 74:1168–74.
15. Simpson JL, Mills JL, Holmes LB, et al. Low fetal loss rates after ultrasound-proved viability in early pregnancy. JAMA 1987; 258:2555–7.
16. Kuleshov NP. Chromosome anomalies of infants dying during the perinatal period and premature newborn. Hum Genet 1976; 31:151–60.
17. Hefler LA, Hersh DR, Moore PJ, et al. Clinical value of postnatal autopsy and genetics consultation in fetal death. Am J Med Genet 2001; 104:165–8.
18. Warburton D, Byrne J, Canik N. Chromosome Anomalies and Prenatal Development: An Atlas. New York: Oxford University Press, 1991.
19. Kalousek DK. Pathology of abortion: chromosomal and genetic correlations. In: Kraus FT, Damjanov IKN, eds. Pathology of Reproductive Failure. Baltimore: Williams & Wilkins, 1991:228.
20. Hassold T, Merrill M, Adkins K, et al. Recombination and maternal age-dependent nondisjunction: molecular studies of trisomy 16. Am J Hum Genet 1995; 57:867–74.
21. Fisher JM, Harvey JF, Morton NE, et al. Trisomy 18: studies of the parent and cell division of origin and the effect of aberrant recombination on nondisjunction. Am J Hum Genet 1995; 56:669–75.
22. Bugge M, Collins A, Petersen MB, et al. Non-disjunction of chromosome 18. Hum Mol Genet 1998; 7:661–9.
23. Hassold TJ. Nondisjunction in the human male. Curr Top Dev Biol 1998; 37:383–406.
24. Henderson SA, Edwards RG. Chiasma frequency and maternal age in mammals. Nature 1968; 217:22–8.
25. Lamb NE, Yu K, Shaffer J, et al. Association between maternal age and meiotic recombination for trisomy 21. Am J Hum Genet 2005; 76:91–9.
26. Hassold T, Abruzzo M, Adkins K, et al. Human aneuploidy: incidence, origin, and etiology. Environ Mol Mutagen 1996; 28:167–75.
27. Savage AR, Petersen MB, Pettay D, et al. Elucidating the mechanisms of paternal non-disjunction of chromosome 21 in humans. Hum Mol Genet 1998; 7:1221–7.
28. Verlinsky Y, Kuliev A. Practical Preimplantation Genetic Diagnosis. London: Springer-Verlag, 2005.
29. Reddy KS. Double trisomy in spontaneous abortions. Hum Genet 1997; 101:339–45.
30. Diego-Alvarez D, Ramos-Corrales C, Garcia-Hoyos M, et al. Double trisomy in spontaneous miscarriages: cytogenetic and molecular approach. Hum Reprod 2006; 21:958–66.
31. Li S, Hassed S, Mulvihill JJ, et al. Double trisomy. Am J Med Genet 2004; 124:96–8.
32. Clouston HJ, Herbert M, Fenwick J, et al. Cytogenetic analysis of human blastocysts. Prenat Diagn 2002; 22:1143–52.
33. Beatty RA. The origin of human triploidy: an integration of qualitative and quantitative evidence. Ann Hum Genet 1978; 41:299–314.
34. Jauniaux E, Burton GJ. Pathophysiology of histological changes in early pregnancy loss. Placenta 2005; 26:114–23.
35. McFadden DE, Robinson WP. Phenotype of triploid embryos. J Med Genet 2006; 43:609–12.
36. Jacobs PA, Angell RR, Buchanan IM, et al. The origin of human triploids. Ann Hum Genet 1978; 42:49–57.
37. Egozcue S, Blanco J, Vidal F, et al. Diploid sperm and the origin of triploidy. Hum Reprod 2002; 17:5–7.
38. McFadden DE, Langlois S. Parental and meiotic origin of triploidy in the embryonic and fetal periods. Clin Genet 2000; 58:192–200.
39. Schluth C, Doray B, Girard-Lemaire F, et al. Prenatal diagnosis of a true fetal tetraploidy in direct and cultured chorionic villi. Genet Couns 2004; 15:429–36.
40. Rosenbusch B, Schneider M. A brief look at the origin of tetraploidy. Cytogenet Genome Res 2004; 107:128–31.
41. Baumer A, Dres D, Basaran S, et al. Parental origin of the two additional haploid sets of chromosomes in an embryo with tetraploidy. Cytogenet Genome Res 2003; 101:5–7.
42. Singh RP, Carr DH. The anatomy and histology of XO human embryos and fetuses. Anat Rec 1966; 155:369–83.
43. Jirasek JE. Principles of reproductive embryology. In: Simpson JL, ed. Disorders of Sex Differentiation: Etiology and Clinical Delineation. San Diego: Academic Press, 1976: 51–110.
44. Simpson JL. Pregnancies in women with chromosomal abnormalities. In: Schulman JD, Simpson JL, eds. Genetic Diseases in Pregnancy. New York: Academic Press, 1981: 439–71.
45. Chandley AC. The origin of chromosomal aberrations in man and their potential for survival and reproduction in the adult human population. Ann Genet 1981; 24:5–11.

46. Warburton D, Kline J, Stein Z, et al. Does the karyotype of a spontaneous abortion predict the karyotype of a subsequent abortion? Evidence from 273 women with two karyotyped spontaneous abortions. Am J Hum Genet 1987; 41:465–83.

47. Hassold TJ, Matsuyama A, Newlands IM, et al. A cytogenetic study of spontaneous abortions in Hawaii. Ann Hum Genet 1978; 41:443–54.

48. Munné S, Sandalinas M, Magli C, et al. Increased rate of aneuploid embryos in young women with previous aneuploid conceptions. Prenat Diagn 2004; 24:638–43.

49. Bianco K, Caughey AB, Shaffer BL, et al. History of miscarriage and increased incidence of fetal aneuploidy in subsequent pregnancy. Obstet Gynecol 2006; 107:1098–102.

50. Drugan A, Koppitch FC, III, Williams JC III, et al. Prenatal genetic diagnosis following recurrent early pregnancy loss. Obstet Gynecol 1990; 75:381–4.

51. Rubio C, Simon C, Vidal F, et al. Chromosomal abnormalities and embryo development in recurrent miscarriage couples. Hum Reprod 2003; 18:182–8.

52. Alberman ED. The abortus as a predictor of future trisomy 21. In: Cruz DI, Gerald PS, eds. Trisomy 21 (Down syndrome). Baltimore: Raven Press, 1981:69.

53. Snijders RJ, Nicolaides KH. Ultrasound Markers for Fetal Chromosomal Defects. New York: Parthenon, 1996.

54. Stern C, Chamley L, Hale L, et al. Antibodies to β_2 glycoprotein I are associated with in vitro fertilization implantation failure as well as recurrent miscarriage: results of a prevalence study. Fertil Steril 1998; 70:938–44.

55. Stephenson MD, Awartani KA, Robinson WP. Cytogenetic analysis of miscarriages from couples with recurrent miscarriage: a case–control study. Hum Reprod 2002; 17:446–51.

56. Carp H, Toder V, Aviram A, et al. Karyotype of the abortus in recurrent miscarriage. Fertil Steril 2001; 75:678–82.

57. Ogasawara M, Aoki K, Okada S, et al. Embryonic karyotype of abortuses in relation to the number of previous miscarriages. Fertil Steril 2000; 73:300–4.

58. Benkhalifa M, Kasakyan S, Clement P, et al. Array comparative genomic hybridization profiling of first-trimester spontaneous abortions that fail to grow in vitro. Prenat Diagn 2005; 25:894–900.

59. Simpson JL. Choosing the best prenatal screening protocol. N Engl J Med 2005; 353:2068–70.

60. Munne S, Fischer J, Warner A, et al. Preimplantation genetic diagnosis significantly reduces pregnancy loss in infertile couples: a multicenter study. Fertil Steril 2006; 85:326–32.

61. Munné S, Escudero T, Colls P, et al. Predictability of preimplantation genetic diagnosis of aneuploidy and translocations on prospective attempts. Reprod Biomed Online 2004; 9:645–51.

62. Fortuny A, Carrio A, Soler A, et al. Detection of balanced chromosome rearrangements in 445 couples with repeated abortion and cytogenetic prenatal testing in carriers. Fertil Steril 1998; 49:774–779

63. Simpson JL, Meyers CM, Martin AO, et al. Translocations are infrequent among couples having repeated spontaneous abortions but no other abnormal pregnancies. Fertil Steril 1989; 51:811–14.

64. De Braekeleer M, Dao TN. Cytogenetic studies in couples experiencing repeated pregnancy losses. Hum Reprod 1990; 5:519–28.

65. Simpson JL, Elias S, Martin AO. Parental chromosomal rearrangements associated with repetitive spontaneous abortions. Fertil Steril 1981; 36:584–90.

66. Goddijn M, Joosten JH, Knegt AC, et al. Clinical relevance of diagnosing structural chromosome abnormalities in couples with repeated miscarriage. Hum Reprod 2004; 19:1013–17.

67. Boue A, Gallano P. A collaborative study of the segregation of inherited chromosome structural rearrangements in 1,356 prenatal diagnoses. Prenat Diagn 1984; 4:45–67.

68. Daniel A, Hook EB, Wulf G. Risks of unbalanced progeny at amniocentesis to carriers of chromosome rearrangements: data from European, USA, and Canadian laboratories. Am J Hum Genet 1988; 43:918 (Abstr 230).

69. Sugiura-Ogasawara M, Ozaki Y, Sato T, et al. Poor prognosis of recurrent aborters with either maternal or paternal reciprocal translocations. Fertil Steril 2004; 81:367–73.

70. Carp H, Feldman B, Oelsner G, Schiff E. Parental karyotype and subsequent live births in recurrent miscarriage. Fertil Steril 2004; 81:1296–301.

71. Carp H, Guetta E, Dorf H, et al. Embryonic karyotype in recurrent miscarriage with parental karyotypic aberrations. Fertil Steril 2006; 85:446–50.

72. Stephenson MD, Sierra S. Reproductive outcomes in recurrent pregnancy loss associated with a parental carrier of a structural chromosome rearrangement. Hum Reprod 2006; 21:1076–82.

73. Mackie OC, Scriven PN. Meiotic outcomes in reciprocal translocation carriers ascertained in 3-day human embryos. Eur J Hum Genet 2002; 10:801–6.

74. Sutherland GR, Gardiner AJ, Carter RF. Familial pericentric inversion of chromosome 19, inv(19)(p13q13) with a note on genetic counseling of pericentric inversion carriers. Clin Genet 1976; 10:54–9.

75. Anton E, Vidal F, Egozcue J, et al. Genetic reproductive risk in inversion carriers. Fertil Steril 2006; 85:661–6.

76. Pettenati MJ, Rao PN, Phelan MC, et al. Paracentric inversions in humans: a review of 446 paracentric inversions with presentation of 120 new cases. Am J Med Genet 1995; 55:171–87.

77. Baek KH. Aberrant gene expression associated with recurrent pregnancy loss. Mol Hum Reprod 2004; 10:291–7.

78. Philipp T, Kalousek DK. Generalized abnormal embryonic development in missed abortion: embryoscopic and cytogenetic findings. Am J Med Genet 2002; 111:43–7.

79. Henderson DJ, Sherman LS, Loughna SC, et al. Early embryonic failure associated with uniparental disomy for human chromosome 21. Hum Mol Genet 1994; 3:1373–6.

80. Lanasa MC, Hogge WA, Kubik C, et al. Highly skewed X-chromosome inactivation is associated with idiopathic recurrent spontaneous abortion. Am J Hum Genet 1999; 65:252–4.

81. Pegoraro E, Whitaker J, Mowery-Rushton P, et al. Familial skewed X inactivation: a molecular trait associated with high spontaneous-abortion rate maps to Xq28. Am J Hum Genet 1997; 61:160–70.

DEBATE

3a. Should fetal karyotyping be performed in RPL? – For

Howard JA Carp

The objective of any investigation in clinical medicine is to reach a diagnosis, inform the patient of the subsequent prognosis, and offer effective treatment (if available), based on these three parameters. Recurrent pregnancy loss is no exception to this basic plan of management. Sixty percent of sporadic miscarriages have been reported to have a chromosomal aberration as the underlying cause.[1–3] Although the incidence of chromosomal aberrations is lower in recurrent than in spontaneous miscarriages, incidences of 25–60% have been reported to be caused by embryonic chromosomal aberrations.[4–8] In fact, embryonic chromosomal aberrations have been found in the presence of other presumptive causes of pregnancy loss. In the antiphospholipid syndrome (APS), two small series, both from Japan, have reported incidences of 20%[9] and 40%.[5] Carp et al[10] have reported four chromosomal aberrations in patients with hereditary thrombophilias. In the series of Carp et al,[6] trisomies were the most common form of aberration, occurring in 66.7% of chromosomally aberrant embryos, with trisomies 21, 16, and 18 being the most common. Monosomy X and triploidies were also seen. Since the publication of that series, chromosomes 1 and 2 trisomies have also been seen. Chromosome 1 and 2 would not normally be sought in a pregestational screening (PGS) program.

The standard banding technique for karyotyping can only assess structural and numerical rearrangements, and is liable to fail due to contamination, culture failure, or overgrowth of maternal cells. Other more sophisticated tests such as comparative genomic hybridization (CGH) or multiplex fluorescence in situ hydridization (M-FISH),[12] may overcome these problems and allow additional genetic diagnoses to be made, such as uniparental disomy or skewed X-chromosome inactivation.[13] It is not possible to reach an accurate diagnosis of cause or recurrent miscarriage unless the chromosomal status of the fetus is determined.

Karyotyping of the abortus allows the patient to be given prognostic information regarding subsequent pregnancy outcomes. Warburton et al[14] summarized 273 women who had had abortuses karyotyped. They concluded that after a previous trisomic miscarriage, the prognosis is favorable. Two subsequent studies[5,6] have examined the outcome of the subsequent pregnancy according to the karyotype of the miscarriage. In the series of Ogasawara et al[5] (Figure 3a.1), there was a statistically significant trend for a patient with an aneuploidic abortion to have a better prognosis. The same trend was apparent in the series of Carp et al[6] However, the smaller numbers in the series of Carp et al[6] precluded the figures from reaching statistical significance (95% confidence interval (CI) 0.85–11.74). In women with three miscarriages and an aneuploidic miscarriage, reassurance of a good prognosis may be sufficient, and may save the patient more extensive investigations and treatment of dubious value. This may not be the case in euploidic abortions. The better prognosis after an aneuploid abortion is entirely logical, as fetal aneuploidy is due to a fetal cause. Hence, there is a greater chance that in a subsequent pregnancy, with

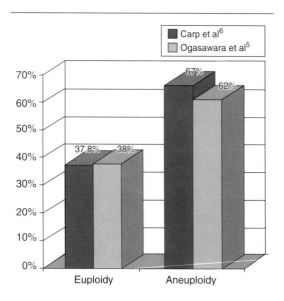

Figure 3a.1 Outcome of subsequent pregnancy according to fetal karyotype. Odds ratio for a live birth after aneuploidic abortion: 3.28 (95% confidence interval 0.94–11.9);[6] 2.62 (1.21–5.67).[5]

a new embryo, the next fetus will be euploid. However, a euploid abortus indicates that the cause of miscarriage is more likely to be maternal; hence, the same problem is liable to return in a subsequent pregnancy, thus worsening the prognosis. Any prognosis is empirical if the karyotype of the abortus is unknown.

Fetal karyotyping has been assessed in a subsequent abortion in the study by Sullivan et al.[8] Of 30 patients with an aneuploid abortion, only 3 (10%) had a subsequent aneuploid abortion. In the present author's series (unpublished), 43 abortuses were found to be aneuploid, and a subsequent abortion was karyotyped. Only 8 of the 43 abortuses were aneuploid (19%). Hence, only approximately 15% of aneuploid abortions will be followed by a subsequent aneuploid abortion. Hence, 85% of patients with an aneuploid abortion can be assured that the prognosis is good, and that the aneuploid abortion may be a chance ocurrence. However, the other 15% may have a recurring cause of fetal aneuploidy, and can be offered PGS.

Fetal karyotyping also directs treatment. If the fetus is karyotypically abnormal, a normal embryo can be provided to the mother by PGS. However, if the fetus is normal, the maternal environment needs treatment. As all previous maternal treatment modalities have ignored the fetal karyotype, the abnormal fetal karyotype has confounded the results. Hence, there are debates in this book as to whether hormone supplementation, thromboprophylaxis, immunopotentiation, etc. should be used. Additionally, the place of surgery for uterine anomalies and treatment of APS are equally debateable. If these therapies had only been used in the patient aborting chromosomally normal embryos, the above-mentioned therapies might be found to be efficacious, and their role might need no debate. Additionally, due to the possibility of fetal chromosomal aberrations, PGS has come into use, in order to provide the patient with a chromosomally normal embryo. When this technique is used on unselected patients with recurrent miscarriage, it has also been reported to be of little value.[15] It is our opinion that PGS has a role to play,[16] but that role is limited to patients with repeat aneuploidies, or those in whom there is a greater likelihood of fetal chromosomal aberrations, such as the older patient.

We have recently seen a 42-year-old patient with three consecutive aneuploid abortions. Her details are given in Table 3a.1. If fetal karyotyping had not been performed, she would have been recommended paternal leukocyte immunization or immunoglobulin in view of her advanced age. However, as the karyotype was available, immunotherapy would probably not have increased her chance of a live birth. In fact, if she had been placed in an immunotherapy trial, the trial might have concluded that immunotherapy was futile. In view of the advanced maternal age, which makes chromosomal aberrations more likely, and as all 23 chromosomes cannot be assessed at PGS, she was recommended ovum donation. These poor-prognosis patients are outside the normal guidelines for treatment, and do not have the good prognosis of 70–75% as other patients. However, they still require appropriate management, which rests on accurate diagnosis.

Table 3a.1 Patient with recurrent aneuploidy

Age: 42

Obstetric history:

1st pregnancy: artificial abortion

2nd pregnancy: normal delivery, ♀ 3400 g

3rd pregnancy: normal delivery, ♂ 3500 g

4th pregnancy: blighted ovum

5th pregnancy: left ectopic pregnancy, treated conservatively with methotrexate

6th pregnancy: blighted ovum

7th pregnancy: terminated artificially at 20 weeks for 47,XXX fetal karyotype

8th pregnancy: biochemical pregnancy

9th pregnancy: missed abortion 10 weeks, after treatment with aspirin and progesterone supplements; fetal karyotyping showed a 48,XX karyotype with both trisomies 14 and 15

10th pregnancy: missed abortion at 10 weeks; fetal karyotyping showed trisomy 22

Previous investigations: showed no maternal cause for miscarriage

Parental karyotype: 46,XX/ 46,XY

Treatment advised: ovum donation in view of advanced maternal age, increasing chance of subsequent aneuploid abortion, impossibility for screening all 23 chromosomes at PGS, and low possibility of conceiving at IVF

There is no substitute for karyotyping the abortus – two techniques have been attempted: karyotyping of the parents and PGS as a diagnostic procedure. Chromosomal aberrations are often suspected to have a recurring basis due to either a structural anomaly, such as a reciprocal or robertsonian translocation, or mosaicism for numerical aberrations. These conditions have been found in 10.8% of recurrently aborting women in the present author's series,[17] but the usually quoted prevalence is 3–5%.[18–20] If a parental chromosomal aberration is found, this is usually assumed to be the cause of recurrent miscarriage. However, parental karyotyping does not provide a diagnosis or prognosis, nor does it direct treatment. Carp et al[21] have karyotyped 39 abortuses from recurrently miscarrying couples with parental karyotypic aberrations. Of the 39, 17 (26%) were euploid. Another 10 (26%) had the same balanced translocation as the parent. Hence, 69% were chromosomally normal. Only 5 (13%) abortuses had unbalanced translocations, whereas 7 (18%) of the abortuses had subsequent abortuses with numerical aberrations unrelated to the

parental chromosomal disorder (5 trisomies and 2 monosomy X).

Parental karyotyping does not provide a prognosis. Three papers have looked at the subsequent live birth rate in patients with recurrent miscarriage and parental chromosomal rearrangements. These are summarized in Table 3a.2. Ogasawara et al[22] have reported a 32% subsequent live birth rate, whereas Carp et al[17] have reported a 44% rate and Goddijn et al[23] a 70% rate. Taken together, the live birth rate was 47.5% for patients with a mean of 3.7 previous miscarriages. This live birth rate of 47.5% is the expected rate for patients with 3.7 abortions, according to numerous series in the literature.[24,25]

Parental karyotyping, in addition to not providing a diagnosis and not providing a prognosis, does not direct us towards treatment. Munné et al[26] have reported 47 PGS cycles in 35 patients with chromosomal rearrangements; 16 subsequent pregnancies resulted in 14 live births. Simopoulou et al[27] have reported 11 PGS cycles in 8 patients with chromosomal rearrangements; euploid embryos were replaced in all 11 cycles. There were four subsequent pregnancies, with three live births and one 'biochemical' pregnancy. Although these results look encouraging, both series only include six patients with recurrent miscarriages. Eleven embryos were replaced, resulting in two pregnancies and one live birth. It is impossible to draw conclusions from one live birth in two pregnancies.

PGS is also problematic as a diagnostic and therapeutic procedure when it is unknown whether the patient loses chromosomally normal or abnormal embryos. As it is impossible to screen for all 23 chromosomes, an embryo can never be said to be

---

Table 3a.2 Subsequent live birth rate with parental chromosomal aberrations

	Ogasawara et al[22]	Goddijn et al[23]	Carp et al[17]
Pregnancies	47	42	75
Live births	15	30	33
Proportion	32%	70%	44%
Mean no. of abortions	2.9	3.9	4.23

normal on PGS – it can only be stated that the most common chromosomal aberrations are absent. The less commonly ocurring aberrations such as trisomy 2 are not usually screened for. Hence, PGS cannot provide a diagnosis, or select patients for treatment of maternal factors.

Therefore, karyotyping of the abortus seems to be the most important single investigation for the assessment of recurrent miscarriage, as recommended by the Royal College of Obstetricians and Gynaecologists in their 1998[28] guideline revised in 2003.[29] We find this test to be invaluable, and its absence in cases where the culture fails or is contaminated leads to an incomplete diagnosis, inaccurate prognosis, and possibly wrong advice as to management.

REFERENCES

1. Boue J, Boue A, Lazar P. The epidemiology of human spontaneous abortions with chromosomal anomalies. In: Blandau RJ, Ed. Aging Gametes. Basel: Karger, 1975:330.
2. Stein Z. Early fetal loss. Birth Defects 1981; 17:95–9.
3. Sanchez JM, Franzi L, Collia F, et al. Cytogenetic study of spontaneous abortions by transabdominal villus sampling and direct analysis of villi. Prenat Diagn 1999; 19:601–3.
4. Stern JJ, Dorfman AD, Gutierez-Najar MD, et al. Frequency of abnormal karyotype among abortuses from women with and without a history of recurrent spontaneous abortion. Fertil Steril 1996; 65:250–3.
5. Ogasawara M, Aoki K, Okada S, et al. Embryonic karyotype of abortuses in relation to the number of previous miscarriages. Fertil Steril 2000; 73:300–4.
6. Carp HJA, Toder V, Orgad S, et al. Karyotype of the abortus in recurrent miscarriage. Fertil Steril 2001; 5:678–82.
7. Stephenson MD, Awartani KA, Robinson WP. Cytogenetic analysis of miscarriages from couples with recurrent miscarriage: a case–control study. Hum Reprod 2002; 17:446–51.
8. Sullivan AE, Silver RM, LaCoursiere DY, et al. Recurrent fetal aneuploidy and recurrent miscarriage. Obstet Gynecol 2004; 104:784–8.
9. Takakuwa K, Asano K, Arakawa M, et al. Chromosome analysis of aborted conceptuses of recurrent aborters positive for anticardiolipin antibody. Fertil Steril 1997; 68:54–8.
10. Carp HJA, Dolitzky M, Inbal A. Thromboprophylaxis improves the live birth rate in women with consecutive recurrent miscarriages and hereditary thrombophilia. J Thromb Hemost 2003; 1:433–8.
11. Daniely M, Aviram-Goldring A, Barkai G, et al. Detection of chromosomal abberation in fetuses arising from recurrent spontaneous abortion by comparative genomic hybridization. Hum Reprod 1998; 13:805–9.
12. Uhrig S, Schuffenhauer S, Fauth C, et al. Multiplex-FISH for pre and postnatal diagnostic applications. Am J Hum Genet 1999; 65:448–62.
13. Lanasa MC, Hogge WA, Kubik C, et al. Highly skewed X chromosome inactivation is associated with idiopathic recurrent spontaneous abortion. Am J Hum Genet 1999; 65:252–4.
14. Warburton D, Kline J, Stein Z, et al. Does the karyotype of a spontaneous abortion predict the karyotype of a subsequent abortion? Evidence from 273 women with two karyotyped spontaneous abortions. Am J Hum Genet 1987; 41:465–83.
15. Platteau P, Staessen C, Michiels A, et al. Preimplantation genetic diagnosis for aneuploidy screening in patients with unexplained recurrent miscarriages. Fertil Steril 2005; 83:393–7.
16. Carp HJA, Dirnfeld M, Dor J, et al. ART in recurrent miscarriage: preimplantation genetic diagnosis / screening or surrogacy? Hum Reprod 2004; 19:1502–5.
17. Carp HJA, Feldman B, Oelsner G, et al. Parental karyotype and subsequent live births in recurrent miscarriage. Fertil Steril 2004; 81:1296–1301.
18. De Braekeleer, M. Dao TN. Cytogenetic studies in couples experiencing repeated pregnancy losses. Hum Reprod 1990; 5:519–28.
19. Portnoi MF, Joye N, van den Akker J, et al. Karyotypes of 1142 couples with recurrent abortion. Obstet Gynecol 1988; 72:31–4.
20. Fortuny A, Carrio A, Soler A, et al. Detection of balanced chromosome rearrangements in 445 couples with repeated abortion and cytogenetic prenatal testing in carriers. Fertil Steril 1988; 49:774–9.
21. Carp HJA, Guetta E, Dorf H, et al. Embryonic karyotype in recurrent miscarriage with parental karyotypic aberrations. Fertil Steril 2006; 85:446–450.
22. Sugiura-Ogasawara M, Ozaki Y, Sato T, et al. Poor prognosis of recurrent aborters with either maternal or paternal reciprocal translocations. Fertil Steril 2004; 81:367–73.
23. Goddijn M, Joosten JH, Knegt AC, et al. Clinical relevance of diagnosing structural chromosome abnormalities in couples with repeated miscarriage. Hum Reprod 2004; 19:1013–17.
24. Knudsen UB, Hansen V, Juul S, et al. Prognosis of a new pregnancy following previous spontaneous abortions. Eur J Obstet Gynecol Reprod Biol 1991; 39:31–6.
25. Carp HJA. Investigation and treatment for recurrent pregnancy loss. In: Rainsbury P, Vinniker D, eds. A Practical Guide to Reproductive Medicine. Carnforth, UK: Parthenon, 1997:337–62.
26. Munné S, Sandalinas M, Escudero T, et al. Outcome of preimplantation genetic diagnosis of translocations. Fertil Steril 2000; 73:1209–18.
27. Simopoulou M, Harper JC, Fragouli E, et al. Preimplantation genetic diagnosis of chromosome abnormalities: implications from the outcome for couples with chromosomal rearrangements. Prenat Diagn 2003; 23:652–62.
28. Royal College of Obstetricians and Gynaecologists, Guideline No. 17. The Management of Recurrent Miscarriage. London: RCOG, 1998.
29. Royal College of Obstetricians and Gynaecologists, Guideline No. 17. The Management of Recurrent Miscarriage. London: RCOG, 2003.

DEBATE

3b. Should fetal karyotyping be performed in RPL ?
– Against

Zvi Borochowitz

Zvi Borochowitz

INTRODUCTION

The first report of a chromosomal abnormality in aborted material was of a triploidy in spontaneous abortion, four decades ago by Penrose and Delhanty.[1] It took several years before cytogenetic analysis of miscarriage became an option in laboratories, due to the difficulties of culturing fetal tissue. The development of techniques that allowed chorionic villi to be used for 'long-term cultures', and later direct preparation of metaphases from villi, revolutionized the cytogenetic analysis of products of conception. There has since been a debate as to whether it is either clinically justifiable or psychologically essential to determine the cause of pregnancy loss for the task of counselling for a further pregnancy. The crucial role of chromosomal imbalance in abnormal early human development is well known. Most of the chromosomal abnormalities result in disordered development incompatible with prolonged intrauterine survival and live birth. The mechanism by which a chromosomal abnormality could lead to regression of the conceptus is unclear. Approximately 50–60% of first-trimester spontaneous abortions have karyotypic abnormalities – mainly numerical chromosomal changes such as autosomal trisomy, monosomy X, and polyploidy. This conclusion is based on the results of cytogenetic studies conducted in laboratories throughout the world.[2]

The term 'spontaneous abortion' refers to a pregnancy that ends spontaneously before the fetus has reached a viable gestational age. The World Health Organization (WHO) defines it as expulsion or extraction of an embryo or fetus weighing 500 g or less from its mother. This typically corresponds to a gestational age of 20–22 weeks. In this chapter, the term 'miscarriage' will be used to mean repeated, recurrent, multiple, or habitual abortion. The prevalence of miscarriage has been estimated as 10–15% of all clinically recognized pregnancies. One of the most remarkable, and as yet unexplained, aspects of the first trimester of pregnancy is the fact that the majority (90%) of karyotypically abnormal pregnancies miscarry in the first trimester, and the majority (93%) of karyotypically normal pregnancies continue.[3] There are various risk factors for miscarriage, including, among others, advanced maternal age, alcohol use, anesthetic gas use (i.e., nitrous oxide), heavy caffeine use, chronic maternal diseases, cigarette smoking, cocaine use, conception 3–6 months after delivery, intrauterine device use, maternal infections, medications, multiple previous elective abortions, toxins (lead, arsenic, ethylene glycol, etc.), and uterine abnormalities. Most chromosomal abnormalities that result in spontaneous abortion are random events and are more likely to be associated with recurrent spontaneous abortion, but are uncommon even where one of the parents is a carrier (4–6% of recurrent miscarriages[4,5]).

CYTOGENETIC ABNORMALITIES

Cytogenetic evaluation of sporadic spontaneous abortions has shown that 50–60% are chromosomally abnormal. This means that about 5–10.5% of all pregnancies result in sporadic abortions caused by chromosomal abnormalities. Pregnancy loss of chromosomal origin, which is the scope of this chapter, is uncommon after 15 weeks' gestation; therefore, this chapter is concerned mainly with first-trimester miscarriages. It is well documented that fetal de novo chromosomal abnormalities are a major cause. These detection rates of chromosomal abnormalities have remained constant over time, and are independent of the culture method used or the culture success rate, which is now reported to be 90%.[2,4,6] The recurrence risk of another miscarriage after an aneuploidic miscarriage is not elevated, or is only slightly so (16%), when compared with the initial risk of all women (10–15%). Thus, routine karyotyping of fetal material in miscarriages is not thought to be worthwhile and is considered unnecessary.[4] Half of the structural abnormalities may be inherited from a parent carrying a balanced chromosome translocation or inversion. This type of chromosomal abnormality would be found by parental karyotyping, which is now a routine procedure in most countries after two (or at most three) missed abortions.

PROGNOSIS

The presence of a cytogenetic abnormality in miscarriages explains the reason for the loss. In most couples with recurrent pregnancy loss (RPL), an evaluation, including parental karyotype testing, will be negative. Therefore, a majority (approximately 50–75%) of couples with RPL will have no certain diagnosis. Live birth rates of 35–85% are commonly reported in couples with unexplained RPL who undertake an untreated or placebo-treated subsequent pregnancy.[7] Meta-analysis of randomized prospective studies suggests that 60–70% of women with unexplained RPL will have a successful next pregnancy.[8]

RPL may be due to an abnormal embryo that is incompatible with life. As the number of miscarriages increases, the prevalence of chromosomal abnormality decreases, and the chance of recurring maternal cause increases.[9] It is thus assumed that in recurrent miscarriage, there is more likely to be a recurring cause leading to RPL. Hence, RPL occurs in up to 1% of the population – which is more than would be expected if recurrent miscarriage occurs as a result of repeated aneuploidy. Many couples will view these data with optimism.

LABORATORY TECHNIQUE

Results of conventional cytogenetic analysis of spontaneous abortions depend strongly on tissue culture and are associated with a significant culture failure rate, which varies from 5% to 42% in different laboratories. The banding technique for karyotyping can only assess structural and numerical rearrangements, and is liable to fail as a result of contamination, culture failure, or overgrowth of maternal cells. The cytogenetic factors of cell death in vitro have not been sufficiently investigated. A possible disadvantage of the (semi)direct preparation is the discrepancy that may occur between embryonic cells and chorionic villi. Such a discrepancy might be due to the fact that mosaicism is found only in placental tissue (i.e., confined placental mosaicism). It is possible to assume that tissue culture failure is a marker of particular genomic imbalances incompatible with normal cell proliferation. If this hypothesis is true, then the standard cytogenetic analysis of spontaneous abortions may underestimate the frequency and diversity of detected chromosomal abnormalities. Thus, the fetal karyotype may not be represented correctly by the villous karyotype. The estimated percentage of mosaicism is 1–2% for (semi)direct chromosome preparation in chorionic villus sampling (CVS). In view of these difficulties, it has been argued that other more sophisticated tests such as comparative genomic hybridization (CGH) or multiplex fluorescence in situ hybridization (M-FISH) may overcome these problems and allow additional genetic diagnoses to be made, such as uniparental disomy or skewed X-chromosome inactivation. However, it appears from these series that there must be an alternative cause for the pregnancy loss in most (71%) of patients. The results of FISH analysis of uncultured cells from spontaneous abortions reveal a high frequency of both intratissue and confined placental mosaicism, and suggest that culture techniques underestimate the incidence of chromosomal anomalies. This observation underlines the fact that early stages of human development are associated with a high rate of mitotic errors, which has been confirmed by data from molecular cytogenetic analyses of cleavage-stage embryos. It is probable that mitotic instability is an important factor in early prenatal selection.[2,4,10,11]

As current rates of chromosomal abnormalities are constant over time, and are independent of the current routine culture method used in most laboratories, as well as the culture success rate, which is now reported to be of 90%,[6] it seems that FISH or CGH techniques have not significantly changed the clinical approach or the psychological benefits. The dubious value of FISH or CGH must be weighed against the highly sophisticated laboratory requirements (still not routinely available in many countries and laboratories) and the high costs involved.

It can be summarized that current laboratory techniques are obstacles in making the karyotyping of abortus material a required routine test. Cytogenetic analysis of fetal tissue is expensive. Formerly, it was thought that the histological features of miscarriage could predict karyotype, and could possibly be an alternative to karyotyping. Examples of such histological features are villous contour, hydropic villi, trophoblastic hyperplasia, trophoblastic lacunae, cisterns, inclusions, and perivillous and intervillous fibrin deposits. So far, hydropic villi, trophoblastic lacunae, trophoblastic hyperplasia, cisterns, and inclusions have shown a significant association with triploidy in only a very few studies. In general, histological features are unhelpful for predicting karyotype.[4]

CONSENSUS REMARKS

AMERICAN COLLEGE OF OBSTETRICIANS AND GYNECOLOGISTS (ACOG)[7]

- 'Many experts obtain a karyotype of the abortus tissue when a couple with recurrent pregnancy loss experiences a subsequent spontaneous abortion. The rationale is that if the abortus is aneuploid, the physician and patient may conclude that a maternal cause of pregnancy loss is excluded. Also, an abnormal abortus karyotype is a legitimate explanation for the loss that may provide a source of comfort to the couple. *However, no published evidence supports these hypotheses, and definite recommendations for routinely obtaining abortus karyotypes cannot be made.*'

ROYAL COLLEGE OF OBSTETRICIANS AND GYNAECOLOGISTS (RCOG)[12]

- 'If the karyotype of the miscarriage pregnancy is abnormal, there is a better prognosis in the next pregnancy. Cytogenetic testing is an expensive tool and may be reserved for patients who have undergone treatment in the index pregnancy or have been participating in a research trial. For them, karyotyping the products of conception provides useful information for counselling and future management.'
- *This statement is under Category C – level IV – which is based solely on expert opinion with no clinical studies of good quality.*

JOINT WORKING PARTY OF THE ROYAL COLLEGE OF PATHOLOGISTS (RCPath) AND THE ROYAL COLLEGE OF OBSTETRICIANS AND GYNAECOLOGISTS (RCOG)[13]

- 'Because of the high failure rate of post-abortal and post-stillbirth karyotyping, the Working Party recommends that multiple samples be collected, usually placenta and full-thickness skin. Consideration should also be given to collecting a specimen in utero before the termination process begins.'

GYNECOLOGISTS, OBSTETRICIANS, AND FERTILITY SPECIALISTS FROM 18 COUNTRIES PARTICIPATING IN A THREE-DAY WORKSHOP HELD IN DENMARK IN 2002[14]

- 'Improved techniques in cytogenetics have permitted more accurate and reliable assessments of the products of conception. Given these improvements in our diagnostic ability, it is even more important that every effort be made to study the products of conception in every case of miscarriage *in therapeutic trials* so that a more valid evaluation can be made regarding the efficacy *of the experimental treatment.*'
- *They do not recommend karyotyping of abortus material.*

CONCLUDING REMARKS

1. The recurrence risk of another miscarriage is not elevated, or is only slightly so (16%), when compared with the initial risk of all women (10–15%), and thus routine karyotyping of fetal material in miscarriages is not thought to be worthwhile in daily practice, and is considered to be unnecessary.
2. More than half of abortuses have normal chromosomes, while most of the abnormal chromosomes are numerical abnormalities (86%), with trisomies of various chromosomes occuring in more than two-thirds of these, giving rise to a randomly occurring incident.
3. With so many possible causes for recurrent miscarriage, it would be tempting to think that the prognosis for those women whose recurrent miscarriages are unexplained is dire. But three-quarters of these women will go on to have a successful pregnancy if offered nothing more, and nothing less, than tender, love and care, and reassurance through ultrasound that nothing is abnormal.[15]
4. The current techniques of tissue culture used in conventional cytogenetic analysis of abortal fetal material are laborious and subject to problems such as external contamination, culture failure,

and selective growth of maternal cells, with success rates varying from 5% to 42%.
5. As rates of chromosomal abnormalities have remained constant over time, and are independent of the culture method used, FISH or CGH techniques have not significantly changed the clinical approach or the psychological benefits.
6. The highly sophisticated laboratory requirements (unavailable in many laboratories), and high costs should be considered.
7. Presently, current laboratory techniques are obstacles in allowing the karyotyping of the abortus to become a routine test.
8. Summary of several major consensus papers:

- ACOG: definite recommendations for routinely obtaining abortus karyotypes cannot be made.[7]
- RCOG: cytogenetic testing is an expensive tool and may be reserved for patients who have undergone treatment in the index pregnancy or have been participating in a research trial.[12]
- Joint Working Party of RCPath and RCOG: because of the high failure rate of post-abortal karyotyping, the Working Party recommends that consideration should also be given to collecting a specimen in utero before the termination process begins.[13]
- International workshop (Denmark, 2002): not as a routine procedure, but in therapeutic trials only.[14]

Hence, one must conclude that there is no clinical justification, nor any psychological benefit, for fetal karyotyping. This conclusion is well noted throughout this in-depth current literature survey, as well in these consensus clinical guidelines of the more important professional societies around the world.

REFERENCES

1. Penrose LS, Delhanty JD. Triploid cell cultures from a macerated foetus. Lancet 1961; i:1261–2.
2. Lebedev IN, Ostroverkhova NV, Nikitina TV, et al. Features of chromosomal abnormalities in spontaneous abortion cell culture failures detected by interphase FISH analysis. Eur J Hum Genet 2004; 12:513–20.

3. Quenby S, Vince G, Farquharson R, et al. Recurrent miscarriage: a defect in nature's quality control? Hum Reprod 2002; 17;1959–63.

4. Goddijn M, Leschot NJ. Genetic aspects of miscarriage. Baillieres Best Pract Res Clin Obstet Gynaecol 2000; 14:855–65.

5. Griebel CP, Halvorsen J, Golemon TB, et al. Management of spontaneous abortion. Am Fam Physician 2005; 72:1243–50.

6. Yusuf RZ, Naeem R. Cytogenetic abnormalities in products of conception: a relationship revisited. Am J Reprod Immunol 2004; 52:88–96.

7. ACOG Practice Bulletin No. 24, Feb. 2001. Management of recurrent early pregnancy loss. Int J Gynecol Obstet 2002; 78:179–90.

8. Jeng GT, Scott JR, Burmeister LF. A comparison of meta-analytic results using literature vs individual patient data. Paternal cell immunization for recurrent miscarriage. JAMA 1995; 274:830–6.

9. Ogasawara M, Aoki K, Okada S, et al. Embryonic karyotype of abortuses in relation to the number of previous miscarriages. Fertil Steril 2000; 73:300–4.

10. Carp H, Toder V, Aviram A, et al. Karyotype of the abortus in recurrent miscarriage. Fertil Steril 2001; 75:678–82.

11. Stephenson MD, Awartani KA, Robinson WP. Cytogenetic analysis of miscarriages from couples with recurrent miscarriage: a case–control study. Hum Reprod 2002; 17:446–51.

12. Royal College of Obstetricians and Gynaecologists, Guideline No. 17. The Management of Recurrent Miscarriage. London: RCOG, 2003.

13. Fetal and Perinatal Pathology: Report of a Joint Working Party – 2005. http://www.rcpath.org.

14. Christiansen OB, Nybo Andersen AM, Bosch E, et al. Evidence-based investigations and treatments of recurrent pregnancy loss. Fertil Steril 2005; 83:821–39.

15. Kavalier F. Investigation of recurrent miscarriages. BMJ 2005; 331:121–2.

DEBATE

3c. Should PGD be performed in RPL?
– For

Howard JA Carp and JG Grudzinskas

Pregnancy loss may be caused by a maternal factor or a fetal factor. Until now, most investigations and treatment have concerned maternal factors causing pregnancy loss or recurrent pregnancy loss (RPL). Preimplantation genetic diagnosis (PGD) is the only strategy available to prevent loss due to aneuploidy of the fetus. While it is difficult to gauge the true incidence of aneuploid fetuses in RPL, various series in which the abortus has been analyzed have quoted that 25–60% of recurrent miscarriages may be caused by embryonic chromosomal aberrations.[1–5] Rubio et al[6] and Platteau et al[7] have together summarized 559 and 413 embryos of RPL patients, respectively. Taken together, there was a 63.4% prevalence of aneuploidy. In the series of Rubio et al[6] the prevalence was 395/559 embryos (70.7%), compared with 97/218 (44.5%) of control embryos. Thus, aneuploid miscarriages account for a significant number of pregnancy losses. Hence, the use of PGD may be appropriate for this significant subgroup of patients with RPL.

Like most other modes of treatment, PGD is not a panacea for all patients with RPL, and to argue the case for using PGD in all patients would show PGD to be ineffective. Rubio et al[6] published a trial of pregestational screening (PGS) in 71 women with two or more pregnancy losses (mean 2.9). There were 19 live births in 23 subsequent pregnancies. This 82% success rate is higher than the 60% that would be expected naturally. However, the series includes patients with two pregnancy losses, which makes the figures difficult to interpret. Our opponents in this debate have published a prospective study of

49 patients with recurrent miscarriage.[7] Fifteen pregnancies ensued from 31 cycles. These 15 pregnancies resulted in 10 live births, 2 miscarriages and 3 biochemical pregnancies. This 66% live birth rate (10 of 15 pregnancies) is often said to be no better than the natural rate of approximately 60%. However, the mean number of miscarriages in the series of Platteau et al[7] was 4.7. In patients with 4.7 miscarriages, a live birth rate of only 35–40% is expected.[8,9] Hence, a 66% live birth rate is an excellent result for this cohort of patients, even when it is considered that there was only a 24% implantation rate (15 pregnancies of 63 embryos in 63 cycles). The results of the paper by Platteau et al[7] indicate the need for a larger trial, rather than arguing that PGD is not worthwhile. If the figures from the series of Platteau et al[7] are pooled with those from Rubio et al[6] then, there is a 76% live birth rate (29 of 38 pregancies) in women with 3.6 losses, which is higher than would be expected by chance. However, it must be remembered that PGD requires assisted reproductive technology (ART). The implantation rate was only 24%, and patients with recurrent miscarriage do not per se have a problem conceiving. Thus, the higher ongoing pregnancy rate may be a reflection of a reduced pregnancy rate.

It is our opinion that PGD is appropriate for a subgroup of women with RPL. If the right patients are selected, further miscarriages can be prevented, and the patient can be saved the heartbreak and agony of having to terminate the pregnancy if aneuploidy should be found by chorionic villus sampling (CVS) or amniocentesis in the later stages of pregnancy. We have published a guideline that gives the possible indications for using ART in RPL.[10] The indications included poor-prognosis patients, those not responding to simpler forms of treatment, repeated fetal aneuploidy, and the older patient. Judgment was reserved in cases of parental chromosomal rearrangements. Some of these conditions are explored in more detail below in order to show that PGD has a definite role to play in RPL.

REPEAT FETAL ANEUPLOIDY

Most fetal chromosomal aberrations are isolated ocurrences. Hence, the patient who loses a chromosomally abnormal fetus has a greater chance of a live birth than the patient losing a euploid embryo (see Figure 3a.1). However, there are a few patients who repeatedly lose aneuploid embryos. Although there is no large series assessing the incidence of repeat aneuploidy in patients with recurrent miscarriage, there are two small series. Repeat fetal aneuploidy has been shown in 3 of 30 patients in the series of Sullivan et al[5] and in 8 of 43 patients in that of Carp et al.[10] If both series are pooled, this indicates that approximately 15% of women with repeated pregnancy loss with fetal aneuploidy will have a repeat aneuploidy. In cases of repeat aneuploidy PGD/PGS should be used. If the repeat aneuploidy involves the same chromosome, PGD can be performed, using the relevant probes. This is important, as the affected chromosome may be one that is not usually sought in standard five-, seven-, or even nine-probe PGS. If different chromosomes are involved each time, it may be necessary to use PGS, screening for the affected chromosomes in past miscarriages. Even in this form of PGS, the screening will be more directed to affected chromosomes than in standard five-, seven-, or nine-probe PGS.

PARENTAL CHROMOSOMAL REARRANGEMENTS

A karyotypic aberration, in either partner, may lead to recurrent miscarriage. However, there is little information on the role of PGD in RPL with parental chromosomal aberrations, as there have been no case–control studies comparing miscarriage rates between PGD and natural pregnancies. There are three series describing PGD in the case of parental chromosomal translocations. Chun et al[11] have described the results of 49 translocation carriers. Of 49 patients, 15 (30.6%) delivered after 70 cycles. However, Chun et al[11] do not state if any of their patients had recurrent miscarriage. Munné et al[12] have summarized 47 PGS cycles in 35 patients. There were 16 pregnancies, with 14 live births. Simopoulou et al[13] carried out 11 PGD cycles in 8 patients. There were three subsequent live births and one 'biochemical' pregnancy. There were only six patients with recurrent miscarriage in both the series of Munné et al[12] and of Simonopoulou et al[13] together. Hence, at present, no conclusions can be drawn about the role of PGD in the presence of parental chromosomal aberrations. In the presence of parental chromosome aberrations, the aberration is passed on to the embryo in 18% of cases (7 of 39 abortuses in the present authors'[14] series. In patients with parental chromosomal aberrations, inherited in an unbalanced form by the embryo, PGD will prevent the subsequent abortion. One such patient is described as Patient No. 4 in Chapter 19.

ADVANCED MATERNAL AGE

With increasing female age, the incidence of chromosomal abnormalities increases. The chromosomal abnormalities seem to mainly originate from female meiosis. The higher incidence of aneuploidy compared with younger patients has been shown both when the abortus is studied[3,5] and when embryos obtained by in vitro fertilization (IVF) were studied.[15,16] In the study by Rubio et al[15] the incidence of chromosomal abnormalities was 63.59% in the group of women above 37 years of age, and was significantly increased compared with 33.1% in a control group of women with sex-linked diseases. In this age group, there was a significant increase ($p < 0.05$) in the prevalence of aberrations for chromosomes 13, 16, 21, and 22. Although there was an increased prevalence of aberrations in chromosome 18 and the sex chromosomes, this difference did not reach statistical significance. Dailey et al[17] used fluorescence in situ hybridization (FISH) studies on IVF patients and showed that nondisjunction seems to mainly affect the smaller chromosomes such as 13, 16, 18, 21, 22, and X in women above 35 years of age. Other studies[18] have found no anomalies regarding chromosomes 1, 9, or 12. Hence, 7-probe PGS should exclude the common aberrations leading to miscarriage, and, although there are no direct figures, PGS should reduce the incidence of miscarriage, and the need to terminate the pregnancy if a chromosome aberration were to be found at a later CVS or amniocentesis.

There are few data available on the effect of PGS in patients of advanced age. The only prospective study is that by Platteau et al.[7] Only one pregnancy of five developed to a live birth after PGD in women aged above 35. Platteau et al[7] use these figures to conclude that 'The future obstetric outcome for the older patients remains grim, whatever treatment is done.' We would contend that one out of five is too small a sample to draw conclusions, as a larger sample is required. Other series have drawn different conclusions to those of Platteau et al.[7] Munné et al[19] have reported 20 infants born to 37 women from 44 PGS cycles. There was a 54% live birth rate in women with a mean of 4.1 miscarriages. The study by Munné et al[19] was retrospective, and the results were compared with a calculated probability of a live birth according to the criteria of Brigham et al[20] for the number of previous miscarriages and maternal age. However, their live birth rate was above the rate expected for women with a similar number of miscarriages and of the same age. Munné et al[19] concluded that 'Our findings indicate that PGD can be recommended to RM [repeated miscarriage] patients who are 35 years and older and show no clear etiology of RM.'

CONCLUSIONS

Both PGD and PGS have a role in the management of RPL. It now remains to develop a screening system for the entire genome that can be used rapidly.

At that point, the rare chromosomal anomalies which are found in RPL can be assessed. Great strides have been made in this field with the introduction of comparative genomic hybridization (CGH),[21] multiplex FISH[22] and isothermal whole-genome amplification.[23] CGH has been used on the abortus[24] and for PGS.[25] However, if CGH is used, whole-ploidy errors such as triploidy cannot be excluded, and the time required in order to obtain a result (up to 3 days) may preclude transfer in the same cycle. The attendant cryopreservation and thawing is associated with loss of embryos. Hence, more work is required on the technique before it can become standard clinical practice. At that point, it may be unnecessary to have a debate such as this. The argument for using PGD/PGS may be obvious.

Currently, we propose that PGS may be helpful to identify the proportion of euploid embryos in couples with RPL with a view to transferring only euploid embryos. Embryos that are deemed screened 'normal' or 'no result' should have follow-up FISH analysis. This strategy should be considered in euploid couples, especially if the woman is 35 years of age or older, as well as couples in whom a balanced translocation have been identified, particularly if the aberrations have been transmitted to the embryo in an unbalanced form. The clinical history of the couple, together with knowledge of the karyotype of the abortus, should be used to determine whether recourse to host surrogacy is indicated, as in the case of the aborted euploid fetus, or PGS is incorporated in the case of aneuploidy of the abortus.

REFERENCES

1. Stern JJ, Dorfman AD, Gutierez-Najar MD, et al. Frequency of abnormal karyotype among abortuses from women with and without a history of recurrent spontaneous abortion. Fertil Steril 1996; 65:250–3.
2. Ogasawara M, Aoki K, Okada S, et al. Embryonic karyotype of abortuses in relation to the number of previous miscarriages. Fertil Steril 2000; 73:300–4.
3. Carp HJA, Toder V, Orgad S, et al. Karyotype of the abortus in recurrent miscarriage. Fertil Steril 2001; 5:678–82.
4. Stephenson MD, Awartani KA, Robinson WP. Cytogenetic analysis of miscarriages from couples with recurrent miscarriage: a case-control study. Hum Reprod 2002; 17:446–51.
5. Sullivan AE, Silver RM, LaCoursiere DY, et al. Recurrent fetal aneuploidy and recurrent miscarriage. Obstet Gynecol 2004;104:784–8.

6. Rubio C, Simon C, Vidal F, et al. Chromosomal abnormalities and embryo development in recurrent miscarriage couples. Hum Reprod 2003; 18:182–8.

7. Platteau P, Staessen C, Michiels A, et al. Preimplantation genetic diagnosis for aneuploidy screening in patients with unexplained recurrent miscarriages. Fertil Steril 2005; 83:393–7.

8. Knudsen UB, Hansen V, Juul S, et al. Prognosis of a new pregnancy following previous spontaneous abortions. Eur J Obstet Gynecol Reprod Biol 1991; 39:31–6.

9. Carp HJA. Investigation and treatment for recurrent pregnancy loss. In: Rainsbury P, Vinniker D, eds. A Practical Guide to Reproductive Medicine. Carnforth, UK: Parthenon, 1997:337–62.

10. Carp HJA, Dirnfeld M, Dor J, et al. ART in recurrent miscarriage: preimplantation genetic diagnosis / screening or surrogacy? Hum Reprod 2004; 19:1502–5.

11. Chun KL, Jin HJ, Dong MM, et al. Efficacy and clinical outcome of preimplantation genetic diagnosis using FISH for couples of reciprocal and robertsonian translocations: the Korean experience. Prenat Diagn 2004; 24:556–61.

12. Munné S, Sandalinas M, Escudero T, et al. Outcome of preimplantation genetic diagnosis of translocations. Fertil Steril 2000; 73:1209–18.

13. Simopoulou M, Harper JC, Fragouli E, et al. Preimplantation genetic diagnosis of chromosome abnormalities: implications from the outcome for couples with chromosomal rearrangements. Prenat Diagn 2003; 23:652–62.

14. Carp HJA, Guetta E, Dorf H, et al. Embryonic karyotype in recurrent miscarriage with parental karyotypic aberrations Fertil Steril 2006; 85:446–50.

15. Rubio C, Rodrigo L, Perez-Cano I, et al. FISH screening of aneuploidies in preimplantation embryos to improve IVF outcome. RBM Online 2005; 11:497–506.

16. Spandorter SD, Davis OK, Barmat LI, et al. Relationship between aternal age and aneuploidy in in vitro fertilization pregnancy loss. Fertil Steril 2004; 8:1265–9.

17. Dailey T, Dall B, Cohen J, et al. Association between nondisjunction and maternal age in meiosis-II human oocytes. Am J Hum Genet 1996; 59:176–84.

18. Cupisti S, Conn CM, Fragouli E, et al. Sequential FISH analysis of oocytes and polar bodies reveals aneuploidy mechanisms. Prenat Diagn 2003; 23:663–8.

19. Munné S, Chen S, Fischer J, et al. Preimplantation genetic diagnosis reduces pregnancy loss in women aged 35 years and older with a history of recurrent miscarriages. Fertil Steril 2005; 3 (Suppl 4):3:31–3.

20. Brigham SA, Colon C, Farquharson G. A longitudinal study of pregnancy outcome following idiopathic recurrent miscarriage. Hum Reprod 1999;14:2868 –71.

21. Kallioniemi A, Kallioniemi OP, Sudar D, et al. Comparative genomic hybridization for molecular cytogenetic analysis of solid tumors. Science 1992; 258:818–21.

22. Uhrig S, Schuffenhauer S, Fauth C, et al. Multiplex-FISH for pre and postnatal diagnostic applications. Am J Hum Genet 1999; 65:448–62.

23. Handyside AH, Robinson MD, Simpson RJ, et al. Isothermal whole genome amplification from single and small numbers of cells: a new era for preimplantation genetic diagnosis of inherited disease. Mol Hum Reprod 2004; 10:767–72.

24. Daniely M, Aviram-Goldring A, Barkai G, et al. Detection of chromosomal abberation in fetuses arising from recurrent spontaneous abortion by comparative genomic hybridization. Hum Reprod 1998; 13:805–9.

25. Wilton L, Williamson R, McBain J, et al. Birth of a healthy infant after preimplantation confirmation of euploidy by comparative genomic hybridization. N Engl J Med 2001; 345:1537–41.

DEBATE

3d. Should PGD be performed in RPL? – Against

Patricio Donoso, Andre Van Steirteghem, and Paul Devroey

INTRODUCTION

The management of recurrent pregnancy loss (RPL) represents an important challenge for reproductive medicine specialists, as we are confronted with a distressed couple in need not only of medical care but also of psychological support, especially when no etiology is found after a complete workup has been performed (50%).[1]

Preimplantation genetic diagnosis (PGD) has been proposed as a treatment for couples suffering from recurrent miscarriage in two situations: unexplained recurrent miscarriage and in the presence of parental chromosome structural rearrangements. A separate analysis is presented for each group.

UNEXPLAINED RECURRENT MISCARRIAGE

Recurrent miscarriage defined as three or more consecutive pregnancy losses occurs in 0.5–3% of women.[2]

Although a high rate of chromosomal abnormalities (50–70%) has been demonstrated in sporadic miscarriage,[3,4] conflicting results are available for unexplained recurrent miscarriage. Carp et al[5] evaluated the karyotypes of 167 abortuses in women with at least three consecutive miscarriages, finding an abnormal result in only 29% of the abortuses. In agreement with these results, a case–control study[6] showed an aneuploidy rate of only 25% in women with two or more consecutive miscarriages. On the other hand, Stern et al[3] found no difference in the chromosomal abnormality rate of the products of conception from women with or without recurrent miscarriage (57%). These discrepancies have been attributed to different inclusion criteria, since an inverse correlation between the number of abortions and the frequency of chromosomal abnormalities has been described.[7]

To date, therapeutic alternatives for unexplained recurrent miscarriage remain empirical and with unproven efficiency. Furthermore, a live birth rate of 70% can be achieved after three consecutive miscarriages merely by performing supportive care.[8] In this study, only age (over 40 years) had an adverse impact on the pregnancy outcome. Similar results have been observed in other trials without further treatment (68% live birth rate).[5]

PGD for aneuploidy screening (PGD-AS) has been proposed as a therapeutic tool for the management of unexplained recurrent miscarriage, since an increased incidence of numerical chromosomal abnormalities (50–60%) has been reported in embryos derived from these patients.[9–13] The hypothesis is that an enhanced embryo selection provided by PGD-AS may improve the chance of a live birth.

Only one randomized trial has included couples with recurrent miscarriage ($n=11$, PGD-AS group; $n=8$, control group).[11] Even though there was a tendency towards a better outcome after PGD-AS (7/11 vs 3/8 pregnancies per embryo transfer), the limited number of patients does not allow definitive conclusions to be drawn. Moreover, miscarriage rates were not reported, although they represent the main outcome to be evaluated in these couples. In addition, this study was excluded from the meta-analysis performed by the Cochrane database on PGD-AS,[13] since it contained insufficient data to assess the methodological quality. The largest observational trial (n=241 cycles) reported similar miscarriage rates after PGD-AS compared with patients undergoing PGD for sex-linked diseases (12.3% PGD-AS vs 8.3% control) in couples with two or more miscarriages.[14] However, patients in the control group did not have recurrent miscarriage, thus making it an inadequate group to compare the pregnancy outcome. A prospective study performed at our center including 49 patients with at least three consecutive recurrent pregnancy losses[12] revealed an ongoing pregnancy rate per embryo transfer of 29% in young women (less than 37 years old). In the case of older women, the results were extremely disappointing, as an ongoing pregnancy rate of 5.5% was recorded. The main reason for this poor outcome is that most of these women also had infertility as a consequence of decreased oocyte quality. Consequently, these patients had significantly more abnormal embryos than did patients under 37 years old (66.9% vs 43.8%, respectively). Another study,[15] however, reported a

significant reduction in the miscarriage rate in women over 35 years old after the performance of PGD-AS compared with the expected probability of miscarriage (12% PGD-AS group vs 45% expected). Table 3d.1 summarizes the available evidence from observational studies on the outcome of these patients after undergoing PGD-AS.

Although it has been suggested that PGD-AS should be offered only to couples with documented aneuploid miscarriages, two studies[5,7] have shown that these patients have a better prognosis than those with euploid miscarriages. Therefore, results obtained from observational studies must be analyzed with caution, since most of these patients, especially young women, already have a good chance of success.

A major drawback to the effectiveness of PGD-AS is the high incidence of mosaicism documented in preimplantation embryos (up to 50%), since it leads to the loss of suitable embryos for replacement.[16] Additionally, the incomplete assessment of the embryo chromosomal constitution performed by fluorescence in situ hybridization (FISH) does not enable the exclusion of aneuploidy.

An alternative approach is to perform PGD-AS with diagnostic purposes, as it has been shown that

Table 3d.1 Summary of observational studies evaluating the pregnancy outcome of couples with unexplained recurrent miscarriage after performing PGD-AS

Study	Study group	Control group	Outcome
Pellicer et al[9]	≥ 3 miscarriages: ≤ 36 years (n=9)	PGD sex-linked disease: ≤ 36 years (n=10); > 36 years (n=6)	Study group: 3 pregnant, 1 miscarriage Control group: ≤ 36 years: 3 pregnancies, 1 miscarriage > 36 years: 0 pregnancies
Rubio et al[10]	≥ 2 miscarriages: < 37 years (n=51); ≥ 37 years (n=20)	PGD sex-linked disease: < 37 years (n=15); ≥ 37 years (n=13)	Study group: < 37 years, 10.5% miscarriage rate ≥ 37 years, 25% miscarriage rate Control group: no miscarriage
Munné et al[15]	≥ 3 miscarriages: < 35 years (n=21) ≥ 35 years (n=37)	Expected pregnancy loss according to Brigham et al 1999	Study group: < 35 years, 23% miscarriage rate ≥ 35 years, 12% miscarriage rate Control group: < 35 years, expected pregnancy loss 29%; ≥ 35 years, expected pregnancy loss 44.5%
Platteau et al[12]	≥ 3 miscarriages: < 37 years (35 cycles) ≥ 37 years (34 cycles)	No	Ongoing pregnancy rate/embryo transfer: < 37 years, 29% ≥ 37 years, 5.5%
Rubio et al[14]	≥ 2 miscarriages: < 37 years (163 cycles); ≥ 37 years (78 cycles)	PGD for sex-linked disease n= 25	Study group: < 37 years, 10% miscarriage rate ≥ 37 years, 20% miscarriage rate Control group: 8.3% miscarriage rate

about 20% of these couples do not develop chromosomally normal embryos.[10] In addition, a high predictability rate of the first PGD cycle towards successive attempts has been described (73%).[17] This valuable information could help some of these couples in their decision to undergo a second cycle of PGD-AS.

In conclusion, conflicting evidence currently exists regarding the contribution of aneuploidy screening in the outcome of these patients, although it seems that PGD-AS does not perform better than expectant management. Therefore, considering the need to undergo in vitro fertilization (IVF) and the high cost associated with aneuploidy screening, this technique should not be performed on a routine basis, unless informed consent is given. These couples should be well informed about the lack of consistency in available evidence to ensure an appropriate decision is made. Only future well-designed randomized trials will be able to establish the definitive value of this technique in unexplained recurrent miscarriage couples.

STRUCTURAL CHROMOSOME DISORDERS

The prevalence of structural rearrangement in couples with recurrent miscarriage is 3–5%, translocations (reciprocal and robertsonian) being the most frequently observed.[18,19] The diagnosis of a translocation is usually made after repeated miscarriages have occurred or a child with a congenital defect has been born as a consequence of an unbalanced rearrangement. In the case of couples with recurrent miscarriage, the chance of having an affected child is lower than that of couples with a sick child already (2–5% vs 20–22%).[20]

Overall, considering translocations, inversions and numeric mosaics, a live birth rate of 45% has been reported after three consecutive miscarriages without treatment.[21] Moreover, a recent case–control study, including couples with two or more miscarriages with a follow-up of 5 years after the diagnosis of the structural chromosome defect, observed no difference between the carrier and the non-carrier groups (83% vs 84%) in the global chance of having a healthy child.[20] This was not the case, however, for the first and second pregnancies, where a significantly lower success rate was encountered in the carrier couples (62% vs 72% and 44% vs 55%, respectively).

Robertsonian translocations have been traditionally associated with a better outcome than reciprocal translocations, since a higher rate of alternate segregation is present in the spermatozoa (88% vs 46%, respectively).[22] Additionally, up to 70% of the embryos from female carriers of reciprocal translocations show unbalanced rearrangements.[23] Furthermore, in a series of 100 couples with recurrent miscarriages, only patients with reciprocal translocations revealed a higher miscarriage rate in the subsequent pregnancy (72% reciprocal translocations vs 36% robertsonian).[24] Nevertheless, after a long-term follow-up, no difference in live births was observed between these two types of translocations (83% reciprocal vs 82% robertsonian).[20]

PGD has been proposed to these couples as an early form of prenatal diagnosis in order to avoid the negative psychological effects of being confronted with repeated miscarriages or the termination of a pregnancy when malformations are diagnosed. Unfortunately, the few data available for analysis are derived from retrospective studies only (Table 3d.2). Munné et al[23] found a significant decrease in the miscarriage rate after performing PGD (from 92% to 12.5%). A correlation between the pregnancy rate and the number of abnormal embryos with a cutoff value of 50% was also found. The ESHRE PGD Consortium Data Collection[25] reported a clinical pregnancy rate per embryo transfer of 24% for robertsonian translocations and 17% for reciprocal translocations. Chun et al[26] found a significant decrease in the miscarriage rate after PGD (from 95.8% to 16.7%). Finally, a multicenter report including 469 PGD cycles performed for translocations showed a pregnancy rate per embryo transfer of 34%.[27]

Overall, these results reveal that PGD does not perform better than expectant management. Furthermore, the risks and costs of IVF and PGD have to be considered in order to make a

Table 3d.2 Pregnancy outcome after performing PGD in translocation carrier patients with recurrent miscarriage

	Munné et al[2]	Harper et al[25]	Chun et al[26]	Verlinsky et al[27]
No. of patients/cycles	35 patients	574 cycles	49 patients	469 cycles
Outcome	Miscarriage rate decrease from 92% to 12.5%	Pregnancy rate/embryo transfer: robertsonian 24%; reciprocal 17%	Delivery rate 32.6%	Pregnancy rate/embryo transfer 34%

well-informed decision. When counselling these patients, multiple variables must be taken into consideration to enable the most appropriate choice to be performed: woman's age, number of previous miscarriages, existence of an affected offspring, type of translocation, and presence of associated infertility. It is also important to perform a complete workup, since antiphospholipid syndrome has been diagnosed in 29% of these patients.[28]

In conclusion, on the basis of currently available evidence, it seems that PGD does not improve the pregnancy outcome in couples who are carriers of structural chromosome rearrangements when compared with expectant management.

REFERENCES

1. Clifford K, Rai R, Watson H, et al. An informative protocol for the investigation of recurrent miscarriage: Preliminary experience of 500 consecutive cases. Hum Reprod 1994; 9:1328–1332.
2. Li TC, Makris M, Tomsu M, et al. Recurrent miscarriage: aetiology, management and prognosis. Hum Reprod Update 2002; 8:463–81.
3. Stern JJ, Dorfman AD, Gutierrez-Najar, et al. Frequency of abnormal karyotype among abortuses from women with and without a history of recurrent spontaneous abortion. Fertil Steril 1996; 65:250–3.
4. Sanchez JM, Franzi L, Collia F, et al. Cytogenetic study of spontaneous abortions by transabdominal villus sampling and direct analysis of villi. Prenat Diagn 1999; 19:601–3.
5. Carp H, Toder V, Aviram A, et al. Karyotype of the abortus in recurrent miscarriage. Fertil Steril 2001; 75:678–82.
6. Sullivan AE, Silver RM, LaCoursiere Y, et al. Recurrent fetal aneuploidy and recurrent miscarriage. Obstet Gynecol 2004; 104:784–8.
7. Ogasawara M, Aoki K, Okada S, et al. Embryonic karyotype of abortuses in relation to the number of previous miscarriages. Fertil Steril 2000; 73:300–4.
8. Clifford K, Rai R, Regan L. Future pregnancy outcome in unexplained recurrent first trimester miscarriage. Hum Reprod 1997; 12:387–9.
9. Pellicer A, Rubio C, Vidal F, et al. In vitro fertilization plus preimplantation genetic diagnosis in patients with recurrent miscarriage: an analysis of chromosome abnormalities in human preimplantation embryos. Fertil Steril 1999; 71:1033–9.
10. Rubio C, Simon C, Vidal F, et al. Chromosomal abnormalities and embryo development in recurrent miscarriage couples. Hum Reprod 2003; 18:182–8.
11. Werlin L, Rodi I, DeCherney A, et al. Preimplantation genetic diagnosis as both a therapeutic and diagnostic tool in assisted reproductive technology. Fertil Steril 2003; 80:467–8.
12. Platteau P, Staessen C, Michiels A, et al. Preimplantation genetic diagnosis for aneuploidy screening in patients with unexplained recurrent miscarriages. Fertil Steril 2005; 83:393–7.
13. Twisk M, Mastenbroeck S, van Wely, et al. Preimplantation genetic screening for abnormal chromosomes (aneuploidies) in in vitro fertilisation or intracytoplasmic sperm injection. Cochrane Database Syst Rev 2006; (1):CD00S291.
14. Rubio C, Rodrigo L, Perez-Cano I, et al. FISH screening of aneuploidies in preimplantation embryos to improve IVF outcome. RBM Online 2005; 11:497–506.
15. Munné S, Chen S, Fischer J, et al. Preimplantation genetic diagnosis reduces pregnancy loss in women aged 35 years and older with a history of recurrent miscarriages. Fertil Steril 2005; 84:331–5.
16. Bielanska M, Lin Tan S, Ao A. Chromosomal mosaicism throughout human preimplantation development in vitro: incidence, type, and relevance to embryo outcome. Hum Reprod 2002; 17:413–19.
17. Munné S, Escudero T, Colls P, et al. Predictability of preimplantation genetic diagnosis of aneuploidy and translocations on prospective attempts. RBM Online 2004; 9:645–51.
18. Stephenson MD. Frequency of factors associated with habitual abortion in 197 couples. Fertil Steril 1996; 66:24–9.
19. De Braekeleer M, Dao TN. Cytogenetic studies in couples experiencing repeated pregnancy losses. Hum Reprod 1990; 5:519–28.
20. Franssen M, Korevaar J, van der Veen F, Leschot NJ, et al. Reproductive outcome after chromosome analysis in couples with two or more miscarriages: index–control study. BMJ 2006; 322:1012.
21. Carp H, Feldman B, Oelsner G, et al. Parental karyotype and subsequent live births in recurrent miscarriage. Fertil Steril 2004; 81:1296–301.
22. Gardner RJM Sutherland GR. Chromosome Abnormalities and Genetic Counseling, 3rd edn. Oxford: Oxford University Press, 2004.
23. Munné S, Sandalinas M, Escudero T, et al. Outcome of preimplantation genetic diagnosis of translocations. Fertil Steril 2000; 73:1209–18.
24. Sugiura-Ogasawara M, Ozaki Y, Sato T, et al. Poor prognosis of recurrent aborters with either maternal or paternal reciprocal translocations. Fertil Steril 2004; 81:367–73.
25. Harper JC, Boelaert K, Geraedts J, et al. ESHRE PGD Consortium Data Collection V: cycles from January to December 2002 with pregnancy follow-up to October 2003. Hum Reprod 2006; 21:3–21.
26. Chun KL, Jin HJ, Dong MM, et al. Efficacy and clinical outcome of preimplantation genetic diagnosis using FISH for couples of reciprocal

and robertsonian translocations: the Korean experience. Prenat Diagn 2004; 24:556–61.

27. Verlinsky Y, Cohen J, Munné S, et al. Over a decade of experience with preimplantation genetic diagnosis: a multicenter report. Fertil Steril 2004; 82:292–4.

28. Stephenson M, Sierra S. Reproductive outcomes in recurrent pregnancy loss associated with a parental carrier of a structural chromosome rearrangement. Hum Reprod 2006; 21:1076–82.

OPINION

3e. Should CVS or amniocentesis be performed in RPL without screening?

Howard Cuckle

Women with recurrent miscarriages are at increased risk of fetal chromosomal abnormalities in subsequent pregnancies. I will argue that this risk is not sufficiently high to automatically justify invasive prenatal diagnosis. Instead, a policy is advocated of continual risk reassessment using a sequential multiple marker antenatal screening protocol. This conclusion is reached in the context of the steady improvement in the efficacy of antenatal screening methods over recent decades.

Screening for chromosomal abnormalities has the simple aim of identifying pregnancies at sufficiently high risk of an affected birth to warrant the hazards and costs of invasive testing. Chorionic villus sampling (CVS) and amniocentesis lead to at least 0.5% fetal losses;[1] procedural and karyotyping costs exceed US$1000.[2] Despite some progress, the occasional fetal cells and abundant free fetal DNA fragments circulating in maternal blood cannot yet be reliably used for non-invasive inexpensive prenatal diagnosis of the common chromosomal abnormalities.[3]

Local policy and national convention on what counts as sufficiently high risk to warrant invasive testing have generally emerged from the push and pull of healthcare providers, reimbursement tariffs, and professional bodies. Chromosomal abnormalities are relatively rare at birth – about 0.6%, excluding mosaics, in 70 000 consecutive newborns karyotyped[4] – so universal unselective invasive testing has never been considered an option; rather, from the earliest days, there was selection based on advanced maternal age and family history of chromosomal abnormality.

The maternal age-specific birth prevalence of Down syndrome increases to 0.11%, 0.26%, 0.98%, and 3.5% by ages 30, 35, 40, and 45, respectively.[5] The estimated risk at term for all common autosomal trisomies – Down, Edwards, and Patau syndromes – is 0.48% and 1.6% at ages 35–39 and 40–44, and for all chromosomal abnormalities, it is 0.81% and 2.4%, respectively.[6] A family history of chromosomal abnormality confers a much higher risk than this when a maternal balanced translocation is found,[7] while for paternal carriers and for non-carrier couples, there is only a modest excess over their maternal age-specific risk. With a Down syndrome proband and non-carrier parents, the excess at midtrimester is 0.54% for the same disorder and 0.24% for other aneuploidies.[8]

Testing these two high-risk groups can have little impact on birth prevalence, as most chromosomal abnormalities occur in young women and are sporadic. This consideration has led to the development of newer methods of selection for invasive testing. Beginning in the mid-1980s, a series of maternal serum markers of aneuploidy was discovered: human chorionic gonadotropin (hCG), the free-β subunit of hCG, α-fetoprotein (AFP), unconjugated estriol (uE₃), inhibin A, and pregnancy-associated plasma protein (PAPP)-A. Meanwhile even more discriminatory ultrasound markers were found – nuchal translucency (NT), nuchal skinfold (NF), nasal bone (NB), tricuspid regurgitation (TR), and ductus venosus (DV) – as well as the weaker so-called 'soft' markers determined by the late second-trimester anomaly scan or genetic sonogram.

Various marker combinations, determined concurrently, formed the basis for the first effective screening protocols. The efficacy of a given policy is generally measured by applying a statistical model to calculate the expected detection rate – the proportion of affected pregnancies selected for invasive testing – and the false-positive rate – the proportion of unaffected pregnancies selected. When applied to all women using a 1 in 250 term risk cut-off (the norm in the UK), the model-predicted Down syndrome detection rate and false-positive rate are 69% and 4.3% for the best second-trimester maternal serum combination (AFP, free β-hCG, uE$_3$, and inhibin), compared with 82% and 2.4%, respectively, for the most widely used first-trimester combination (PAPP-A and free β-hCG at 10 weeks and NT at 11 weeks).[9] In the USA, where a 1-in-270 midtrimester risk cut-off is favored, equivalent to about 1 in 350 at term, the corresponding rates are 73%, 6.0%, 84%, and 3.3%, respectively. The same markers can also detect a large proportion of other common autosomal trisomies; in the second trimester, this requires a separate risk cut-off for these disorders, but in the first-trimester, most are detected because of increased Down syndrome risks. Many of the remaining severe but non-lethal chromosomal abnormalities are also detected incidentally because of high trisomy risk or an extreme NT level. In Down syndrome (and possibly other chromosomal abnormalities), NF detects fewer affected pregnancies than does NT; nevertheless, with a 1-in-250 term cut-off risk, the model-predicted detection rate and false-positive rate for NF as a single marker are 53% and 3.5%.[9] The soft markers are generally much less powerful, but incorporating them into the risk calculation could substantially increase the efficacy.

Screening was not initially applied to all women but only to those not already regarded as high risk based on age and history, which is inefficient, since some with potentially low risks receive invasive testing. However, it was argued that women in the traditional high-risk groups expect to be provided with a diagnostic testing and the offer of a less definitive screening alternative was unfair. This case was made most forcefully in the USA, where the notion of a 'standard of care' is important and may have implications for litigation. Now, most countries have abandoned this hybrid policy, having realized that universal screening would yield a very high detection rate in the older women and substantially reduce the need for invasive testing. For example, the first-trimester combined test described above with a 1-in-250 term cut-off risk would detect 91% of the Down syndrome pregnancies in women aged 35 or older, while selecting only 8.4% of older women for invasive testing. Similar considerations apply to those with a family history.

Although women with recurrent miscarriages are at an increased risk of a fetal chromosomal abnormality in subsequent pregnancies, this increased risk is not very great. A recent study of almost 47 000 women having invasive prenatal diagnosis found a steadily increasing trend in aneuploidy risk according to the number of previous miscarriages.[10] After adjustment for age, parity, and the indication for testing, the odds ratio compared with no miscarriages was 1.21, 1.26, and 1.51 for one, two, and three or more miscarriages, respectively. For a woman aged 30 with recurrent miscarriages, this would barely increase the risk to that of women aged 35, who are no longer considered automatic candidates for invasive testing.

A large proportion of couples with recurrent miscarriages are carriers of structural chromosomal rearrangements. And subsequent pregnancies are more likely to miscarry: in one study, the proportion of pregnancies ending in a live birth among 73 carrier and 588 non-carrier couples was 45% and 55% respectively;[11] another study of 49 carriers found 52% miscarriages, compared with 28% in a large series of non-carriers.[12] However, fetal unbalanced translocations neither account for the excess of miscarriages nor contribute much to the overall chromosomal abnormality risk. In one study of subsequent abortuses among 39 carrier couples, only 4 had unbalanced translocations;[13] in a study of pregnancies among 239 carriers, just 4 unbalanced karyotypes were found.[14]

Thus, purely in terms of aneuploidy risk, there is no compelling reason to offer invasive testing automatically to women with recurrent miscarriages.

However, there may be an argument in favor of more intensive antenatal screening than is currently provided routinely. Sequential screening protocols are being developed that considerably increase the detection rate for Down syndrome and the other common trisomies. Attendance for screening is required on two or more occasions, which is easier to arrange for women with recurrent miscarriages, who already receive continual surveillance. The simplest protocol starts with the first-trimester combined test described above, but adopts an extremely high cut-off risk, selecting a small number for immediate CVS. The remainder then have the second-trimester test described above, except that all seven first- and second-trimester marker levels are incorporated into the risk calculation. The model-predicted Down syndrome detection rate and false-positive rate with a 1 in 250 term risk cut-off are 91% and 1.9%, respectively. Incorporating the newer first-trimester ultrasound markers (NB, TR, and DV) would substantially enhance detection both of the common trisomies and of other chromosomal abnormalities. For example, based on the latest parameters,[15] routinely adding NB to the risk calculation would improve the above rates to 95% and 1.1%, respectively. A further extension of the protocol could also be envisaged by incorporating into the risk calculation NF and the soft markers, determined at the anomaly scan, possibly after using a more extreme cut-off to select for amniocentesis at the second stage. As well as increasing detection generally, it would, by definition, be more focused on the non-lethal disorders.

Screening is a public health activity, and as such requires the definition of cut-off levels in order to predict use of resources. In practice, though, there is often less than strict adherence to the cut-off, which is merely taken to be a guide to action. Given the high chance of pregnancy failure and the associated anxiety among women with recurrent miscarriages, it might be particularly appropriate to have a loose interpretation. Seen in this way, the screening protocol that I have outlined here is a form of risk reassessment, by turns reassuring many and focusing concerns on a few with extreme risks.

REFERENCES

1. Evans MI, Wapner RJ. Invasive prenatal diagnostic procedures 2005. Semin Perinatol 2005; 29:215–18.
2. Cusick W, Buchanan P, Hallahan TW, et al. Combined first-trimester versus second-trimester serum screening for Down syndrome: a cost analysis. Am J Obstet Gynecol 2003; 188:745–51.
3. Hahn S, Huppertz B, Holzgreve W. Fetal cells and cell free fetal nucleic acids in maternal blood: new tools to study abnormal placentation? Placenta 2005; 26:515–26.
4. Hook EB, Hammerton JL. The frequency of chromosome abnormalities detected in consecutive newborn studies; differences between studies; results by sex and severity of phenotypic involvement. In: Hook EB, Porter IH, eds. Population Cytogenetics: Studies in Humans. New York: Academic Press, 1977:63–79.
5. Cuckle HS, Wald NJ, Thompson SC. Estimating a women's risk of having a pregnancy associated with Down's syndrome using her age and serum alpha-fetoprotein level. Br J Obstet Gynaecol 1987; 94:387–402.
6. Hook EBH. Chromosomal abnormalities: prevalence, risks and recurrence. In: Brock DJH, Rodeck CH, Ferguson-Smith MA, eds. Prenatal Diagnosis and Screening. Edinburgh: Churchill Livingstone, 1992: 351–92.
7. Boué A, Gallano P. A collaborative study of the segregation of inherited chromosome arrangements in 1356 prenatal diagnoses. Prenat Diagn 1984; 4:45–67.
8. Arbuzova S, Cuckle H, Mueller R, et al. Familial Down syndrome: evidence supporting cytoplasmic inheritance. Clin Genet 2001; 60:456–62.
9. Cuckle H, Benn P, Wright D. Down syndrome screening in the first and/or second trimester: model predicted performance using meta-analysis parameters. Seminars Perinatology 2005; 29:252–7.
10. Bianco K, Caughey A, Shaffer BL, et al. Spontaneous abortion and aneuploidy Obstet Gynecol 2006; 107:1098–102.
11. Carp H, Feldman B, Oelsner G, et al. Parental karyotype and subsequent live births in recurrent miscarriage. Fertil Steril 2004; 81:1296–301.
12. Sugiura-Ogasawara M, Ozaki Y, Sato T, et al. Poor prognosis of recurrent aborters with either maternal or paternal reciprocal translocations. Fertil Steril 2004; 81:367–73.
13. Carp H, Guetta E, Dorf H, et al. Embryonic karyotype in recurrent miscarriage with parental karyotypic aberrations. Fertil Steril 2006; 85:446–50.
14. Franssen MTM, Korevaar JC, van der Veen F, et al. Reproductive outcome after chromosome analysis in couples with two or more miscarriages: case–control study. BMJ 2006; 332:759–63.
15. Cicero S, Rembouskos G, Vandecruys H, et al. Likelihood ratio for trisomy 21 in fetuses with absent nasal bone at the 11–14-week scan. Ultrasound Obstet Gynecol 2004; 23:218–23.

4. Does the maternal immune system regulate the embryo's response to teratogens?

Arkady Torchinsky and Vladimir Toder

INTRODUCTION

Maternal factors have long been known to determine the embryo's resistance to teratogens. Research originally focused on the role of the maternal endocrinal, cardiovascular, and nervous systems. The maternal immune system was only investigated with regard to the teratogenic potential of autoimmune phenomena or vaccines. It is only since the beginning of the 1990s that the immune responses operating in the embryonic microenvironment have been recognized to be vital for pregnancy to develop successfully.[1] In addition to their role in regulating embryonic development, there is much evidence implicating these immune responses in determining the tolerance of the embryo to environmental teratogens.[2] This chapter summarizes the data dealing with the susceptibility of the embryo to teratogens, and the possible mechanisms whereby immune responses may affect the ability of the embryo to resist teratogenic insults.

FETOMATERNAL IMMUNOREACTIVITY AND EMBRYONIC DEVELOPMENT

As early as in the mid-1960s, studies were performed that demonstrated that immune responses had a regulatory role in embryonic development. Mean litter size and mean placental weight were found to be higher in allogeneic than in syngeneic pregnancies.[3,4] The survival of transplanted embryos was also shown to be significantly higher when there was a difference in major histocompatibility complex (MHC) antigens between the parents.[5] It has since been observed that the litter size and placental weights were higher in mice preimmunized with allogeneic paternal strain lymphocytes.[6] However, in mice, immunization with syngeneic splenocytes prior to syngeneic mating results in perinatal and postnatal mortality and an increased number of malformations among the progeny.[7] Additionally, it has been shown that the sera of habitually aborting women who were immunized with paternal leucocytes improved blastocyst development in culture and reversed the embryotoxic effect of sera from non-immunized women with recurrent miscarriages.[8]

Finally, stimulation of the maternal immune response has been shown to improve the reproductive performance of mice with a high degree of spontaneous postimplantation embryonic loss. In the CBA/J × DBA/2J mouse mating combination, which is prone to resorption of pregnancies, alloimmunization of the female with leukocytes of paternal haplotype significantly decreased the proportion of resorbed pregnancies from approximately 40% to 10–15%.[9,10] The same effect has been achieved with non-specific immunostimulation of mice with complete Freund's adjuvant (CFA).[11,12]

FETOMATERNAL IMMUNOREACTIVITY AND TERATOLOGIC SUSCEPTIBILITY

The above studies, which have demonstrated that survival of the embryo depends on immune responses acting in the embryonic microenvironment, have initiated research into whether these responses are also involved in determining the susceptibility of the embryo to developmental toxicants. Torchinsky et al[13] have compared the effects of two teratogens, cyclophosphamide (CP) and 2,3-quinoxalinedimethanol-1,4-dioxide (CAS 17311-31-8)[14] in syngeneically and allogeneically mated CBA/J and

C57Bl/6 mice. Both strains had almost identical sensitivities to these teratogens, and both strains also showed a higher sensitivity to both teratogens after syngeneic mating than allogeneic mating. However, the design of these experiments precluded the authors from assessing the effect of genetic differences between inbred and F1 (CBA/J × C57Bl/6) embryos on the different response to the teratogens. Therefore, further experiments were performed in C57Bl/6 females whose immune responses were either depressed by removing the paraaortic lymph nodes or activated by intrauterine immunization with allogeneic paternal splenocytes.[15,16] It has been observed[15] that suppression of the maternal immune response significantly increases the sensitivity of F1 (C57Bl/6 × CBA/J) embryos to both teratogens and almost eliminates the different responses between allogeneically and syngeneically mated females. Thus, in mice undergoing extirpation of draining lymph nodes, CP produced a resorption rate of approximately 20%, and a malformation rate of 77%, whereas in sham-operated females these indices were 6% and 31%, respectively. In contrast, females primed with allogeneic paternal splenocytes before allogeneic mating showed enhanced tolerance to both teratogens.[16]

The response to the above teratogens has also been tested in the second pregnancy of C57Bl/6 mice.[16] It has been observed that the degree of embryotoxicity induced by both teratogens depends on the type of mating (allogeneic or syngeneic) in the first and second pregnancy, and that embryos of females mated twice allogeneically demonstrate a significantly higher resistance to both teratogens than do embryos of allogeneically mated primigravid mice. These results suggested that the exposure of the maternal immune system to paternal antigens in the first pregnancy may modify the teratogenic response of embryos in repeated pregnancies.

Nomura et al[17] have observed that embryos of ICR mice pretreated with synthetic (Pyran copolymer) or biological (bacillus Calmette–Guerin (BCG) vaccine) agents that are known to activate macrophages exhibit increased tolerance to teratogens such as urethane, N-methyl-N-nitrosourea, and ionizing radiation. Nomura et al[17] also reported

that injection of Pyran-activated macrophages to CL/Fr mice, which have a high incidence of cleft lip and palate, decreased the incidence of these anomalies. Torchinsky et al[18] have also shown that immunostimulation of ICR mice with a non-specific immune trigger (xenogeneic rat splenocytes) increases the tolerance of embryos to CP-induced teratogenic effects (Figure 4.1). Furthermore, it has been found that immunization performed twice (21 days before mating and on day 1 of pregnancy) has a greater influence on the teratogenic response to CP than a single inoculation.[18]

The influence of the immune response on the susceptibility to teratogens has also been investigated in type 1 ('insulin-dependent') diabetes mellitus (IDM) and heat shock. Meticulous metabolic control of diabetes has significantly decreased the risk of gross structural malformations in newborn infants. Nevertheless, the incidence of fetal malformations in women with type 1 IDM (6–10%) is still three to five times higher than in non-diabetic women.[19] In our studies,[20] in laboratory animals, streptozocin (STZ) was used to induce diabetes in ICR mice treated with rat splenocytes 21 days before mating. In STZ-induced diabetic ICR mice, approximately 9% of embryos show gross structural anomalies and the incidence of litters with malformed embryos reaches 63%.[21] Immunostimulation resulted in a decrease of both indices: only 18% of litters had malformed fetuses and the incidence of malformed embryos was approximately 2%. Moreover, immunostimulation was followed by in an increase in the pregnancy rate: approximately 70%, compared with 44% in non-immunized diabetic females.

Heat shock-induced teratogenic effects in rodents are associated with the occurrence of anomalies in the brain and eye.[22] Our experiments in ICR mice[23] have shown that immunization with rat splenocytes significantly decreases the proportion of fetuses with exencephaly and open eyes. Also, the resorption rate in immunized mice was similar to that seen in intact ICR mice (approximately 6%–10%), whereas in non-immunized mice exposed to heat shock, it exceeded 20%.[23]

Recently, a number of studies have been published that concur with the above observations.

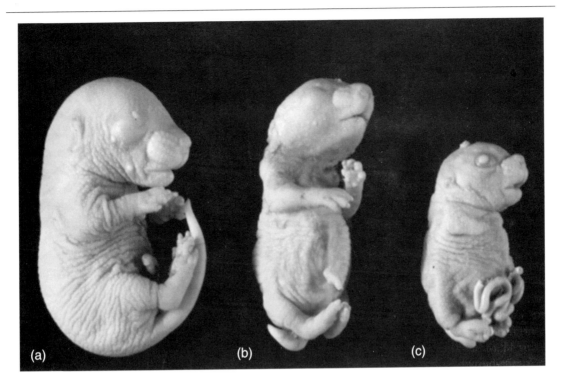

Figure 4.1 The teratogenic response of embryos of cyclophosphamide (CP)-treated intact and immunostimulated mice. CP induces a specter of gross structural anomalies, such as open eyes, digit and limb reduction anomalies, exencephaly, gastroschisis, and growth retardation, in a dose-dependent fashion. Immunostimulation of females with xenogeneic rat splenocytes is followed by a decrease in the incidence and severity of these anomalies and an increase in fetal weight. (a) Fetus of an intact mouse. (b) Fetus of an immunostimulated CP-treated mouse. (c) Fetus of a non-immunostimulated CP-treated mouse.

Holladay et al[24] showed that immune stimulation of pregnant mice with Pyran copolymer, attenuated BCG, or CFA increased the resistance of embryos to teratogens such as 2,3,7,8-tetrachlorodibenzo-p-dioxin (TCDD, 'dioxin'), urethane, N-methyl-N-nitrosourea, and valproic acid. This group also found that maternal immune stimulation with CFA, granulocyte–macrophage colony-stimulating factor (GM-CSF), or interferon-γ (IFN-γ) protects murine embryos against diabetes-induced teratogenic effects.[25] In our studies,[26] maternal immunostimulation with GM-CSF increased the resistance of murine embryos to CP.

The effect of maternal immunostimulation has also been demonstrated in mice exposed to ultrasonic and restraint stresses, neither of which has a teratogenic effect but both of which do induce postimplantation embryonic death.[27] It has been shown[28] that immunization of C3H/HeJ female mice with allogeneic paternal splenocytes of DBA/2J mice 7 days before mating reduces the number of restraint stress-induced embryonic losses. Immune stimulation of CBA/J female mice with paternal splenocytes of DBA/2J males 2 weeks before mating decreases the number of ultrasonic stress-induced resorptions. Finally, Hatta et al[29] have reported that stimulation of female mice with the biostimulators PSK and OK432 decreased the susceptibility of embryos to the teratogen 5-azacytidine, whereas injection of interleukin-1 (IL-1) decreased the tolerance of embryos to this teratogen.

The above studies provide evidence that immune responses occurring between mother and fetus may influence the susceptibility of embryos to both environmental teratogens and detrimental stimuli generated by the mother. The mechanisms underlying this phenomenon remain largely undefined. However, research in reproductive immunology, developmental biology, and teratology may outline some of the mechanisms involved. Some possible mechanisms are described below.

POSSIBLE MECHANISMS OF INTERACTIONS BETWEEN IMMUNE RESPONSES AND DEVELOPMENTAL TOXINS

MOLECULES REGULATING APOPTOSIS IN THE EMBRYO

Most teratogens act on the embryo itself. Therefore, some of the mechanisms that determine the response of embryonic cells to teratogens must be affected by maternal immune stimulation modifying teratological susceptibility. These mechanisms are mainly associated with the mechanisms regulating programmed cell death (apoptosis) in embryos responding toteratogenic stress.[30] A comprehensive review of the literature addressing this topic is clearly beyond the scope of this chapter. Suffice it to say that apoptosis plays a crucial role in normal embryogenesis. Apoptosis is involved in eliminating abnormal, misplaced, non-functional, or harmful cells, sculpting structures, eliminating unwanted structures, and controlling cell numbers.[31] Teratological studies have shown that many of the chemical and physical developmental toxicants that induce structural anomalies also induce excessive apoptosis in embryonic structures, which are subsequently malformed.[32,33] Toder et al[34] investigated whether maternal immune stimulation affects the degree of teratogen-induced apoptosis, and reported that immune stimulation of females with xenogeneic rat splenocytes did indeed decrease the intensity of CP-induced excessive apoptosis in embryonic structures.

Apoptosis is a genetically regulated process that is realized by the activation of both death signaling cascades and prosurvival pathways acting to suppress the process of apoptosis.[35] A number of molecules have been suggested to be key components of the machinery of apoptosis and have also been implicated as powerful determinants of teratogenic susceptibility.[30] It may be that teratogen-induced alterations in the expression of these molecules may be normalized by maternal immune potentiation. The tumor suppressor protein p53, which is activated by various cellular stresses that induce DNA damage, is presently considered to be a key regulator of apoptosis.[36] It is thought that p53, which targets several steps in the apoptotic process, increases the probability that the process goes forward, and ensures a well-coordinated program once the process is initiated.[36] Evidence is accumulating that suggests that p53 regulates the response of embryos to teratogens such as benzo[a]pyrene,[37] 2-chloro-2-deoxyadenosine,[38] ionizing radiation,[39,40] diabetes,[41] and CP.[42] Our team[43] has shown that a CP-induced teratogenic insult was followed by the accumulation of p53 protein in embryonic structures, and that maternal immune stimulation with xenogeneic rat splenocytes, or GM-CSF, while increasing the tolerance of murine embryos to the teratogen, partially normalized the expression of the protein.[26] Sharova et al[44] have shown that mice exposed to the teratogen urethane (which induces cleft palate in mice), injection of CFA or IFN-γ was followed by a decreased incidence of malformed fetuses and that CFA also normalized the urethane-induced alterations in the expression of the gene TP53 encoding for p53. Sharova et al[44] also reported that maternal immune stimulation also normalized the expression of the BCL2 gene, which is thought to encode one of the key antiapoptotic proteins, BCL-2.[45]

Other proteins considered to be the main executors of apoptosis are the caspases, which belong to the family of cysteine proteases.[46] Caspases are divided into two groups: initiator and effector caspases. The activation of initiator caspases takes place after their binding to adapter molecules, and mature initiator caspases activate effector caspases. The initiator caspase 9 (and possibly caspase 2) operates in the mitochondrial proapoptotic pathway, whereas the initiator caspases 8 and 10 act in the death-receptor proapoptotic pathway. Both pathways use effector caspases (caspases 3, 6, and 7).[47] It has been reported[30] that at least one of the main initiator caspases 8 or 9 and/or the main effector caspase 3 are involved in the response to teratogens such as diabetes, ionizing radiation, heat shock, CP, sodium arsenite, and retinoic acid.[30] The possibility that maternal immune stimulation may modify teratological susceptibility by affecting the process of teratogen-induced activation of caspases has been supported by our recent study.[48] The levels of active caspases 3, 8, and 9 were lower in the embryos of immunostimulated CP-treated mice than in embryos of mice exposed to the teratogen alone.[48]

The transcription factor, nuclear factor κB (NF-κB) is also thought to be a key molecule preventing cell death via the activation of genes whose products function as antiapoptotic proteins.[49] NF-κB is transcriptionally active in embryos during organogenesis. One subunit of NF-κB, p65, has been shown to be indispensable for the protection of the embryonic liver against the physiological apoptosis induced by tumor necrosis factor α (TNF-α).[50] There are a number of studies implicating NF-κB as a regulator of the response to teratogens such as thalidomide,[51] phenytoin,[52] and CP.[53] Our recent study[48] has shown that NF-κB may be a target for immune responses operating in the embryonic microenvironment. The results suggested that intrauterine immunostimulation with rat splenocytes attenuates the CP-induced suppression of NF-κB DNA-binding activity in mouse embryos.

The above data suggest some of the mechanisms by which maternal immune stimulation might alter teratological susceptibility. However, these mechanisms operate in the embryo, and the pathways by which maternal immune stimulation affects these mechanisms remain elusive. Therefore, we have only presented data that should be taken consideration in research dealing with this topic.

CYTOKINES AND GROWTH FACTORS OPERATING AT THE FETOMATERNAL INTERFACE

There is considerable evidence that the establishment of a balanced cytokine milieu is a necessary condition for maternal–fetal immune tolerance.[54–56] There are data indicating that cytokine imbalances that precede or accompany embryonic death induce various stresses and are also involved in some of the mechanisms regulating the susceptibility of the embryo to detrimental stimuli.[57] Additionally, teratogenic insults may also be accompanied by dysregulation of the cytokines operating in the embryo. We have observed that CP-induced teratogenesis is accompanied by an increase in TNF-α and decreases in transforming growth factor-β2 (TGF-β2) and macrophage colony-stimulating factor (M-CSF; colony-stimulating factor 1, CSF-1) expression at the fetomaternal interface.[58–60] Increased TNF-α and decreased TGF-β2 expression have also been described in the uterus of diabetic mice.[61–63]

Studies in TNF-α knockout mice have shown no alterations in litter size, sex ratio, weight gain, or structural anomalies, indicating that TNF-α probably does not play an essential role in regulating normal embryogenesis.[64] Early studies addressing the functional role of TNF-α in reproduction implied that TNF-α may be a trigger of embryonic death caused by developmental toxins, various stresses, and maternal metabolic and immunological imbalances.[64] Subsequently, TNF-α was shown to activate both apoptotic and antiapoptotic signaling cascades,[65] which suggests that TNF-α may regulate the response of the embryo to various stresses. Indeed, in our experiments with CP, the incidence and severity of CP-induced gross structural craniofacial and limb anomalies were found to be higher in TNF-α-knockout fetuses than in their TNF-α-positive counterparts.[66] TNF-α-knockout embryos have also been found to be sensitive to diabetes-induced teratogenic stimuli.[67]

TGF-β, a multipotent growth factor, has been reported to be involved in regulating cell growth, differentiation, and migration, and extracellular matrix deposition.[68] TGF-β family isoforms such as TGF-β1, TGF-β2, and TGF-β3 seem to be indispensable for normal embryogenesis. Indeed, TGF-β1-null embryos die before day 11 of pregnancy, whereas 25% of TGF-β2-knockout fetuses and 100% of TGF-β3-knockout fetuses exhibit cleft palate.[69] A number of studies have reported that TGF-β may be involved in the mechanisms of induced teratogenesis. In experiments with the teratogen TCDD, which induces cleft palate in mouse embryos, TGF-β3 was shown to counteract the effect of TCDD in blocking palatal fusion.[70] Additionally, TGF-β2-knockout embryos have been found to be more sensitive to retinoid-induced teratogenesis than their TGF-β2-positive counterparts.[71]

The above data imply that TNF-α and TGF-β are determinants of the teratological susceptibility of embryos. Maternal immune stimulation, in addition to increasing the resistance of embryos to teratogenic stress, also tends to normalize the expression of these cytokines at the fetomaternal interface,[58,59,61,62] implicating maternally derived TNF-α and TGF-β in pathways through which maternal immune stimulation modifies the responses of the embryo to teratogens. Although effective reciprocal signaling has been demonstrated between the uterus and preimplantation and periimplantation embryos,[72,73] the effectiveness of reciprocal signaling during organogenesis (the period of greatest sensitivity to teratogens) remains undetermined. Nevertheless, the mechanisms thought to ensure maternal–fetal immune tolerance – cytokines and growth factors acting in the embryonic microenvironment – may be acting primarily as mediator through which the maternal immune system regulates the response of the embryo to environmental teratogens. The above data suggest a model depicting a possible pathway by which maternal immunostimulation may modify teratological susceptibility (Figure 4.2). Within the context of this model, modification of teratological susceptibility by maternal immunostimulation depends on both the type of teratogen and the type of immune stimulator.

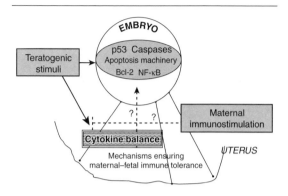

Figure 4.2 A simplified model depicting a possible pathway for maternal immunostimulation-induced modification of teratologic susceptibility. A teratogen affects the function of molecules regulating the teratogenic response (i.e., those regulating apoptosis) directly and, possibly, indirectly, via an imbalance of cytokines operating in the embryonic vicinity. Maternal immunostimulation influences the teratological susceptibility via modifying the expression pattern of these cytokines.

immune system may modify the embryo's sensitivity not only to maternally derived immune abortifacient stimuli, but also to environmental teratogens. These mechanisms may also be relevant in interpreting the mechanisms underlying 'occult' pregnancy loss[74] and for developing therapy aimed at prevention of pregnancy loss.

CONCLUSIONS

This review has provided data indicating that maternal immune responses may be involved in mechanisms determining the resistance of the embryo to teratogens. An important implication of this paradigm is that modulation of the maternal

REFERENCES

1. Hunt JS. Immunology of pregnancy. Curr Opin Immunol 1992; 4:1153–6.
2. Toder V, Torchinsky A. Immunoteratology: where we are and where to go. Am J Reprod Immunol 1996; 35;114–17.
3. Billingham RE. Transplantation immunity and the maternal–fetal relation. N Engl J Med 1964; 270:667–72.
4. Billington WD. Influence of immunologic dissimilarity of mother and foetus on size placenta in mice. Nature 1964; 202:317–18.
5. Kirby DKS. Transplantation and pregnancy. In: Rapoport FT, Dausser J, eds. Human Transplantation. New York: Grune and Stratton, 1968: 565–8.
6. Beer AE, Scott JR, Billingham RE. Histocompatibility and maternal immune status as determinants of fetoplacental and litter weights in rodents. J Exp Med 1975; 142:180–98.
7. Pechan PA. Syngeneic spleen immunization induces high mortality among progeny in mice. Teratology 1986; 33:239–41.
8. Zigril M, Fein A, Carp H, Toder V. Immunopotentiation reverses the embryotoxic effect of serum from women with pregnancy loss. Fertil Steril 1991; 56:653–69.
9. Chaouat G, Kiger N, Wegmann TG. Vaccination against spontaneous abortion in mice. J Reprod Immunol 1983; 5:389–92.

10. Chaouat G, Menu E, Bonneton C, et al. Immunological manipulation in animal pregnancy and models of pregnancy failure. Curr Opin Immunol 1989; 1:1153–6.

11. Toder V, Strassburger D, Irlin Y, et al. Nonspecific immunopotentiators and pregnancy loss: complete Freund adjuvant reverses high fetal resorption rate in CBA/J × DBA/2 mouse combination. Am J Reprod Immunol 1990; 24:63–6.

12. Szekeres-Bartho J, Kinsky R, Kapovic M, et al. Complete Freund adjuvant treatment of pregnant females influences resorption rates in CBA/J × DBA/2 matings via progesterone-mediated immunomodulation. Am J Reprod Immunol 1991; 26:82–3.

13. Torchinsky AM, Chirkova EM, Koppel MA, et al. Dependence of the embryotoxic action of dioxidine and cyclophosphamide on the immunoreactivity of the maternal–fetal system in mice. Farmakol Toksikol 1985; 48:69–73. [in Russian]

14. Sweet DV. Registry of Toxic Effects of Chemical Substances. 1985–1986 Edition. Washington: US Government Printing Office, 1986; 5:4305.

15. Torchinsky A, Fein A, Toder V. Immunoteratology: I. MHC involvement in the embryo response to teratogens in mice. Am J Reprod Immunol 1995; 34:288–98.

16. Torchinsky A, Fein A, Carp H, et al. MHC-associated immunopotentiation affects the embryo response to teratogen. Clin Exp Immunol 1994; 98:513–19.

17. Nomura T, Hata S, Kusafuka T. Suppression of developmental anomalies by maternal macrophages in mice. J Exp Med 1990; 172:1325–30.

18. Torchinsky A, Fein A, Toder V. Modulation of mouse sensitivity to cyclophosmamide-induced embryopathy by nonspecific intrauterine immunopotentiation. Toxicol Meth 1995; 5:131–41.

19. Reece EA, Homko CJ, Wu YK. Multifactorial basis of the syndrome of diabetic embryopathy. Teratology 1996; 54:171–83.

20. Torchinsky A, Toder V, Carp H, et al. In vivo evidence for the existence of a threshold for hyperglycemia-induced major fetal malformations: relevance to the etiology of diabetic teratogenesis. Early Pregnancy 1997; 3:27–33.

21. Torchinsky A, Toder V, Savion S, et al. Immunopotentiation increases the resistance of mouse embryos to diabetes-induced teratogenic effect. Diabetologia 1997; 40:635–40.

22. Edwards MJ, Shiota K, Smith MRS, et al. Hyperthermia and birth defects. Reprod Toxicol 1995; 9:411–25.

23. Yitzhakie D, Torchinsky A, Savion S, et al. Maternal immunopotentiation affects the teratogenic response to hyperthermia. J Reprod Immunol 1999; 45:49–66.

24. Holladay SD, Sharova L, Smith BJ, et al. Nonspecific stimulation of the maternal immune system. I. Effects on teratogen-induced fetal malformations. Teratology 2000; 62:413–19.

25. Punareewattana K, Holladay SD. Immunostimulation by complete Freund's adjuvant, granulocyte macrophage colony-stimulating factor, or interferon-γ reduces severity of diabetic embryopathy in ICR mice. Birth Defects Res A Clin Mol Teratol 2004; 70:20–7.

26. Savion S, Kamshitsky-Feldman A, Ivnitsky I, et al. Potentiation of the maternal immune system may modify the apoptotic process in embryos exposed to developmental toxicants. Am J Reprod Immunol 2003; 49:30–41.

27. Scialli AR. Is stress a developmental toxin? Reprod Toxicol 1988; 1:163–72.

28. Clark DA, Banwatt D, Chaouat G. Stress-triggered abortion in mice is prevented by alloimmunization. Am J Reprod Immunol 1993; 29:141–7.

29. Hatta A, Matsumoto A, Moriyama K, et al, Opposite effects of the maternal immune system activated by interleukin-1β vs. PSK and OK432 on 5-azacytidine-induced birth defects. Congenit Anom (Kyoto) 2003; 43:46–56.

30. Torchinsky A, Fein A, Toder V. Teratogen-induced apoptotic cell death: Does the apoptotic machinery act as a protector of embryos exposed to teratogens? Birth Defects Res C Embryo Today 2005; 75:353–61.

31. Jacobson MD, Weil M, Raff MC. Programmed cell death in animal development. Cell 1997; 88:347–54.

32. Knudsen TV. Cell death. In: Kavlock RJ, Daston GP, eds. Drug Toxicity in Embryonic Development I. Berlin; Springer-Verlag, 1997:211–44.

33. Mirkes PE. 2001 Warkany Lecture: To die or not to die, the role of apoptosis in normal and abnormal mammalian development. Teratology 2002; 65:228–39.

34. Toder V, Savion S, Gorivodsky M, et al. Teratogen-induced apoptosis may be affected by immunopotentiation. J Reprod Immunol 1996; 30:173–85.

35. Danial NN, Korsmeyer SJ. Cell death: critical control points. Cell 2004; 116:205–19.

36. Fridman JS, Lowe SW. Control of apoptosis by p53. Oncogene 2003; 22:9030–40.

37. Nicol CJ, Harrison ML, Laposa RR, et al. A teratologic suppresser role for p53 in benzo[a]pyrene-treated transgenic p53-deficient mice. Nat Genet 1995; 10:181–7.

38. Wubah JA, Ibrahim MM, Gao X, et al. Teratogen-induced eye defects mediated by p53-dependent apoptosis. Curr Biol 1996; 6:60–9.

39. Norimura T, Nomoto S, Katsuki M, et al. p53-dependent apoptosis suppresses radiation-induced teratogenesis. Nat Med 1996; 2:577–80.

40. Wang B, Ohyama H, Haginoya K, et al. Prenatal radiation-induced limb defects mediated by Trp53-dependent apoptosis in mice. Radiat Res 2000; 154:673–9.

41. Pani L, Horal M, Loeken MR. Rescue of neural tube defects in Pax-3-deficient embryos by p53 loss of function: implications for Pax-3-dependent development and tumorigenesis. Genes Dev 2002; 16:676–80.

42. Moallem SA, Hales BF. The role of p53 and cell death by apoptosis and necrosis in 4-hydroperoxycyclophosphamide-induced limb malformations. Development 1998; 125:3225–34.

43. Torchinsky A, Ivnitsky I, Savion S, et al. Cellular events and the pattern of p53 protein expression following cyclophosphamide-initiated cell death in various organs of developing embryo. Teratog Carcinog Mutagen 1999; 19:353–67.

44. Sharova LV, Sura P, Smith BJ, et al. Non-specific stimulation of the maternal immune system. I. Effects on fetal gene expression. Teratology 2000; 62:420–8.

45. Tsujimoto Y, Shimizu S. Bcl-2 family: life-or-death switch. FEBS Lett 2000; 466:6–10.

46. Degterev A, Boyce M, Yuan J. A decade of caspases. Oncogene 2003; 22:8543–67.

47. Pommier Y, Antony S, Hayward RL, et al. Apoptosis defects and chemotherapy resistance: molecular interaction maps and networks. Oncogene 2004; 23:2934–49.

48. Torchinsky A, Gongadze M, Zaslavsky Z, et al. Maternal immunopotentiation affects caspase activation and NF-κB DNA-binding activity in embryos responding to an embryopathic stress. Am J Reprod Immunol 2006; 55:36–44.

49. Karin M, Lin A. NF-κB at the crossroad of life and death. Nat Immunol 2002; 3:221–7.

50. Beg AA, Sha WC, Bronson RT, et al. Embryonic lethality and liver degeneration in mice lacking the RelA component of NF-κB. Nature 1995; 376:167–70.

51. Hansen JM, Harris C. A novel hypothesis for thalidomide-induced limb teratogenesis: redox misregulation of the NF-κB pathway. Antioxid Redox Signal 2004; 6:1–14.

52. Kennedy JC, Memet S, Wells PG. Antisense evidence for nuclear factor-κB-dependent embryopathies initiated by phenytoin-enhanced oxidative stress. Mol Pharmacol 2004; 66:404–12.

53. Torchinsky A, Gongadze M, Savion S, et al. Differential teratogenic response of TNFα$^{+/+}$ and TNFα$^{-/-}$ mice to cyclophosphamide: the possible role of NF-κB. Birth Defects Res A Clin Mol Teratol 2006; 76:437–44.

54. Raghupathy R. Pregnancy: success and failure within the Th1/Th2/Th3 paradigm. Semin Immunol 2001; 13:219–27.

55. Niederkorn JY. See no evil, hear no evil, do no evil: the lessons of immune privilege. Nat Immunol 2006; 7:354–9.

56. Trowsdale J, Betz AG. Mother's little helpers: mechanisms of maternal–fetal tolerance. Nat Immunol 2006; 7:241–6.

57. Arck PC. Stress and pregnancy loss: role of immune mediators, hormones and neurotransmitters. Am J Reprod Immunol 2001; 46:117–23.

58. Gorivodsky M, Zemliak I, Orenstein H, et al. Tumor necrosis factor α mRNA and protein expression in the uteroplacental unit of mice with pregnancy loss. J Immunol 1998; 160:4280–8.

59. Gorivodsky M, Torchinsky A, Zemliak I, et al. TGFβ2 mRNA expression and pregnancy failure in mice. Am J Reprod Immunol 1999; 42:124–33.

60. Gorivodsky M, Torchinsky A, Shepshelovich J, et al. Colony-stimulating factor-1 (CSF-1) expression in the uteroplacental unit of mice with spontaneous and induced pregnancy loss. Clin Exp Immunol 1999; 117:540–9.

61. Fein A, Kostina E, Savion S, et al. Expression of tumor necrosis factor-α in the uteroplacental unit of diabetic mice: effect of maternal immunopotentiation. Am J Reprod Immunol 2001; 46:161–8.

62. Fein A, Magid N, Savion S, et al. Diabetes teratogenicity in mice is accompanied with distorted expression of TGF-β2 in the uterus. Teratog Carcinog Mutagen 2002; 22:59–71.

63. Pampfer S. Dysregulation of the cytokine network in the uterus of the diabetic rat. Am J Reprod Immunol 2001; 45:375–81.

64. Toder V, Fein A, Carp H, et al. TNF-α in pregnancy loss and embryo maldevelopment: a mediator of detrimental stimuli or a protector of the fetoplacental unit? J Assist Reprod Genet 2003; 20:73–81.

65. Baud V, Karin M. Signal transduction by tumor necrosis factor and its relatives. Trends Cell Biol 2001; 11:372–7.

66. Torchinsky A, Shepshelovich J, Orenstein H, et al. TNF-α protects embryos exposed to developmental toxicants. Am J Reprod Immunol 2003; 49:159–68.

67. Torchinsky A, Gongadze M, Orenstein H, et al. TNF-α acts to prevent occurrence of malformed fetuses in diabetic mice. Diabetologia 2004; 47:132–9.

68. Massague J. How cells read TGF-β signals. Nat Rev Mol Cell Biol 2000; 1:169–78.

69. Nawshad A, LaGamba D, Hay ED. Transforming growth factor β (TGF-β) signalling in palatal growth, apoptosis and epithelial mesenchymal transformation (EMT). Arch Oral Biol 2004; 49:675–89.

70. Thomae TL, Stevens EA, Bradfield CA. Transforming growth factor-β3 restores fusion in palatal shelves exposed to 2,3,7,8-tetrachlorodibenzo-p-dioxin. J Biol Chem 2005; 280:12742–6.

71. Nugent P, Pisano MM, Weinrich MC, et al, Increased susceptibility to retinoid-induced teratogenesis in TGF-β2 knockout mice. Reprod Toxicol 2002; 16:741–7.

72. Diaz-Cueto L, Gerton GL. The influence of growth factors on the development of preimplantation mammalian embryos. Arch Med Res 2001; 32:619–26.

73. Dominguez F, Pellicer A, Simon C. Paracrine dialogue in implantation. Mol Cell Endocrinol 2002; 186:175–81.

74. Clark DA, Chaouat G, Gorczynski RM. Thinking outside the box: mechanisms of environmental selective pressures on the outcome of the materno-fetal relationship. Am J Reprod Immunol 2002; 47:275–82.

5. Fetal structural malformations – embryoscopy

Thomas Philipp

INTRODUCTION

Most pregnancy losses are spontaneously aborted when the conceptus is undergoing embryonic development. Pregnancy loss is a significant health concern in economically advanced societies, where traditional early reproduction is replaced by a social trend towards establishing the mother's career before starting reproduction. As the whole reproductive period may be shortened to 5–7 years, each pregnancy becomes precious. Finding the cause of pregnancy loss is essential for prognosis, recurrence risk counselling, and management of future pregnancies. Approximately 1% of fertile couples will experience recurrent early pregnancy losses.[1] Although recurrent early pregnancy losses have been associated with maternal factors such as maternal thrombophilic disorders, structural uterine anomalies, maternal immune dysfunction, endocrine abnormalities, and parental chromosomal anomalies (as described in other chapters of this book), approximately 50% of recurrent miscarriages are classified as idiopathic following maternal investigation. For affected couples, idiopathic pregnancy loss creates a great deal of grief and anxiety about the outcome of future pregnancies. It is currently unclear whether embryonic maldevelopment is a contributiory factor in these cases. Investigations of the dead embryo are rare.[2,3] Demised embryos cannot be investigated for several practical reasons. Most losses occur when the conceptus is undergoing embryonic development. The small size of the embryo precludes detailed examination, either by ultrasound (due to limitations of resolution) or by pathological techniques. Both instrumental evacuation and spontaneous passage damage the embryo. It is rarely retrieved whole due to its minute size and fragility.[4]

Transcervical embryoscopy permits visualization of the embryo in utero, without the damage caused by instrumental evacuation or spontaneous passage.[5] Embryoscopy in early spontaneous abortions allows visualization of subtle morphological abnormalities undetectable by ultrasound (Figure 5.1), and the diagnostic potential of transcervical embryoscopy in early failed pregnancies is just beginning to unfold.

TECHNIQUE OF TRANSCERVICAL EMBRYOSCOPY IN EARLY SPONTANEOUS OR MISSED ABORTIONS

Transcervical embryoscopy requires an average of 10 minutes (range 3–25 minutes) and is performed by us under intravenous general anesthesia, it can be organized into five different steps:

1. *Insertion of hysteroscope and exploration of the uterine cavity.* The patient is placed in a dorsal lithotomy position. A speculum is inserted into the vagina, which is cleaned with Betadine solution. After careful dilatation of the cervix, a rigid hysteroscope (12° angle of view, with both biopsy and irrigation working channels, Circon Ch 25–8 mm) is passed through the cervix under direct vision. If vision is lost, the hysteroscope is withdrawn slightly, and reinserted. A continuous normal saline flow is used throughout the procedure (pressure 40–120 mmHg) to help distend and clean the cervical canal and endometrial cavity, and thus provide a clear view. In failed first-trimester pregnancies, the decidua capsularis and parietalis have not yet fused, so the uterine cavity can be assessed. (The uterine cavity is obliterated in

(a)

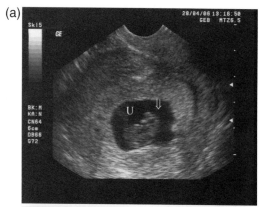

(b)

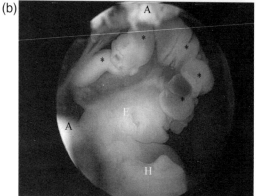

Figure 5.1 (a) Endovaginal sonography prior to embryoscopy. The embryo, of 17 mm crown–rump length, showed no heartbeat. No abnormalities were identified sonographically. The arrow marks the head of the embryo. U, umbilical cord. (b) Embryoscopic lateral view of the upper portion revealed a well-preserved embryo with anencephaly. The exposed brain tissue (*) is still intact (exencephaly). The digital rays of the hand (H) are notched. Parts of the external ear (E) are clearly discernable. Remnants of the amnion are labeled (A). A normal karyotype (46,XX) was diagnosed cytogenetically.

Table 5.1 Incidence of acquired and congenital uterine abnormalities diagnosed by transcervical embryo-hysteroscopy in missed abortion

Uterine pathology	No. of cases	Percentage
Acquired	33	64.7
Adhesions	26	51
Polyp	6	11.8
Fibroid	1	2
Congenital	18	35.3
Didelphys uterus[a]	1	2
Unicornuate uterus[a]	1	2
Septate uterus[a]	7	13.7
Arcuate uterus	4	7.8
Unclassified	5	9.8
Total	51	100

[a]Ascertained by laparoscopy/laparotomy investigating the external uterine contour.

is opened with microscissors (CH 7–2 mm), due to its opacity, and the embryo is first viewed through the amnion. The small size of the embryo makes high demands on image resolution. At the end of the 8th week, it measures 30 mm, but already possesses several thousand named structures. Therefore, the embryoscope should be advanced as close as possible to the embryo in order to document the minute developing structures such as the limbs (Figure 5.2). The amnion usually obscures vision by reflecting light. In failed pregnancies, there is no need to avoid amniotic rupture. Hence, the hysteroscope is inserted into the amniotic cavity after opening the membrane with microscissors. Documentation of the embryo's details can be better achieved from within the amniotic cavity.

3. *Morphological evaluation of the embryo.* A complete examination of the conceptus includes visualization of the head, face, dorsal and ventral walls, limbs, and umbilical cord. The incidence of developmental defects is particularly high in early abortion specimens.[6,7] The development of the human embryo is a dynamic process, with constantly changing anatomy and hence appearance. Early diagnosis of developmental defects by embryoscopy requires basic knowledge of the anatomy of the developing human embryo.

midtrimester by fusion of the decidua capsularis with the decidua parietalis.) At this stage, congenital and acquired uterine defects can be diagnosed. Table 5.1 shows the spectrum of uterine defects that we have been able to diagnose by this technique in early failed pregnancies.

2. *Localization of the gestational sac and incision of chorion and amnion.* After inspection of the uterine cavity, the gestational sac is localized. The chorion

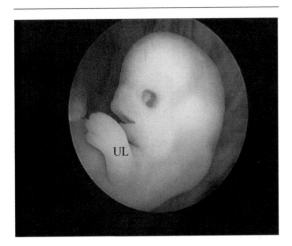

Figure 5.2 Embryoscopic lateral view of the upper portion of a triploid embryo (69,XXY) 18 mm in length. The upper limb (UL) shows characteristics of the 7th week of development. The digital rays of the hands are notched. The elbow region is appearing. The microcephalic embryo shows a poorly developed cranium. The frontal area has lost the usual bulge expected in embryos of this size.

Therefore, the investigator must develop the ability to evaluate the developmental age of embryos accurately, as the diagnosis of an embryonic defect is dependent on precise staging.[8,9] The term 'gestational age', which is used in clinical and ultrasound terminology, should not used for studying missed abortions, as most of these specimens are usually retained in utero after embryonic demise. The actual developmental age (DA) is derived from the crown–rump length (CRL), measured by ultrasonography, and from the developmental stage assessed by embryoscopy.[8]

4. *Tissue sampling.* In couples with recurrent miscarriage, and in cases of phenotypically abnormal embryos (see 'Etiology of developmental defects in early missed abortions', below), accurate cytogenetic analysis of pregnancy tissue is essential.[10,11] The value of karyotyping early abortion specimens is limited by frequent false-negative results, caused by maternal tissue contamination. The finding of a 46,XX karyotype in the curettage material is not

always a reliable result.[12] Transcervical embryoscopy allows selective and reliable sampling of chorionic tissues with minimal potential for maternal contamination.[13] Direct chorion biopsies can be taken embryoscopically at the end of the morphological examination[13,14] (Figure 5.3). In our service, direct chorionic villus sampling (CVS) is performed under direct vision, through the hysteroscope using a microforceps (CH 7–2 mm). At the end of the procedure, chorionic villi are placed in normal saline and carefully dissected. The chorionic villi are then placed in culture medium and immediately forwarded to the cytogenetic laboratory for further processing. In our service, the tissue is subsequently cultured and analyzed cytogenetically, using standard G-banding cytogenetic techniques. Figure 5.4 shows the distribution of chromosome anomalies in our series of 359 specimens with an abnormal karyotype.

5. *Instrumental evacuation of the uterus.* At the end of the procedure, instrumental evacuation of the uterus is performed.

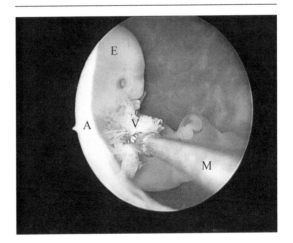

Figure 5.3 Direct chorionic villus sampling is performed under visual monitoring using a microforceps (M). Note the chorionic villi (V) at the tip of the microforceps. 'A' marks the remnants of the amnion. A microcephalic 45,XO embryo (E) with a crown–rump length of 28 mm is visible in the background of the picture.

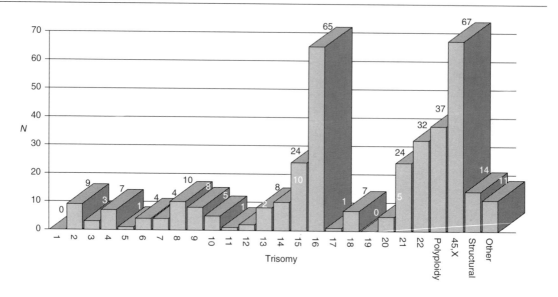

Figure 5.4 Frequency of trisomy for each chromosome, polyploidy, monosomy X, and structural chromosome anomalies among 359 specimens with an abnormal karyotype.

COMMON MORPHOLOGICAL DEFECTS IN EARLY ABORTION SPECIMENS DIAGNOSED EMBRYOSCOPICALLY

This section provides an overview of developmental defects that we have been able to diagnose using this technique of transcervical embryoscopy. Abnormal embryonic development can be local or general. General embryonic maldevelopment is known as 'embryonic growth disorganization'. There are four grades, which are based on the degree of abnormal embryonic development.[15] An empty or anembryonic sac is known as grade 1 (GD1). The amnion, if present, is usually closely adherent to the chorion (fusion of the amnion to the chorion is abnormal prior to 10 weeks of gestation). GD2 conceptuses show embryonic tissue of 3–5 mm in size, but with no recognizable external embryonic landmarks and no retinal pigment. It is not possible to differentiate caudal and cephalic poles (Figure 5.5). The embryo is often directly attached to the chorionic plate. GD3 embryos are up to 10 mm long. They lack limb buds, but retinal pigment is often present. A cephalic and a

caudal pole can be differentiated. GD4 embryos have a CRL > 10 mm, with a discernible head, trunk, and limb buds. The limb buds show marked retardation in development and the development of the facial structures is highly abnormal.

In our experience, growth-disorganized embryos show a high frequency (92%) of autosomal trisomies, trisomy 16 being the most common, accounting for 46% of abnormal karyotypes.[16]

LOCALIZED DEFECTS

Localized defects may be isolated or combined. Morphologically they are similar to developmental defects seen in fetuses. Malformations that have external manifestation and that we have been able to diagnose embryoscopically include the following.

HEAD DEFECTS

Microcephaly, anencephaly, encephalocele, facial dysplasia, cleft lip, cleft palate, fusions of the face to

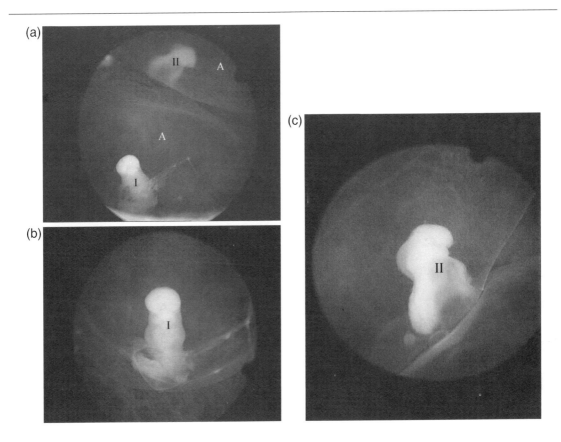

Figure 5.5 Endovaginal sonographic and embryoscopic examination (a) shows a monochorionic diamniotic twin pregnancy with two intact amniotic sacs (A). The crown–rump lengths of the embryos (without cardiac activity) were 4 and 3 mm. Close-ups of twin I (b) and twin II (c) showed two growth-disorganized embryos (GD2) with no recognizable external embryonic landmarks and no retinal pigment after the amnion (A) was opened. Trisomy 16 (47,XY,+16) was diagnosed in this case.

the chest, absence of eyes, unfused eye globes, and proboscis are some of the defects that we have seen.

Microcephalic embryos may be seen on embryoscopy with a poorly developed cranium with loss of normal vascular markings. In particular, the usual bulge of the frontal area, which is expected in embryos of this size, is absent (Figure 5.2). Embryos with a *dysplastic face* show poorly developed branchial arches and midface structures on embryoscopic examination. Microcephaly and facial dysplasia are usually observed in combination. Chromosomal anomalies are the most common cause of these developmental defects. *Encephaloceles* present as a bulge in the cranium, often

covered by adherent discolored skin on embryoscopy. Embryoscopy has identified encephaloceles in the frontal and parietal regions of the embryonic head, unlike the situation in the fetus, where the defect usually occurs in the occipital area. Encephaloceles may range from small defects to large ones involving most of the cranium.[11,17]

In *anencephalic embryos*, the brain tissue may still be present, and this condition is called *exencephaly* (Figure 5.1b). The developing cerebral structures subsequently undergo varying degrees of destruction, leaving a mass of vascular structures and degenerated neural tissue. *Neural tube defects* (anencephaly, encephalocele, and spina bifida) can be multifactorial in origin, caused by a lethal gene defect or non-genetic mechanisms such as amniotic bands. Chromosomal anomalies are the most common cause of embryonic neural tube defects.[11,17,18–20] The most common associations with chromosomal abnormalities are triploidy with spina bifida,[21] and 45,XO and trisomies 9 and 14 with encephalocele.[22]

Lateral and median cleft lip can be distinguished embryoscopically. Lateral clefts may be unilateral or bilateral. Cleft lip occurs when the maxillary prominence and the united medial nasal prominences fail to fuse. The midline cleft lip represents a fusion defect of the median nasal swellings (Figure 5.6). In the embryo, cleft lip cannot be diagnosed until after 7 weeks of development, since fusion does not occur until that time. Cleft lip may be part of a malformation syndrome. Irregular clefting may be caused by amniotic bands. In embryos, clefting defects occur commonly with chromosomal aberrations, especially trisomy 13. *Cleft palate* occurs if the primary anterior palate, lateral palatine processes, and nasal septum fail to unite. Cleft palate can only be diagnosed in the fetal period, since fusion is completed after the 10th week of development.

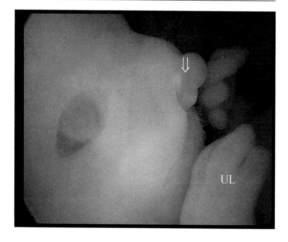

Figure 5.6 Close-up of the face of an embryo with a crown–rump length of 27 mm. A median cleft lip (arrow) is present. 'UL' marks the right upper limb. Trisomy 9 (47,XY,+9) was diagnosed.

TRUNK DEFECTS

Trunk defects include spina bifida, omphalocele, and gastroschisis. The phenotype of *spina bifida* is different in the early developmental stages than the well-known appearance in the fetus or neonate. In the embryo, spina bifida is frequently observed as a plaque-like protrusion of neural tissue over the caudal spine.[23] It is not clear whether the spina bifida seen in the embryo is due to a different cause to that seen in the fetus, or whether it is merely a precursor to the lesion observed in the fetus. *Myeloceles* vary in size and location. The most common site in the embryo is the lumbar and sacral regions. Chromosomal aberrations are the most common cause of embryonic myeloceles.

Physiological midgut herniation is a macroscopically visible process which starts in the 6th week after fertilization. The midgut only fully returns to the abdominal cavity at the end of the 10th week of development. Herniation is still physiological at 8 weeks of development; hence *omphalocele* can only be diagnosed in the fetal period. *Gastroschisis* differs from the physiological herniation of the midgut, as the umbilical cord is not involved and no sac is present. Gastroschisis is rarely observed in the embryo, and occurs when the bowel protrudes from a defect that is generally located to the right side of the umbilicus. The pathogenesis of this defect is controversial, with a variety of different theories having been proposed.[24–26] The theory of abdominal wall disruption as a result of an 'in utero' vascular accident has gained most acceptance. Thus, gastroschisis is considered to be a sporadic event with a negligible risk of recurrence. Since the defect is usually not associated with chromosome aberrations, it is rarely observed in early spontaneous abortions.

LIMB DEFECTS

Polydactyly, syndactyly, split-hand/split-foot malformation, and transverse limb reduction defects are the most commonly observed malformations.

Polydactyly is one of the most common limb abnormalities found in the embryo. It may be on the radial (preaxial) or ulnar (postaxial) side of the limb. Polydactyly may occur as an isolated malformation

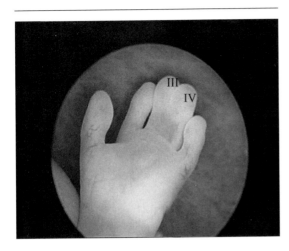

Figure 5.7 An early fetus, of 60 mm crown–rump length, is shown with syndactyly of digits III and IV. The karyotype showed triploidy (69,XXX).

or may be part of a malformation syndrome. Postaxial polydactyly is common in trisomy 13.[27] In *syndactyly*, two or more of the fingers or toes are joined together. At the end of the 8th week of development fingers become free and syndactyly can be diagnosed embryoscopically (Figure 5.7). Syndactyly may be part of a malformation syndrome. Syndactyly of digits III and IV is common in triploidy.[27,28]

The *split-hand/split-foot malformation* involves ectrodactyly. The hand is divided into two parts, which are opposed like a lobster claw. In the second anatomical type, the radial rays are absent, with only the fifth digit remaining.[29] Split hand can be a part of numerous syndromes. In embryos with split-hand malformation, trisomy 15 can often be found. In the *transverse limb reduction defect*, distal structures of the limb are absent, with proximal parts being more or less normal. These limb defects are regarded as a disruption sequence that is presumed to be a result of peripheral ischemia.[30] The recurrence risk in future pregnancies is minimal.[27]

UMBILICAL CORD DEFECTS

The following complications may affect the umbilical cord: knots, torsion, stricture, cysts, and abnormal thin and/or short cords. The mechanical lesions of the cord (*knots, torsion,* and *stricture*) are rarely observed embryoscopically. *Torsion of the umbilical cord* can often be found in macerated specimens, but is usually a postmortem artifact. *Umbilical cord cysts* and *abnormal thin* and/or *short cords* are usually found in chromosomally abnormal embryos.

DUPLICATION ANOMALIES

Chorangiopagus parasiticus (CAPP), or *acardiac conjoined twins*, and other conjoined twins have been observed. The most severe defect in the *acardiac conceptus* is usually seen at the cranial pole. The parasitic twin is usually seen as a markedly edematous mass. The upper portion of the conceptus has missing or highly abnormal facial structures. Usually, only remnants of the upper extremities, are present, but the lower limbs are often well developed. The 'pump' twin is also usually developmentally abnormal.[31,32] The circulation is through the normal pump twin by a return reversed flow from artery directly to artery, or vein to vein, via anastomoses of the cord, or via chorionic surface vessels. The observed anomalies of the parasitic twin are presumed to be caused by a combination of a primary developmental defects and decreased oxygenation of the recipient twin, with disruption of organogenesis.

Conjoined twinning is the result of late and incomplete twin formation at the latest possible moment when the embryonic axis is being laid down (between 13 and 15 days postconception). Most classifications are descriptive and based on the anatomical zones of coalescence. Fusion of the thorax (thoracopagus) is most commonly (70%) reported.

The importance of identifying these rare duplication anomalies cannot be overemphasized; parents can be reassured that the anomalies are accidental sequela of twinning, with no additional risk of recurrence in future pregnancies.[28]

AMNION RUPTURE SEQUENCE

The pathogenesis of amniotic bands is still being debated. There are numerous theories.[33] The theory of early amnion rupture, as proposed by Torpin,[34] has gained most acceptance. Amniotic rupture leads to subsequent amniotic band formation, which interferes with normal embryonic development by causing malformations or disruptions. This sequence of events is known as the amnion rupture sequence (ARS).[35] Although this sequence is uncommon in liveborn infants, its frequency may be as high as 1 in 56 in previable fetuses. Bands that constrict the umbilical cord are recognized as the main cause of death in this sequence.[36] ARS may cause abnormalities that are detectable by embryoscopy, such as encephaloceles, cleft lip, and amputations. When aberrant sheet or bands of tissue are seen on embryoscopy, which are attached to the conceptus with characteristic deformities in a non-embryological distribution, a diagnosis of amniotic band syndrome or ARS can be made.[37] Amniotic bands can occur as a result of abdominal trauma,[38] CVS,[39] and connective tissue abnormalities.[40] However, in most cases of ARS, no such cause can be identified. Therefore, most authors consider ARS to be a sporadic event with a negligible risk of recurrence.

ETIOLOGY OF DEVELOPMENTAL DEFECTS IN EARLY MISSED ABORTIONS

Table 5.2 provides a general description of 514 cases studied by transcervical embryoscopy. The correlations between the morphology and specific cytogenetic findings are shown in Table 5.3. It can be seen from Table 5.2 that no external abnormalities were found in 58 cases (11.3%), whereas abnormal development was seen in 456 (88.7%) cases of missed abortion. Among the abnormal cases, embryonic growth disorganization (GD1–4) was seen in 237 (46.1%) cases. One hundred and ninety-eight cases (38.5%) showed no disorganization of development, but had severe combined localized defects. There were isolated localized developmental defects in 21 specimens. Cytogenetic evaluation was successfully performed in 495 (96.3%) of the 514 cases. Three hundred and fifty-nine (73%) specimens were abnormal, of which 230 (64.1%) were trisomic, 67 (18.7%) showed monosomy X, 37 (10.3%) were polyploid, and 14 (3.9%) were structural chromosomal anomalies. Trisomies were observed for all chromosomes except chromosomes 1 and 19 (Figure 5.4). The highest incidence of chromosomal anomalies was found in the 198 conceptuses with combined developmental defects. In this subgroup, cytogenetic evaluation was successful in 193 cases (97.3%). Chromosomal abnormalities were found in 166 cases (86%; Table 5.2). Of the 237 grossly disorganized embryos, 225 (95%) were analyzed cytogenetically. Of these, 156 (69.3%) were cytogenetically abnormal. The lowest incidence of chromosomal abnormalies was found in phenotypically normal specimens and in specimens with isolated

Table 5.2 Specimen morphology and karyotype of 514 missed abortions

Morphology	Total specimens		Total specimens successfully karyotyped		Specimens with abnormal karyoytype	
	No.	%[a]	No.	%[b]	No.	%[c]
Normal	58	11.3	56	96.2	23	41.1
Growth disorganization	237	46.1	225	95	156	69.3
Combined defects	198	38.5	193	97.3	166	86.0
Isolated defects	21	4.1	21	100	14	66.7
Total	514	100	495	96.3	359	72.5

[a]Percentage of total number of specimens with that morphology.
[b]Percentage of each morphological category successfully karyotyped.
[c]Percentage of each morphological category with an abnormal karyotype.

Table 5.3 Summary of cytogenetic findings

Karyotype	No. of external embryonic abnormalities	Growth disorganization	Combined developmental defects	Isolated
46,XY/46,XX	33	69	27	7
Trisomy 2		9		
Trisomy 3		3		
Trisomy 4		3	4	
Trisomy 5			1	
Trisomy 6		4		
Trisomy 7		2	1	1
Trisomy 8		8	2	
Trisomy 9			8	
Trisomy 10		5		
Trisomy 11		1		
Trisomy 12		2		
Trisomy 13	1		6	1
Trisomy 14		1	9	
Trisomy 15		3	21	
Trisomy 16		65		
Trisomy 17		1		
Trisomy 18	1	3	3	
Trisomy 20	1	4		
Trisomy 21	16	1	7	
Trisomy 22		18	14	
Triploidy	2	3	19	4
Tetraploidy		6	3	
45,X		1	58	8
Structural defect	2	3	9	
Other		10	1	
No cytogenetic results availabale	2	12	5	
Total	58	237	198	21

This series comprises 58 embryos with normal external features, 237 growth-disorganized embryos, 198 embryos with combined localized developmental defects, and 121 embryos with isolated localized developmental defects.

defects (Table 5.2). Of 58 cases with normal external features, 56 could be analyzed cytogenetically, with 23 cases (41.1%) showing cytogenetically abnormal results. Of 21 specimens with isolated defects, 14(66.7%) showed chromosomal abnormalities.

In summary, aneuploidy/polyploidy is the major factor affecting normal embryonic development in early intrauterine deaths, and may explain why spontaneous abortion is usually a sporadic event in a patient's reproductive history although the incidence of developmental defects is high. Most (95%) of the observed chromosomal mutations are not hereditary and carry no increased risk for future pregnancies. They originate 'de novo' either in gametogenesis (trisomy and monosomy) or from polyspermic fertilization or failure of normal cleavage (triploidy and tetraploidy). Therefore, all embryoscopic findings should be supplemented by the results of cytogenetic analysis to distinguish between non-chromosomal and chromosomal causes of anomalies. Aneuploidy/polyploidy provides a causal explanation for these developmental defects in cases of phenotypically abnormal embryos, and also indicates that the recurrence risk for the observed developmental defect and chromosomal abnormality in these couples is not increased.[41]

CLINICAL SIGNIFICANCE AND IMPLICATIONS OF DETAILED MORPHOLOGICAL AND CYTOGENETIC EVALUATION OF EARLY SPONTANEOUS ABORTION

A detailed embryoscopic examination of the dead embryo is likely to be useful in couples who have experienced recurrent abortion or have reproductive loss after in vitro fertilization (IVF).[14] Table 5.4 provides a general description of embryoscopic and cytogenetic findings of 53 patients with recurrent miscarriages (three or more consecutive miscarriages). Of these cases, 32 of 50 (64%) had an abnormal embryonic karyotype. Fourteen embryos had a morphological defect with a normal karyotype, while no embryonic or chromosomal abnormality could be diagnosed in four cases. The Royal College of Obstetricians and Gynaecologists[42] recommends fetal karyotyping in the investigation of recurrent miscarriage. The value of karyotyping early abortion specimens is limited by frequent false-negative results caused by maternal contamination. A 46,XX karyotype in the curettage material is therefore not a reliable result.[12] In missed abortions, transcervical embryoscopy allows selective and reliable sampling of chorionic tissue with minimal maternal contamination.[13] In addition, uterine malformations can be diagnosed at the same time. Isolated or combined localized developmental defects with an apparently normal karyotype might be heterogeneous or multifactorial in origin, and may be caused be a single gene defect or non-genetic mechanisms such as amniotic bands, duplication anomalies, vascular disruptions, etc. An accurate description of these specimens is essential, as it helps identify the specific mechanism leading to the defect. This information would be completely lost if morphological examination of the demised embryo had not been carried out and the particular developmental defects remained undetected.

The recurrence rate of these defects differs according to the etiology. If the observed defects are multifactorial in origin, then the risk of recurrence is approximately 2–5%. The recurrence rate may be much higher for autosomal dominant or recessive genes, or not significantly increased if non-genetic mechanisms (amniotic bands, duplication anomalies, or vascular disruptions) are responsible for abnormal embryonic development. Multiple localized developmental defects without a chromosomal anomaly are rare, and may indicate a single-gene defect.[28] In these cases, a high recurrence rate cannot be excluded. Diagnosis of a specific syndrome is usually not possible at these early stages.

Expert first-trimester ultrasonographic examination has become standard management for women at increased risk of hereditary conditions. An accurate description of specific developmental defects by embryoscopy complements and aids early prenatal ultrasonographic examination in excluding a recurrence in subsequent pregnancies reaching the second trimester.

Table 5.4 Morphology and karyotype in 53 patients with recurrent miscarriage

Morphology	Total specimens		Total specimens successfully karyotyped		Specimens with abnormal karyotype	
	No.	%[a]	No.	%[b]	No.	%[c]
Normal	8	15.1	7	87.5	3	42.9
Growth disorganization	26	49.1	24	92.3	15	62.5
Combined defects	18	34	18	100	13	72.2
Isolated defects	1	1.9	1	100	1	100
Total	53	100	50	94.3	32	64

[a]Percentage of embryos with the specific morphology.
[b]Percentage of each morphological category successfully karyotyped.
[c]Percentage of each morphological category with an abnormal karyotype.

If single-gene defects exist in chromosomally normal abortions with multiple localized developmental defects, this would explain why a normal karyotype is usually interpreted as a poor prognostic sign in early-abortion specimens.[43,44] The embryoscopic diagnosis of embryonic growth disorganization is less informative. Chromosomal abnormalities can be found in 70% of cases, with autosomal trisomies forming 92% of the 70%.[16] Most of the chromosomal abnormalities found in growth-disorganized embryos are non-viable (Table 5.3), and their presence explains the minimal embryonic development observed embryoscopically. Embryonic growth disorganization and a normal karyotype, which has a similar embryoscopic appearance to growth disorganization resulting from an aneuploidy/polyploidy, suggests that some cases of growth disorganization may be genetic in origin, but undetectable by current cytogenetic techniques. Routine cytogenetic analysis of the abortus is hampered by contamination of the culture with maternal tissues and by the limits of chromosome resolution. Submicroscopic chromosomal rearrangements have only recently been considered to be etiologically related to pregnancy loss.[45,46] The presence of submicroscopic chromosomal rearrangements challenges the prevailing assumption that if no routine laboratory test confirms the presence of a genetic disorder, then non-genetic causes should be sought. The advent of whole-genome screening technologies has introduced new opportunities for screening chromosomally normal pregnancy losses with developmental defects for previously undetectable submicroscopic chromosomal abnormalities. Embryoscopy identifies subtle morphological abnormalities undetectable by ultrasound, and may identify a highly characterized cohort of abortion specimens with apparently normal chromosomes as a starting point for further detailed genetic studies. Such studies are required in order to reach a better understanding of embryopathogenesis, and consequently of early and recurrent pregnancy loss.

ACKNOWLEDGMENT

I am grateful to a wonderful embryopathologist and teacher, who introduced me to embryopathology, Prof. Dr DK Kalousek.

REFERENCES

1. Salat-Baroux J. Recurrent spontaneous abortions. Reprod Nutr Dev 1988; 28:1555–68.
2. Kalousek DK, PantzarT, Tsai M, et al. Early spontaneous abortion: morphologic and karyotypic findings in 3912 cases. Birth Defects 1993; 29:53–61.
3. Warburton D, Byrne J, Canki N. Chromosome Anomalies and Prenatal Development: An Atlas. New York. Oxford University Press, 1991.
4. Kalousek DK. Anatomical and chromosomal abnormalities in specimens of early spontaneous abortions: seven years experience. Birth Defects 1987; 23:153–68.
5. Philipp T, Kalousek DK. Transcervical embryoscopy in missed abortion. J Assist Reprod Genet 2001; 18:285–90.
6. Philipp T, Philipp K, Reiner A, Beer F, Kalousek DK. Embryoscopic and cytogenetic analysis of 233 missed abortions: factors involved in the pathogenesis of developmental defects of early failed pregnancies. Hum Reprod 2003; 18:1724–32.
7. Shiota K. Development and intrauterine fate of normal and abnormal human conceptuses. Cong Anom 1991; 31:67–80.
8. Moore KL. The Developing Human – Clinically Orientated Embryology, 5th edn. Philadelphia: WB Saunders Co., 1993.
9. Philipp T. Atlas der Embryologie. Embryoskopische Aufnahmen der normalen und abnormen Embryonalentwicklung. Vienna: Facultas Verlag, 2004.
10. Wolf GC, Horger EO. Indication for examination of spontaneous abortion specimens: a reassessment. Am J Obstet Gynecol 1995; 5:1364–7.
11. Philipp T, Kalousek DK. Neural tube defects in missed abortions – embryoscopic and cytogenetic findings. Am J Med Genet 2002; 107:52–7.
12. Bell KA, Van Deerlin PG, Haddad BR, et al. Cytogenetic diagnosis of 'normal 46,XX' karyotypes in spontaneous abortions frequently may be misleading. Fertil Steril 1999; 71:334–41.
13. Ferro J, Martinez MC, Lara C, et al. Improved accuracy of hysteroembryoscopic biopsies for karyotyping early missed abortions. Fertil Steril 2003; 80:1260–4.
14. Philipp T, Feichtinger W, Van Allen M, et al. Abnormal embryonic development diagnosed embryoscopically in early intrauterine deaths after in vitro fertilization (IVF): a preliminary report of 23 cases. Fertil Steril 2004; 82:1337–42.
15. Poland BJ, Miller JR, Harris M, et al. Spontaneous abortion: a study of 1961 women and their conceptuses. Acta Obstet Gynecol Scand 1981; 102(Suppl):5–32.
16. Philipp T, Kalousek DK. Generalized abnormal embryonic development in missed abortion: embryoscopic and cytogenetic findings. Am J Med Genet 2002; 111:41–7.
17. Mc Fadden DE, Kalousek DK. Survey of neural tube defects in spontaneously aborted embryos. Am J Med Genet 1989; 32:356–8.
18. Bell JE, Gosden CM. Central nervous system abnormalities – contrasting patterns in early and late pregnancy. Clin Genet 1978; 13:387–96.
19. Coerdt W, Miller K, Holzgreve W, et al. Neural tube defects in chromosomally normal and abnormal human embryos. Ultrasound Obstet Gynecol 1997; 10:410–15.
20. Creasy MR, Alberman ED. Congenital malformations of the central nervous system in spontaneous abortions. J Med Genet 1976; 13:9–16.
21. Philipp T, Grillenberger K, Separovic ER, Philipp K, Kalousek DK. Effects of triploidy on early human development. Prenat Diagn 2004; 242:276–81.

22. Canki N, Warburton D, Byrne J. Morphological characteristics of monosomy X in spontaneous abortions. Ann Genet 1988; 31:4–13.

23. Patten BM. Overgrowth of the neural tube in young human embryos. Anat Rec 1952; 113:381–93.

24. Shaw A. The myth of gastroschisis. J Pediatr Surg 1975; 10:235–44.

25. De Vries PA. The pathogenesis of gastroschisis and omphalocele. J Pediatr Surg 1980; 15:245–51.

26. Hoyme H, Higginbottom MC, Jones KL. The vascular pathogenesis of gastrochisis: intrauterine interruption of the omphalomesenteric artery. J Pediatr 1981; 98:228–3l.

27. Ramsing M, Duda V, Mehrain Y, et al. Hand malformations in the aborted embryo: An informative source of genetic information. Birth Defects 1996; 30:79–94.

28. Dimmick JE, Kalousek DK. Developmental Pathology of the Embryo and Fetus. Philadelphia: JB Lippincott, 1992.

29. Birch-Jensen A. Congenital Deformities of Upper Extremities. Copenhagen: Munksgaard, 1949.

30. Golden CM, Ryan LM, Holmes LB. Chorionic villus sampling: a distinctive teratogenic effect on fingers. Birth Defects Res 2003; 67:557–62.

31. Philipp T, Separovic ER, Philipp K, et al. Trancervical fetoscopic diagnosis of structural defects in four first trimester monochorionic twin intrauterine deaths. Prenat Diagn 2003 ; 12:964–9.

32. Napolitani FD, Schreiber I. The acardiac monster. A review of the world literature and presentation of two cases. Am J Obstet Gynecol 1960; 82:708–11.

33. Evans MI. Amniotic bands. Ultrasound Obstet Gynecol 1997; 10:307–8.

34. Torpin R. Amniochorionic mesoblastic fibrous strings and amniotic bands. Associated constricting fetal anomalies or fetal death. Am J Obstet Gynecol 1965; 91:65–75.

35. Kalousek DK, Bamforth S. Amnion rupture sequence in previable fetuses. Am J Med Genet 1988; 3:63–73.

36. Hong CY, Simon MA. Amniotic bands knotted about umbilical cord. A rare cause of fetal death. Obstet Gynecol 1963; 222:667–70.

37. Philipp T, Kalousek DK. Amnion rupture sequence in a first trimester missed abortion. Prenat Diagn 2001; 21:835–8.

38. Ossipoff V, Hall BD. Etiologic factors in the amniotic band syndrome. A study of 24 patients. Birth Defects 1977; 13:117–32.

39. Firth HV, Boyd PA, Chamberlain P, et al. Severe limb abnormalities after chorion villus sampling at 56–66 days gestation. Lancet 1991; 337:762–3.

40. Young ID, Lindenbaum RH, Thompsen EM, Pemburg ME. Amniotic bands in connective tissue disorders. Arch Dis Child 1985; 60:1061–3.

41. Warburton D, Kline J, Stein Z, et al. Does the karyotype of a spontaneous abortion predict the karyotype of a subsequent abortion? Evidence from 273 women with two karyotyped spontaneous abortions. Am J Hum Genet 1987; 41:465–83.

42. Royal College of Obstetricians and Gynaecologists, Guideline No. 17. The Management of Recurrent Miscarriage. London: RCOG, 2003.

43. Osagawara M, Aoki K, Okada S, et al. Embryonic karyotype of abortuses in relation to the number of previous miscarriages. Fertil Steril 2000; 73:300–4.

44. Stephenson M, Awartani KA, Robinson WP. Cytogenetic analysis of miscarriages from couples with recurrent miscarriage: a case control study. Hum Reprod 2002; 17:446–51.

45. Schaeffer AJ, Chung J, Heretis K, et al. Comparative genomic hybridization-array analysis enhances the detection of aneuploidies and submicroscopic imbalances in spontaneous miscarriages. Am J Med Genet 2004; 6:1168–74.

46. Le Caignec C, Boceno M, Saugier-Veber P, et al. Detection of genomic imbalances by array based comparative genomic hybridisation in fetuses with multiple malformations. J Med Genet 2005; 2:121–8.

6. Endocrinology of pregnancy loss

Stefano Luisi, Lucia Lazzeri, and Andrea Riccardo Genazzani

INTRODUCTION

Following implantation, the maintenance of pregnancy is dependent on a multitude of endocrinological events that will eventually aid in the successful growth and development of the fetus. Although the great majority of pregnant women have no preexisting endocrine abnormalities, a small number can have certain endocrine alterations that could potentially lead to recurrent pregnancy losses.

It is estimated that approximately 8–12% of all pregnancy losses are the result of endocrine factors. During the preimplantation period, the uterus undergoes important developmental changes stimulated by estrogen and, more importantly, progesterone. Progesterone is essential for successful implantation and maintenance of pregnancy. Therefore, disorders related to inadequate progesterone secretion by the corpus luteum are likely to affect the outcome of the pregnancy. Luteal phase deficiency (LPD), hyperprolactinemia, and polycystic ovary syndrome (PCOS) are some examples. Several other endocrinological abnormalities, such as thyroid disease, hypoparathyroidism, uncontrolled diabetes, and decreased ovarian reserve, have been implicated as etiologic factors for recurrent pregnancy loss. Inhibins and activins are nonsteroidal glycoproteins thought to have important roles in reproductive physiology, and have been proposed as markers of fetal viability.

LUTEAL PHASE DEFICIENCY AND PREGNANCY LOSS

Progesterone secreted by the corpus luteum plays a paramount role in the maintenance of early pregnancy. Immediately after implantation, under the influence of human chorionic gonadotropin (hCG)

secreted by the trophoblast, the corpus luteum receives a signal to continue producing 17α-progesterone along with estradiol, estrone, and relaxin. Relaxin is a member of the insulin-like growth factor family, and its increase parallels that of hCG, suggesting a synergistic effect with progesterone in maintaining myometrial quiescence.[1,2]

The corpus luteum maintains its capacity to synthesize progesterone almost throughout pregnancy, but at approximately 7 weeks of gestation, its functional ability decreases markedly, at the start of the luteoplacental transition. Excission of the corpus luteum before the 8th week of gestation results in abortion, whereas after the 9th week it does not.[3]

Abnormalities of the luteal phase have been reported to occur in up to 35% of women with recurrent pregnancy loss (RPL).[4] There are several causes for LPD, including stress, exercise, weight loss, hyperprolactinemia, and menstrual cycles at the onset of puberty or perimenopause. The mechanisms by which LPD occurs are unclear, but could be associated with decreased progesterone production by the corpus luteum, decreased follicle-stimulating hormone (FSH) levels in the follicular phase, abnormal pattern of luteinizing hormone (LH) secretion, and a decreased response to progesterone by the endometrium. Many studies suggest that LPD originates as a preovulatory event. LPD may be secondary to abnormal follicle formation, associated with poor oocyte quality.[5,6]

The methods used to diagnose LPD are controversial and not universally accepted. For the diagnosis of LPD, both serum progesterone and the use of endometrial biopsy are advocated.[7,8] Serum progesterone levels greater than 10 ng/ml in the midluteal phase are rarely associated with an abnormal luteal phase when a targeted endometrial biopsy is performed.[9,10] The endometrium is considered to be out of phase when the histological dating lags behind the menstrual dating by 2 days or more; as determined from the subsequent day of menses, the diagnosis requires endometrial biopsies in a minimum of two cycles. Endometrial biopsy, with evaluation of the morphological changes, has been considered superior to serum progesterone determinations because of the pulsatile nature of progesterone secretion. More importantly, the morphological changes in the endometrium better represent the cumulative effect of cycle-specific patterns of corpus luteum function.[11] Despite the above-mentioned rationale, there is considerable inter- and intraobserver variation in the interpretation of the endometrial biopsies.

Epidemiological studies of RPL appear to support the concept that LPD is in fact an etiological factor. This is documented by studies demonstrating that hormone treatment to enhance progesterone production or supplementation is associated with an increased chance of a term pregnancy in women with RPL.[12]

The treatment of LPD may include the use of ovulation-induction agents such as clomiphene citrate, alone or in combination with gonadotropins. These agents enhance progesterone secretion by creating more than one follicle, resulting in multiple sites for progesterone production; 5000 or 10 000 units of hCG injected at the time of expected ovulation have also been used. Progesterone supplementation after ovulation, with or without the use of ovulation-induction agents, can also be used 2–3 days after the basal body temperature increases (or after a positive urinary LH test) and continued up to 7–11 weeks of gestation.[13]

Progesterone supplementation can be administered by intravaginal suppositories (25–100 mg twice daily), by intramuscular injection of progesterone in oil (50 mg daily), or as oral micronized progesterone (100 mg two or three times daily). Bromocriptine or cabergoline are recommended to treat luteal phase deficiency associated with hyperprolactinemia.[14] The subject of LPD and its association with RPL continues to be controversial. A meta-analysis of randomized trials of pregnancies treated with progestational agents failed to find any

evidence for a positive effect on the maintenance of pregnancy.[15]

HYPERPROLACTINEMIA AND PREGNANCY LOSS

The role of prolactin (PRL) in human ovarian steroidogenesis remains unclear. PRL may participate in the regulation of ovarian steroidogenesis; but, in pathological states with high PRL levels, it may interfere with corpus luteum function. In vitro studies have revealed that progesterone secretion by cultured granulosa cells obtained from human ovarian follicles is almost completely inhibited by high PRL concentrations (100 ng/ml), but not by lower concentrations (10–20 ng/ml).[16] These observations suggest the possibility that high PRL concentrations in the early phase of follicular growth may inhibit progesterone secretion, resulting in luteal phase defects. The precise cellular mechanism of PRL action in the human ovary remains to be elucidated; furthermore, a recent study of 64 hyperprolactinemic women with RPL treated with bromocriptine was associated with a higher rate of successful pregnancy, and PRL levels were significantly higher in women who miscarried.[17]

In conclusion, normal PRL levels may play an important role in the growth and maintenance of early pregnancy.

THYROID ABNORMALITIES AND PREGNANCY LOSS

HYPERTHYROIDISM

Excess production of thyroid hormone is not usually correlated with infertility or RPL. Women with subclinical or mild hyperthyroidism have evidence of ovulation when endometrial sampling is performed. Although hyperthyroidism has been associated with poor pregnancy outcomes, including preterm delivery, abruptio placentae, maternal heart failure, fetal growth restriction, and stillbirth,[18,19] it has not been reported commonly as an independent cause of RPL. RPL has been associated with Graves disease in a case report;[20] however, the patient was also diagnosed with antiphospholipid syndrome, which is an independent cause of RPL. However, a recent retrospective study[21] has suggested that excess exogenous thyroid hormone is associated with an elevated rate of fetal loss. This study was performed in a unique population of patients with a genotype (Arg243Gln mutation in the thyroid hormone receptor β gene) showing resistance to thyroid hormone, and a high serum concentration of free thyroxine and triiodothyronine without suppressed thyrotropin. These women maintain a euthyroid state despite high thyroid hormone levels. Patients were analyzed in three different groups: affected mothers ($n = 9$), affected fathers ($n = 9$), and unaffected relatives ($n = 18$). The mean miscarriage rates were 22.9, 2.0, and 4.4%, respectively ($\chi^2 = 8.66$; $p = 0.01$). Affected mothers had an increased rate of miscarriage ($z = 3.10$; $p = 0.002$, by Wilcoxon rank-sum test).[21]

HYPOTHYROIDISM

The causes of thyroid dysfunction include autoimmunity, severe iodine deficiency, postpartum thyroiditis, and drug-induced hypothyroidism as a result of radical treatment of hyperthyroidism. Autoimmune thyroid disease is the most prevalent associated etiology in patients of reproductive age. There seems to be no doubt that hypoactive thyroid hormone is associated with infertility.

Thyroid hormones have an impact on oocytes at the level of the granulosa and luteal cells that interfere with normal ovulation.[22] Low thyroxine levels have a positive feedback on thyrotropin-releasing hormone (TRH). Elevations in TRH have been associated with PRL elevation.[23] It is believed that elevated PRL alters the pulsatility of gonadotropin-releasing hormone (GnRH) and interferes with normal ovulation.

Therefore, severe forms of hypothyroidism rarely complicate pregnancy, because they are associated with anovulation and infertility. However, in mild hypothyroidism, pregnancies can occur, and are associated with higher rates of pregnancy loss and maternal complications.[24] Even if an association

exists between low thyroid function and pregnancy loss, direct evidence for a causal role is missing.[25] One postulated explanation for this relationship is that luteal phase defects have been linked to thyroid hypofunction. Given that the production of progesterone is a pivotal element of a successful pregnancy, it is conceivable that RPL could be related to deficient corpus luteum action. Given the methodological flaws in the diagnosis of luteal phase defects,[26,27] and the lack of evidence to recommend the use of exogenous progesterone supplementation in early gestation,[28] their existence is controversial at best.

We believe that it is prudent to screen for thyroid disease and normalize thyroid function prior to conception when function is found to be abnormal. Even if there is no clear cause–effect relationship between hypothyroidism and RPL, there is some evidence that subclinical hypothyroidism is correlated with poor maternal outcome as well as prematurity and reduced intelligence quotient in the offspring.[24] There is disagreement as to the suitable upper limit of normal serum thyroid-stimulating hormone (TSH) in order to make the diagnosis of subclinical hypothyroidism. There is a trend with the new TSH assays to decrease the upper limit of the normal TSH range (4.5–5.0 mU/l) to 2.5 mU/l. This upper limit is recommended by the National Academy of Clinical Biochemistry guidelines, and is based on the fact that 2.5 mU/l represents more than two standard deviations above the level in meticulously screened euthyroid volunteers.[29] Clearly, this new upper limit will significantly increase the number of patients diagnosed with subclinical hypothyroidism, and its clinical benefit remains questionable.

ANTITHYROID ANTIBODIES

Thyroid peroxidase and thyroglobulin are two key players in the biosynthesis of thyroid hormone. The former is an enzyme involved in the coupling of iodine residues and in the iodination of thyroid residues. The role of thyroglobulin is in the storage and synthesis of thyroid hormones. Both can be involved in auto-antigenicity in thyroid immune disease.[30] Although patients with RPL have a higher prevalence of antithyroid antibodies (ATA: 158 of 700 (22.5%)) when compared with controls (29 of 200 (14.5%)), they are found with equal frequency in patients undergoing artificial reproductive technology (ART: 162 of 688 (19.2%)).[31] In theory, it is feasible that patients with ATA have inferior reproductive outcomes; however, the relationship between RPL and ATA remains speculative. In a prospective cohort study, 134 RPL patients who were positive for ATA and had normal thyroid functions were compared with 710 patients with RPL but negative for ATA. No treatment was offered to either group, and both groups yielded a live birth rate of 58%.[32] The above findings suggest that in the presence of normal thyroid function, ATA have no impact on pregnancy outcome. How can we explain the association between RPL and ATA? One possibility is that positive ATAs coincide with other autoimmune disorders, suggesting an immunoregulatory dysfunction as the underlying etiology of the reproductive losses. Up to 45.5% of patients with active systemic lupus erythematosus have positive ATAs. Another possibility is that ATA are markers of poor ovarian reserve and signal a diminished oocyte cohort. Up to one-third of patients with premature ovarian failure have been reported to be ATA-positive,[33] whereas only 10% of the adult female population carry these antibodies.[34]

Given that reproductive failure cannot be improved significantly by egg donation, another interesting explanation may lie within the endometrium of these patients. Activated T cells in the endometrium of patients with ATA may produce cytokines disrupting implantation. Stewart-Akers et al[35] found a significant increase in the endometrial T-cell population in women with ATA compared with that of controls. The relative abundance of interleukin 4 (IL-4) and IL-10 was decreased in women with ATA compared with controls, whereas interferon-γ (IFN-γ) was increased. Stewart-Akers et al[35] found that the source of cytokine production for IL-4, IL-10, and IFN-γ was endometrial leukocytes. Finally, a teleological explanation proposes that the RPL in women with elevated titers of

ATA is an attempt to minimize the transmission of autoimmune genes to the offspring.[36]

A recent evidence-based review[37] of investigations and treatments of RPL concluded that the association between ATA and RPL is doubtful. This report also found it doubtful that ATA is a cause of RPL.

The above data may suggest that the association between ATA and RPL represents an immune disorder rather than an endocrinological abnormality. Nevertheless, patients with positive ATA and euthyroidism are at an increased risk for hypothyroidism during and after pregnancy. These individuals should have their TSH screened during each trimester of pregnancy and postpartum for thyroiditis.

DIABETES MELLITUS AND PREGNANCY LOSS

Patients with type 1 ('insulin-dependent') diabetes mellitus (DM) with normal or near-normal glycemic control are not at higher risk for RPL. A well-designed prospective cohort study by the National Institute of Child Health and Human Development included 386 women with type 1 DM and 432 women without diabetes before or within 21 days after conception and observed both groups prospectively.[38] The rate of spontaneous abortion was similar in both groups when the mothers had adequate glycemic control. In this same study, the efficacy of strict glycemic control was demonstrated. For the subgroup of patients who had elevated values for glycosylated hemoglobin in the first trimester, each increase of one standard deviation above the normal range was associated with an increase of 3.1% in the rate of pregnancy loss (95% confidence interval (CI), 0.6–5.6). The importance of glycemic control in the period of conception and early pregnancy cannot be overemphasized. There is a direct correlation between the glycosylated hemoglobin (HbA1c) values and the incidence of pregnancy loss and congenital malformations. In a study of 303 pregnant type 1 DM patients, the risk of spontaneous abortion was found to be 12.4% with first-trimester HbA1c ≤ 9.3%, and 37.5% with HbA1c > 14.4% (risk ratio (RR) 3.0;

95% CI 1.3–7.0). The risk for major malformations was 3.0% with HbA1c ≤ 9.3% and 40% with HbAlc > 14.4% (RR 13.2; 95% CI 4.3–40.4).[39] The improvements in pregnancy outcome due to glycemic control have been confirmed by a well-conducted meta-analysis[40] of 14 studies comparing the HbA1c of diabetic pregnant women receiving preconception care compared with diabetic patients without care. The risk of malformations was 2.1% and 6.5%, respectively (RR 0.36; 95% CI 0.22–0.59). The increased rate of RPL in poorly controlled diabetic patients may be due to several pathophysiological processes, such as maternal vascular disease including uteroplacental deficiency and perhaps immunological causes.

In summary, poorly controlled diabetes mellitus is associated with more frequent pregnancy losses, and adequate control will normalize the rate of miscarriages. To prevent most of the pregnancy losses in diabetic patients, it is recommended to have a prepregnancy level of HbAlc ≤ 7.5%.[41] However, in addition to miscarriages, other adverse pregnancy outcomes can be avoided if the glycosylated hemoglobin is less than 6.6%.[42]

POLYCYSTIC OVARY SYNDROME, INSULIN RESISTANCE, AND PREGNANCY LOSS

Patients with PCOS have an increased rate of pregnancy loss (>50%), predominantly during early gestation.[43] The underlying causes of RPL in PCOS patients may involve several contributing and interrelated factors. These include obesity, hyperinsulinemia, hyperandrogenemia, insulin resistance, poor endometrial receptivity, and elevated levels of LH.

One of the working hypotheses for the association between PCOS and pregnancy loss is that PCOS causes hypofibrinolysis modulated by the 4G4G mutation of the plasminogen activator inhibitor 1 gene, as well as elevated levels of its products, plasminogen activator inhibitor activity (PAI-Fx).[44] Furthermore, in uncontrolled trials, PCOS patients given metformin during pregnancy exhibit a reduced rate of early losses[45] and the high

insulinemia and PAI-Fx are reversed to those of normal controls.[46] Others have suggested that the association between PCOS and early pregnancy loss may be due to increased LH, which stimulates a highly androgenic milieu and affects reproductive outcome.[47,48]

There are several studies confirming the findings of LH hypersecretion in RPL.[49] One study found that over 80% of patients with RPL had polycystic ovaries, and that 81% of the PCOS women had elevated LH levels. The relevance of LH hypersecretion in RPL is controversial.[50] Interestingly, extreme suppression of LH has been linked to a high miscarriage rate in ART, but no cause-and-effect relationship has been studied.[51] Moreover, a randomized controlled trial[52] in which 106 patients with RPL, PCOS, and elevated LH were allocated preconception to either receive GnRH to suppress LH, or allowed to conceive naturally, failed to show any advantage in the treatment arm in terms of either pregnancy rates or miscarriage rates.

Hyperinsulinemia and insulin resistance have been claimed to be a potential cause of the high rate of RPL in patients with PCOS and have been linked to many of the metabolic and endocrine abnormalities potentially associated with the physiopathology of RPL. The prevalence of insulin resistance, as diagnosed by fasting insulin and glucose measurements using glucose-to-insulin ratios and HOMA (homeostasis model assessment) scores, has been found approximately three times higher in an unselected population of women with RPL when compared with an age-, race-, and body mass index-matched group of controls.[53] Metformin bas been the main treatment advocated to reduce RPL in PCOS patients. Although some studies have demonstrated promising results with metformin, it is essential to have a well-randomized controlled trial with appropriate power before metformin can be recommended as effective therapy. Given that metformin is a pregnancy category B drug, and clinical practice is always ahead of evidence-based practice, some investigators consider that the potential benefits of metformin outweigh its risks and advocate its use to reduce miscarriages.[54]

ELEVATED FSH AND PREGNANCY LOSS

The underlying challenge present in certain women with unexplained RPL may reside in the quality and quantity of their oocytes. In a retrospective comparative analysis, Trout and Seifer[55] measured FSH levels on day 3 of the cycle and estradiol (E2) in 36 patients with unexplained RPL and in 21 control RPL patients with a known etiology. These finding were reproduced subsequently in a similar analysis of 58 patients with RPL and unknown etiology.[56] Women with unexplained RPL were found to be more likely to have abnormal ovarian reserve. Among the 36 patients with unexplained RPL, 11 (31%) had elevated FSH, 14 (39%) had elevated E2, and 21 (58%) had abnormal results for one or both tests, In the 20 patients of the control group, the findings were that 1 patient had elevated FSH (5%), 3 (14%) had elevated E2, and 4 (19%) had abnormal results for one or both tests. In a different study, Hofmann et al[57] performed a clomiphene challenge test in 44 patients with RPL and found a similar incidence of diminished ovarian reserve when compared with 648 general infertility patients.

Women with abnormal ovarian reserve testing and unexplained RPL may have a higher incidence of chromosomal abnormalities in their miscarriages. Thus, we believe that it is prudent to incorporate ovarian reserve testing in the workup of patients with RPL. However, we must acknowledge that any assessment of ovarian reserve is not a diagnostic test, but rather a screening tool. An abnormal test does not preclude the possibility of a live birth. Decreased ovarian reserve should not be presented to the patient as an absolute. Extensive counselling is recommended, given that no treatment (other than egg donation) is available.

INHIBINS AND PREGNANCY LOSS

Inhibins are non-steroidal glycoproteins thought to play important roles in reproductive physiology. Inhibin A has a molecular weight of 34 kDa, and comprises an α-subunit linked by a disulfide bond to a highly homologous βA subunit. Inhibin B is a similar dimeric glycoprotein with α and βB subunits. Non-bioactive forms of the α subunit include the amino-terminally extended product named inhibin pro-αC. Inhibin A is the major circulating bioactive inhibin found in early pregnancy. Inhibin B is not detectable in early pregnancy in the human.[58] Although the major function of inhibins is in the negative feedback control of gonadotropin secretion, their function in pregnancy may possibly be the promotion and modulation of placental secretary activity and placental immune modulation.

Circulating levels of inhibin A and pro-αC have been implicated in the process of implantation and early pregnancy development.[59] Inhibins have also been proposed as markers of fetal viability. In the non-pregnant female, inhibins are secreted and synthesized by both the developing graafian follicle and corpus luteum.[60,61] Inhibins are also involved in the control of the fetomaternal communication required to maintain pregnancy. Human placenta, decidua, and fetal membranes are the major sites of production and secretion of inhibins A and B in maternal serum, amniotic fluid, and cord blood.[62]

The corpus luteum has been shown to be the major site of inhibin A production. Production of inhibin A continues within the corpus luteum as pregnancy is established. During early pregnancy, mRNA for inhibins α, βA and βB have been demonstrated in the corpus luteum.[63] However, inhibins are also synthesized and secreted by the developing human placenta. Both α- and βA-subunit mRNAs and proteins[64] have been localized in the human placenta, the major expression being from the syncytiotrophoblast.

The local actions during placental growth and differentiation are mirrored by changes in the circulating levels of dimeric inhibins and inhibin pro-αC as pregnancy progresses.[65] Concentrations of inhibin A in the circulation increase progressively in early pregnancy.[66] There is a transient fall in circulating concentration at approximately 12 weeks of gestation, followed by further increases in concentration from midgestation onwards.[59] Studies demonstrating lower levels of inhibin A in failing pregnancies have implicated inhibin A in the

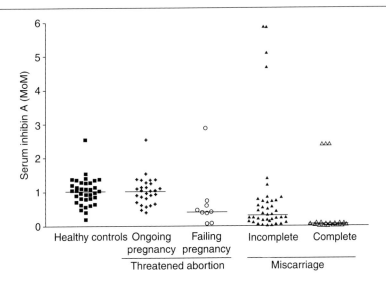

Figure 6.1 Maternal serum inhibin A levels in healthy pregnant women (control), patients with threatened abortion with ongoing and failing pregnancy, and incomplete and complete miscarriage. Individual values are plotted (expressed as mean of mean) and horizontal bars represent the group medians. $*p < 0.05$; $**p < 0.001$; $***p < 0.001$ versus healthy controls and threatened abortion with ongoing pregnancy. MoM is multiples of the median.

processes of successful implantation and early pregnancy development.[67]

Recently, inhibin A concentrations have been measured in the maternal circulation of healthy spontaneously pregnant women progressing to deliver a healthy term singleton baby, in patients with missed abortion (either absence of fetal heart activity or an anembryonic gestational sac) and with complete miscarriage (an empty uterus with a history of passage of products of conception),[62] in order to ascertain whether inhibin A measurement might provide a rapid and useful marker of early pregnancy viability, in comparison with hCG levels. Patients with complete miscarriage had the lowest hCG and inhibin A levels, followed by patients with missed abortion, where the highest levels were seen in ongoing pregnancies (Figure 6.1).

The potential value of inhibin A as a marker of early pregnancy problems should be examined in conjunction with other established biochemical markers such as serum β-hCG, progesterone, and glycodelin. Muttukrishna et al[68] found a statistically significant correlation between serum concentrations of inhibin A and β-hCG (the degree of correlation varied according to the population group: normal controls $r = 0.55$, sporadic miscarriage $r = 0.79$, and recurrent miscarriage $r = 0.66$). In their study, Muttukrishna et al[68] confirmed a statistically significant positive correlation between inhibin A and β-hCG in women who had live births ($r = 0.46$, $p = 0.4$), but not in those who had a miscarriage. Given the small size of this and previous studies, it is not possible at this stage to establish whether serum inhibin A is a better marker than β-hCG, or whether combined inhibin A and β-hCG measurement is superior to β-hCG alone. Further studies are required to address these two questions.[69]

REFERENCES

1. Szlachter N, O'Byrne E, Goldsmith L, et al. Myometrial inhibiting activity of relaxin containing extracts of human corpora lutea of pregnancy. Am J Obstet Gynecol 1980; 136:584–6.
2. Bigazzi M, Nardi E. Prolactin and relaxin: antagonism on the spontaneous motility of the uterus. J Clin Endocrinol Metab 1981; 53:665–7.

3. Csapo AL, Pulkkinen MO, Wiest WG. Effects of lutectomy and progesterone replacement in early pregnant patients. Am J Obstet Gynecol 1973; 115:759–64.

4. Insler V. Corpus luteum defects. Curr Opin Obstet Gynecol 1992; 4:203–11.

5. Tuckerman E, Laird SM, Stewart R, et al. Markers of endometrial function in women with unexplained recurrent pregnancy loss. Hum Reprod 2004; 19:196–205.

6. Jacobs MH, Balash J, Gonzalez-Merlo JM. Endometrial cytosolic and nuclear progesterone receptors in the luteal phase defect. J Clin Endocrinol Metab 1987; 64:472–8.

7. Rosenfeld DL, Garcia CR. A comparison of endometrial histology with simultaneous plasma progesterone determinations in infertile women. Fertil Steril 1976; 27:1256–66.

8. Koninckx PR, Goddeeries PG, Lauweryns JM, et al. Accuracy of endometrial biopsy dating in relation to the mid-cycle luteinizing hormone peak. Fertil Steril 1977; 28:443–5.

9. Hensleigh PA, Fainstat T. Corpus luteum dysfunction: serum progesterone levels in the diagnosis and assessment of therapy for recurrent and threatened abortion. Fertil Steril 1979; 32:396–400.

10. Cumming DC, Honore LH, Scott JZ, et al. The late luteal phase in infertile women: comparison of simultaneous endometrial biopsy and progesterone levels. Fertil Steril 1985; 43:715–19.

11. Coutifaris C, Myers ER, Guzick DS, et al. Histological dating of timed endometrial biopsy tissue is not related to fertility status. Fertil Steril 2004; 82:1264–72.

12. Daya S. Efficacy of progesterone support for pregnancy in women with recurrent miscarriage: a meta-analysis of controlled trials. Br J Obstet Gynaecol 1989; 96:275–80.

13. Karamardian LM, Grimes DA. Luteal phase deficiency effect of treatment on pregnancy rates. Am J Obstet Gynecol 1992; 167:1391–8.

14. Roberts CP, Murphy AA. Endocrinopathies associated with recurrent pregnancy loss. Semin Reprod Med 2000; 18:357–62.

15. Byrne JL, Ward K. Genetic factors in recurrent abortion. Clin Obstet Gynecol 1994; 37:693–704.

16. McNatty KP, Sawers RS. Relationship between the endocrine environment within the graafian follicle and the subsequent secretion of progesterone by human granulosa cells in culture. J Endocrinol 1975; 66:391–400.

17. Hirahara F, Andoh N, Sawai K, et al. Hyperprolactinemic recurrent miscarriage and results of randomized bromocriptine treatment trials. Fertil Steril 1998; 70:246–52.

18. Kriplani A, Buckshee K, Bhargava VL, et al. Maternal and perinatal outcome in thyrotoxicosis complicating pregnancy. Eur J Obstet Gynecol Reprod Biol 1994; 54:159–63.

19. Daniels GH. Thyroid disease and pregnancy: a clinical overview. Endocr Pract 1995; 1:287–301.

20. Nakayama T, Yamamoto T, Kanmatsuse K, et al. Graves' disease associated with anticardiolipin antibody positivity and acquired protein S deficiency. Rheumatol Int 2003; 23:198–200.

21. Anselmo J, Cao D, Karrison T, et al. Fetal loss associated with excess thyroid hormone exposure. JAMA 2004; 292:691–5.

22. Wakim AN, Polizotto SL, Buffo MJ, et al. Thyroid hormones in human follicular fluid and thyroid hormone receptors in human granulosa cells. Fertil Steril 1993; 59:1187–90.

23. Steinberger E, Nader S, Rodriguez-Rigau L, et al. Prolactin response to thyrotropin-releasing hormone in normoprolactinemic patients with ovulatory dysfunction and its use for selection of candidates for bromocriptine therapy. J Endocrinol Invest 1990; 13:637–42.

24. Casey BM, Dashe JS, Wells CE, et al. Subclinical hypothyroidism and pregnancy outcomes. Obstet Gynecol 2005; 105:239–45.

25. Clifford K, Rai R, Watson H, et al. An informative protocol for the investigation of recurrent miscarriage: preliminary experience of 500 consecutive cases. Hum Reprod 1994; 9:1328–32.

26. Coutifaris C, Myers ER, Guzick DS, et al. Histological dating of rimed endometrial biopsy tissue is not related to fertility status. Fertil Steril 2004; 82:1264–72.

27. Kazer RR. Endometrial biopsy should be abandoned as a routine component of the infertility evaluation. Fertil Steril 2004; 82:1297–8.

28. Oates-Whitehead RM, Haas DM, Carrier JA, et al. Progestogen for preventing miscarriage. Cochrane Database Syst Rev 2003; (4):CD003511.

29. Baloch Z, Carayon P, Conte-Devolx, et al. Guidelines Committee, National Academy of Clinical Biochemistry. Laboratory Medicine Practice Guidelines. Laboratory support: for the diagnosis and monitoring of thyroid disease. Thyroid 2003; 13:3–126.

30. Weetman AP. Autoimmune thyroid disease. Autoimmunity 2004; 37:337–40.

31. Kutteh WH, Yetman DL, Carr AC, et al. Increased prevalence of antithyroid antibodies identified in women with recurrent pregnancy loss but not in women undergoing assisted reproduction. Fertil Steril 1999; 71:843–8.

32. Rushworth FH, Backos M, Rai R, et al. Prospective pregnancy outcome in untreated recurrent miscarriers with thyroid autoantibodies. Hum Reprod 2000; 15:1637–9.

33. Santoro N. Research on the mechanisms of premature ovarian failure. J Soc Gynecol Investig 2001; 8:S10–12.

34. Hak AE, Pols HA, Visser TJ, et al. Subclinical hypothyroidism is an independent risk factor for atherosclerosis and myocardial infarction in elderly women: the Rotterdam Study. Ann Intern Med 2000; 132:270–8.

35. Stewart-Akers AM, Krasnow JS, Brekosky J, et al. Endometrial leukocytes are altered numerically and functionally in women with implantation defects. Am J Reprod Immunol 1998; 39:1–11.

36. Matalon ST, Blank M, Ornoy A, et al. The association between antithyroid antibodies and pregnancy loss. Am J Reprod Immunol 2001; 45:72–7.

37. Christiansen OB, Nybo Andersen AM, Bosch E, et al. Evidence-based investigations and treatments of recurrent pregnancy loss. Fertil Steril 2005; 83:821–39.

38. Mills JL, Simpson JL, Driscoll SG, et al. Incidence of spontaneous abortion among normal women and insulin-dependant diabetic women whose pregnancies were identified within 21 days of conception. N Engl J Med 1988; 319:1617–23.

39. Greene MF, Hare JW, Cloherty JP, et al. First-trimester hemoglobin Al and risk for major malformation and spontaneous abortion in diabetic pregnancy. Teratology 1989; 39:225–31.

40. Ray JG, O'Brien TE, Chan WS, et al. Preconception care and the risk of congenital anomalies in the offspring of women with diabetes mellitus: a meta-analysis. QJM 2001; 9:435–44.

41. Temple R, Aldridge V, Greenwood R, et al. Association between outcome of pregnancy and glycaemic control in early pregnancy in type 1 diabetes: population based study. BMJ 2002; 325:1275–6.

42. Nielsen GL, Sorensen HT, Nielsen PH, et al. Glycosylated hemoglobin as predictor of adverse fetal outcome in type 1 diabetic pregnancies. Acta Diabetol 1997; 34:217–22.

43. Glueck CJ, Wang P, Fontaine RN, et al. Pregnancy outcomes among women with polycystic ovary syndrome treated with metformin. Hum Reprod 2002; 17:2858–64.

44. Glueck CJ, Wang P, Fontaine RN, et al. Plasminogen activator inhibitor activity: an independent risk factor for the high miscarriage rate during pregnancy in women with polycystic ovary syndrome. Metabolism 1999; 48:1589–95.

45. Glueck CJ, Phillips H, Cameron D et al. Continuing metformin throughout pregnancy in women with polycystic ovary syndrome appears to safely reduce first-trimester spontaneous abortion: a pilot study. Fertil Steril 200l; 75:46–52.

46. Velazquez EM, Mendoza SG, Wang P, Glueck CJ. Metformin therapy is associated with a decrease in plasma plasminogen activator inhibitor-1, lipoprotein(a), and immunoreactive insulin levels in patients with the polycystic ovary syndrome. Metabolism 1997; 46:454–7.

47. Wang JX, Davie MJ, Norman RJ, et al. Polycystic ovarian syndrome and the risk of spontaneous abortion following assisted reproductive technology treatment. Hum Reprod 2001; 16:2606–9.

48. Tuckerman EM, Okon MA, Li T, et al. Do androgens have a direct effect on endometrial function? An in vitro study. Fertil Steril 2000; 74:771–9.

49. Regan L, Owen EJ, Jacobs HS, et al. Hypersecretion of luteinising hormone, infertility, and miscarriage. Lancet 1990; 336:1141–4.

50. Nardo LG, Rai R, Backos M, et al. High serum luteinizing hormone and testosterone concentrations do not predict pregnancy outcome in women with recurrent miscarriage. Fertil Steril 2002; 77:348–52.

51. Westergaard LG, Laursen SB, Andersen CY. Increased risk of early pregnancy loss by profound suppression of luteinizing hormone during ovarian stimulation in normogonadotrophic women undergoing assisted reproduction. Hum Reprod 2000; 15:1003–8.

52. Clifford K, Rai R, Watson H, et al. Does suppressing lureinising hormone secretion reduce the miscarriage rare? Results of a randomised controlled trial. BMJ 1996; 312:1508–11.

53. Craig LB, Ke RW, Kutteh WH. Increased prevalence of insulin resistance in women with a history of recurrent pregnancy loss. Fertil Steril 2002; 78:487–90.

54. Stadtmauer LA, Wong BC, Oehninger S. Should patients with polycystic ovary syndrome be treated with metformin? Benefits of insulin sensitizing drugs in polycystic ovary syndrome – beyond ovulation induction. Hum Reprod 2002; 17:3016–26.

55. Trout SW, Seifer DB. Do women with unexplained recurrent pregnancy loss have higher day 3 serum FSH and estradiol values? Fertil Steril 2000; 74:335–7.

56. Gurbuz B, Yalti S, Ozden S, et al. High basal estradiol level and FSH/LH ratio in unexplained recurrent pregnancy loss. Arch Gynecol Obstet 2004; 270:37–9.

57. Hofmann GE, Khoury J, Thie J. Recurrent pregnancy loss and diminished ovarian reserve. Fertil Steril 2000; 74:1192–5.

58. Illingworth PJ, Groome NP, Duncan WC, et al. Measurement of circulating inhibin forms during the establishment of pregnancy. J Clin Endocrinol Metab 1996; 81:1471–5.

59. Muttukrishna S, George L, Fowler PA, et al. Measurement of serum concentration of inhibin A (α-βA dimer) during human pregnancy. Clin Endocrinol 1995; 42:391–7.

60. Groome NP, Illingworth PJ, O'Brien M, et al. Detection of dimeric inhibin throughout the human menstrual cycle by two site enzyme immunoassay. Clin Endocrinol 1994; 40:717–23.

61. Muttukrishna S, Fowler P, Groome NP, et al. Serum concentrations of dimeric inhibin during the spontaneous human menstrual cycle and after treatment with exogenous gonadotrophin. Hum Reprod 1994; 9:1634–42.

62. Luisi S, Florio P, Reis F, et al. Inhibins in female and male reproductive physiology: role in gametogenesis, conception, implantation and early pregnancy. Hum Reprod Update 2005; 11:123–35.

63. Roberts VJ, Barth S, el-Roeiy A, et al. Expression of inhibin/activin subunits and follistatin messenger ribonucleic acids and proteins in ovarian follicles and corpus luteum during the human menstrual cycle. J Clin Endocrinol Metab 1993; 77:1402–10.

64. Petraglia F, Garuti C, Calza L, et al. Inhibin subunits in human placenta: localization and messenger ribonucleic acids during pregnancy. Am J Obstet Gynecol 1991; 165:750–8.

65. Ledger W. Measurement of inhibin A and activin A in pregnancy – possible diagnostic applications. Mol Cell Endocrinol 2001; 180:117–21.

66. Lahiri S, Anobile CJ, Stewart P, et al. Changes in circulating concentrations of inhibins A and pro-α C during first trimester medical termination of pregnancy. Hum Reprod 2003; 18:744–8.

67. Florio P, Lombardo M et al. Activin A, corticotrophin-releasing factor and prostaglandin F2α increase immunoreactive oxytocin release from cultured human placental cells. Placenta 1995; 17:307–11.

68. Muttukrishna S, Jauniaux E, Greenwold N, et al. Circulating levels of inhibin A, activin A and follistatin in missed and recurrent miscarriages. Hum Reprod 2002; 17:3072–8.

69. Prakash A, Laird S, Tuckerman S, et al. Inhibin A and activin A may be used to predict pregnancy outcome in women with recurrent miscarriage Fertil Steril 2005; 83:1758–63.

DEBATE

6a. Should progesterone supplements be used?
– For

Jerome H Check

In pregnant women, a 34 kDa protein has been identified that can block natural killer (NK)-cell-mediated lysis of K562 tumor cells.[1,2] Because the expression of this protein by CD8[+] T lymphocytes (γ/δ T cells) requires progesterone exposure for expression, it was called the progesterone-induced blocking factor (PIBF).[3] PIBF may induce a shift from Th1 to Th2 cytokines.[2,4] Progesterone receptors (PgR) have not been demonstrated in normal T lymphocytes, yet these receptors are found in normal pregnancy, but at a lower density than other progesterone target receptor tissues.[5–7] Liver transplants and blood transfusions have been shown to induce PgR on γ/δ T cells, even in males.[8] Paternal lymphocyte injection prior to ovulation has been shown to increase PIBF expression in the mid to late luteal phase in women exposed to embryo transfer.[9]

These data support the following hypothesis as to one way the fetus escapes immune rejection by NK cells. The fetal semi-allograft induces PgR in γ/δ T cells following trophoblast invasion. The interaction with high concentration of progesterone causes the expression of PIBF by γ/δ T cells with induced PgR. The PIBF is only made at the maternal–fetal interface, because that is where there is an adequate progesterone concentration. PgR are made in γ/δ T cells throughout the body, but the progesterone level is insufficient to cause PIBF expression by γ/δ T cells that are not situated at the maternal–fetal interface. The PIBF inhibits NK-cell cytologic activity at least partially by inhibiting the release of perforin from storage granules of NK cells.[10] PIBF also inhibits Th1 cytokines and favors Th2 cytokines, thus inhibiting cellular immune response and promoting humoral responses. The suppression of the cellular immune system is limited to the maternal–fetal interface, and this constitutes selective immune tolerance.

Much less PIBF expression was found in women who eventually lost their pregnancies than in healthy pregnant women, thus supporting this hypothesis.[11,12] However, no such difference was found in aborters or non-aborters in patients aggressively treated with progesterone.[13] Surgical removal of the ovary with the corpus luteum of pregnancy prior to 8 weeks will lead to spontaneous abortion.[14] Donor oocytes do not work unless progesterone is supplemented for at least 8 weeks.

The difficulty in determining the role of progesterone in preventing recurrent pregnancy loss is due to difficulty in determining who has progesterone deficiency and in establishing the diagnosis. Also, the question arises as to whether the problem starts in the luteal phase or whether a need for more progesterone can arise after the pregnancy is more advanced. Are some women more prone to have ovulatory dysfunction or corpus luteum of pregnancy dysfunction – but not in every cycle – leading to a higher frequency of miscarriage in any given pregnancy but possibly without causing recurrent miscarriages? If one performs chromosome analysis on an aborted fetus and aneuploidy is found, does that prove that the woman would not have lost the pregnancy due to progesterone deficiency anyhow?

There is no question that the standard tests of luteal phase defect (LPD) – for example the mid-luteal phase serum progesterone level (or multiple integrated levels during the luteal phase) or an out-of-phase endometrial biopsy in mid or late luteal phase – lack sensitivity and specificity. Multiple flaws exist – such as variability of serum progesterone assays, lack of standardization of what focal point should be used to obtain a serum progesterone level, and lack of standardization of the histological findings on the endometrial biopsy, so that different pathologists may interpret the dating of the biopsy differently. If the need for extra progesterone supplementation occurred in only one-third of pregnancies, would it not be worthwhile to use such supplementation in every cycle to eliminate a 33% miscarriage rate?

I have considered that there may be a spectrum of progesterone deficiency with effects ranging from prevention of embryonic implantation, through successful implantation but with early loss leading to a chemical pregnancy only, through sufficient progression to allow ultrasound evidence of at least a gestational sac with either a non-viable fetal pole or an empty sac (so-called blighted ovum), through fetal viability but death before the end of the first trimester, through second-trimester loss, and finally pre-term delivery.

The question arises, however, as to whether there are any data to confirm this 'spectrum theory'. It is known that estradiol (E2) induces PgR in the human endometrium.[15,16] Women with regular menses who do exhibit a rise in progesterone during the luteal phase may actually not generate a sufficient peak serum E2 level to induce adequate PgR in the endometrium. We performed a study (unpublished) on fertile women seeking contraception, and found that the great majority attained an average follicle diameter of a minimum 18 mm and a serum E2 level of 200 pg/ml or more. We evaluated 100 women with a minimum of 1 year's infertility with an out-of-phase late luteal phase endometrium, and found that 42 did not achieve a mature follicle. They were randomized into three treatment regimens. Only 3 of 12 (25%) conceived within 6 months following exclusive treatment with luteal phase progesterone (but there were no miscarriages), versus 7 of 10 women (70%) with follicle-maturing

drugs (but 4 of these 7 (57.1%) miscarried), versus 14 of 20 (70%) conceiving with the combination of follicle-maturing drugs and progesterone (with only 1 miscarriage (7.1%)).[17] These data suggest that women not producing mature follicles before egg release need more than luteal phase support to achieve pregnancies, but follicle-maturing drugs may not fully correct the luteal phase, so that progesterone supplementation is needed to inhibit miscarriage.[17] These data are consistent with another prospective study where 50 women conceiving after follicle-maturing drugs who were given progesterone supplementation in the luteal phase had a miscarriage rate of 6%, versus 28% in controls not given progesterone.[18]

There were 58 women in the infertility study with LPD who did attain a mature follicle.[17] They were randomized into a group receiving only progesterone supplementation in the luteal phase and a group receiving only follicle-maturing drugs. Of the women taking only progesterone, 24 (77.4%) conceived within 6 months of therapy and 1 (4.1%) miscarried.[17] In comparison, only 3 of 27 (11.1%) conceived with clomiphene citrate or human menopausal gonadotropin and 2 (66.7%) miscarried.[17] Interestingly, 25 women failing to have successful pregnancies with follicle-stimulating drugs were treated exclusively with progesterone supplementation during the next 6 months, and 16 (64%) conceived, with only 1 (6.2%) miscarriage.[17] These data show that, at least in infertile women with apparent luteal phase defects, progesterone therapy can reduce the risk of miscarriage. But what about the group of women who can conceive without help but then miscarry? A study was performed where women seeking help because of previous miscarriage(s) without delivery were offered progesterone therapy starting in the luteal phase and continued through the first trimester, but were warned about the possible risk of birth defects. Of the 100 progesterone-treated women, 10 (10%) had a first-trimester miscarriage, compared with 10 of 24 (41.6%) who elected not to be treated with progesterone.[19]

There is no question that low serum progesterone levels are associated with poor pregnancy outcome. One study found that 17 of 18 women with serum progesterone less than 15 ng/ml lost their pregnancy.[20] The authors even suggested that, given the near inevitability of pregnancy loss, women at risk for possible ectopic pregnancy should have a dilatation and evacuation, and, in the event of products of conception being found, evaluation for ectopic pregnancy should be discontinued, while in the absence of such products, serial ultrasound scans and β human chorionic gonadotropin (β-hCG) determinations should be carried out.[20]

However, it is not clear whether the low progesterone is a result of a dying or dead fetus, reflecting degeneration of the corpus luteum and/or placenta or whether the low progesterone could be etiological. The fact that one study found that 70% (19/27) of women with serum progesterone below 15 ng/ml successfully completed the first trimester with aggressive progesterone therapy strongly implies that low serum progesterone can be a correctable cause of miscarriage.[21] Another study found that 60% of intrauterine pregnancies could be salvaged with a serum progesterone below 8 ng/ml.[22] The pure scientist may argue that many of the 'controlled' studies in support of progesterone therapy were too small or lacked placebo controls or were not double-blinded. The data convince me that I would empirically treat any woman with a previous miscarriage with extra progesterone even if the aforementioned studies of the efficiency of such treatment are not scientifically convincing beyond a shadow of doubt. I would rather give a woman a benign treatment that is later found not be effective than not treat her, have her miscarry, and later find studies showing unequivocally that with such treatment definitely reduces the risk of miscarriage. Possibly, sometimes progesterone may be needed but may not be sufficient – for example if the fetal semi-allograft fails to induce sufficient PgR in γ/δ T cells. Possibly, injection of lymphocytes may also be needed in some cases to maximize the benefit of progesterone therapy by allowing adequate production of immunomodulatory proteins (e.g., PIBF).[7,9,23–25]

REFERENCES

1. Pence H, Petty WM, Rocklin RE. Suppression of maternal responsiveness to paternal antigens by maternal plasma. J Immunol 1975; 114:525–8.

2. Szekeres-Bartho J, Kilar F, Falkay G, et al. The mechanism of the inhibitory effect of progesterone on lymphocyte cytotoxicity: I. Progesterone-treated lymphocytes release a substance inhibiting cytotoxicity and prostaglandin synthesis. Am J Reprod Immunol Microbiol 1985; 9:15–18.

3. Szekeres-Bartho J, Autran B, Debre P, et al. Immunoregulatory effects of a suppressor factor from healthy pregnant women's lymphocytes after progesterone induction. Cell Immunol 1989; 122:281–94.

4. Szekeres-Bartho J, Barakonyi A, Polgar B, et al. The role of γ/δ T cells in progesterone-mediated immunomodulation during pregnancy: a review. Am J Reprod Immunol 1999; 42:44–8.

5. Szekeres-Bartho J, Csernus V, Hadnagy J. The blocking effect of progesterone on lymphocyte responsiveness is receptor-mediated. Biol Immunol Reprod 1989; 15:36.

6. Szekeres-Bartho J, Szekeres Gy, Debre P, et al. Reactivity of lymphocytes to a progesterone receptor specific monoclonal antibody. Cell Immunol 1990; 125:273–83.

7. Chiu L, Nishimura M, Ishii Y, et al. Enhancement of the expression of progesterone receptor on progesterone treated lymphocyte after immunotherapy in unexplained recurrent spontaneous abortion. Am J Reprod Immunol 1996; 35:552–7.

8. Szekeres-Bartho J, Weill BJ, Mike G, et al. Progesterone receptors in lymphocytes of liver-transplanted and transfused patients. Immunol Lett 1989; 22:259–61.

9. Check JH, Arwitz M, Gross J, et al. Lymphocyte immunotherapy (LI) increases serum levels of progesterone induced blocking factor (PIBF). Am J Reprod Immunol 1997; 37:17–20.

10. Faust Z, Laskarin G, Rukavina D, et al. Progesterone induced blocking factor inhibits degranulation of NK cells. Am J Reprod Immunol 1999; 42:71–5.

11. Szekeres-Bartho J, Varga P, Retjsik B. ELISA test for detecting a progesterone-induced immunological factor in pregnancy serum. J Reprod Immunol 1989; 16:19–29.

12. Szekeres-Bartho J, Faust Z, Varga P. The expression of a progesterone-induced immunomodulatory protein in pregnancy lymphocytes. Am J Reprod Immunol 1995; 34:342–8.

13. Check JH, Ostrzenski A, Klimek R. Expression of an immunomodulatory protein known as progesterone induced blocking factor (PIBF) does not correlate with first trimester spontaneous abortions in progesterone supplemented women. Am J Reprod Immunol 1997; 37:330–4.

14. Csapo AI, Pulkkinen M. Indispensability of the human corpus luteum in the maintenance of early pregnancy: lutectomy evidence. Obstet Gynecol Surv 1978; 3:69–81.

15. Lessey BA, Killam AP, Metzger DA, et al. Immunohistochemical analysis of human estrogen and progesterone receptors throughout the menstrual cycle. J Clin Endocrinol Metab 1988; 67:334–40.

16. Bergquist A, Ferno M. Oestrogen and progesterone receptors in endometriotic tissue and endometrium: comparison of different cycle phases and ages. Hum Reprod 1993; 8:2211–17.

17. Check JH, Nowroozi K, Wu CH, et al. Ovulation inducing drugs versus progesterone therapy for infertility in patients with luteal phase defects. Int J Fertil 1988; 33:252–6.

18. Check JH, Chase JS, Wu CH, et al. The efficacy of progesterone in achieving successful pregnancy: I. Prophylactic use during luteal phase in anovulatory women. Int J Fertil 1987; 32:135–8.

19. Check JH, Chase JS, Nowroozi K, et al. Progesterone therapy to decrease first-trimester spontaneous abortions in previous aborters. Int J Fertil 1987; 32:197–9.

20. Yeko TR, Gorrill MJ, Hughes LH, et al. Timely diagnosis of early ectopic pregnancy using a single blood progesterone measurement. Fertil Steril 1987; 48:1048–50.

21. Check JH, Winkel CA, Check ML. Abortion rate in progesterone treated women presenting initially with low first trimester serum progesterone levels. Am J Gynecol Health 1990; 4:33–4.

22. Choe JK, Check JH, Nowroozi K, et al. Serum progesterone and 17-hydroxyprogesterone in the diagnosis of ectopic pregnancies and the value of progesterone replacement in intrauterine pregnancies when serum progesterone levels are low. Gynecol Obstet Invest 1992; 34:133–8.

23. Check JH, Tarquini P, Gandy P, et al. A randomized study comparing the efficacy of reducing the spontaneous abortion rate following lymphocyte immunotherapy and progesterone treatment versus progesterone alone in primary habitual aborters. Gynecol Obstet Invest 1995; 39:257–61.

24. Check JH, Liss JR, Check ML, et al. Lymphocyte immunotherapy can improve pregnancy outcome following embryo transfer (ET) in patients failing to conceive after two previous ET. Clin Exp Obstet Gynecol 2005; 32:21–2.

25. Check JH, Liss J, Check ML, Diantonio A, Choe JK, Graziano V. Leukocyte immunotherapy improves live delivery rates following embryo transfer in women with at least two previous failures: A retrospective review. Clin Exp Obst Gyn 2005; 32:85–8.

DEBATE

6b. Should progesterone supplements be used?
– Against

Shazia Malik and Lesley Regan

INTRODUCTION

The role of progesterone in the mammalian reproductive cycle is well described and undisputed. Its pharmacodynamics have been extensively studied, and progesterone has been synthesized and commercially available since 1935. However, despite the putative role of progesterone in ameliorating unexplained recurrent pregnancy loss (RPL), the evidence base for its use in this setting is lacking, despite decades of clinical use. With this in mind, we argue that the use of progesterone supplementation for women in whom no identifiable cause for three or more successive pregnancy losses prior to 20 weeks of gestation has been identified is currently unjustified.

SCIENTIFIC BASIS

LUTEAL PHASE DEFECT

Removal of the corpus luteum before the end of the 7th week of amenorrhoea leads to miscarriage. Rescue can be achieved with progesterone therapy, but not with estrogen.[1] Corpus luteum deficiency, or luteal phase defect (LPD), has been cited as the underlying pathology in 35–40% of unexplained recurrent pregnancy loss, manifesting in low serum progesterone levels and out-of-phase endometrial biopsies.[2,3] However, women with no history of recurrent miscarriage exhibit an endometrial histology suggestive of LPD in up to 50% of single menstrual cycles and 25% of sequential cycles.[4] A prevalence study of out-of-phase endometrial biopsy specimens[5] failed to show any significant difference between fertile and infertile patients and recurrent pregnancy loss, which calls the role of this intervention into question. In a series of 74 women with recurrent miscarriage before 10 weeks of gestation, there was no difference in pregnanediol excretion curves between those women who either miscarried or went on to have a successful pregnancy.[6] In fact estriol was a better prognostic indicator, showing lower values in those destined to miscarry. In 1993, Quenby and Farquharson[7] audited 203 consecutive couples attending their clinic and found that, compared with any other predictor, oligo-amenorrheic women were most likely to have a further miscarriages, and further, that they exhibited low luteal phase estradiol levels but normal luteal progesterone and normal luteinizing hormone (LH) profiles throughout the cycle. A more recent study found that a mid-luteal progesterone level of less than 10 ng/ml (as a marker of luteal phase deficiency) did not predict a future pregnancy loss in women with two successive unexplained first-trimester miscarriages.[8]

PROGESTERONE AND IMMUNOMODULATION IN EARLY PREGNANCY

There is increasing evidence that progesterone is a key modulator in the immune response required to achieve a successful pregnancy outcome. The complexities of the adaptation between the maternal immune system and the semi-allograft of the fetoplacental unit are not clearly understood. The presence of progesterone and an upregulation of its receptors on decidual natural killer (NK) and placental lymphocytes appears to be required to defend the developing trophoblast from the maternal immune reaction.[9] These activated cells then synthesise progesterone-induced blocking factor (PIBF), mediating both the immunomodulatory and antiabortive effects of progesterone.[10] In addition to the shift towards Th2 cytokine production, NK cytolytic activity in human pregnancy is inversely related to the levels of PIBF-positive lymphocytes,[11] and neutralization in pregnant mice results in NK-cell-mediated abortion.[10] The cellular T-cell system, in particular the Th1 cells, modulates this immune response, releasing either Th1 cytokines (e.g., tumor necrosis factor α, TNF-α) that induce cytotoxic and inflammatory reactions, or Th2 cytokines (e.g., interleukin-10, IL-10) associated with B-cell production.[12] Serum cytokine profiles demonstrate a shift towards Th2 in normal pregnancy, whereas in recurrent miscarriage sufferers, the Th1 response predominates.[13] A recent study has reported that the administration of intramuscular progesterone injections to recurrent miscarriage patients restored levels of soluble TNF receptors to values seen in women with no such history.[14] However, the treatment only commenced at 8 weeks of gestation, included women up to 40 years of age, and, furthermore, showed that in some of the cases no response in terms of receptor levels was seen in pregnancies that then went on to miscarry. PIBF appears to be the main modulator of the actions of progesterone, with significantly lower expression in recurrent miscarriage patients compared with those with a healthy pregnancy.[15] Conversely, Check et al[16] treated women in the first trimester aggressively with progesterone, but found no differences in PIBF expression by lymphocytes. However Th1 and Th2 cytokines were not measured in this study, and could not be correlated either with PIBF levels or with any given response to progesterone supplementation in specific patients.

Murine experiments have shown a poor correlation between Th1/Th2 cytokine ratios and abortion rates, implicating environmental selective pressures in eliminating 'genetically weaker' embryos in early pregnancy.[17] While some rodent data are enticing, PIBF data in human pregnancy are scanty, and the mechanisms underlying immune-mediated pregnancy loss remain incompletely elucidated.[18]

CLINICAL DATA

The uterine decidual and systemic levels of progesterone necessary to maintain an early pregnancy in humans are not known.[19] Hence, clinical studies must, by definition, employ arbitrary doses/mode of delivery of drug. Hill[20] has proposed study criteria that should be fulfilled when designing a treatment trial for unexplained RPL (Table 6b.1). To date, there are no trials that fulfil these criteria having systematically evaluated the role of progesterone treatment in recurrent pregnancy loss. Two meta-analyses published in the same journal reported conflicting results regarding the value of progesterone supplementation in miscarriage patients. Goldstein et al[21] included trials of women with a 'high-risk' pregnancy, including a history of previous

---

Table 6b.1 Study criteria for recurrent pregnancy loss treatments[20]

- Scientifically sound rationale
- Power calculation ensuring sufficient numbers under reasonable assumptions (e.g., 60% success without and 80% success with treatment)
- Exclusion of patients with less than three unexplained clinical pregnancy losses
- Exclusion of patients with presumed causes for prior pregnancy losses
- Prospective study design
- Prestratification of participants by age and number of prior losses (both of which are independent risk factors for subsequent loss)
- Effective randomization after prestratification
- Placebo-controlled
- Double-blinded
- No concomitant therapy
- Karyotype of subsequent losses
- Follow-up to ensure safety

miscarriage, stillbirth, or current preterm labour. In addition, the authors used different preparations commenced at varying gestations, and not surprisingly no benefit of treatment was identified. They subsequently recommended that randomized trials should be the only setting for the use of progestational agents in pregnancy. In contrast, Daya[22] presented a meta-analysis of controlled trials studying the efficacy of progesterone support for pregnancy in women with a history of recurrent miscarriage. Although the odds ratio (OR) for pregnancies reaching at least 20 weeks of gestation was 3.09 (95% confidence interval (CI) 1.28–7.42), even he concluded that recurrent miscarriage patients with LPD should have the efficacy of progesterone assessed in prospective double-blind randomized controlled trials. Closer inspection reveals why this conclusion was reached: only three studies met the inclusion/exclusion criteria, and, as the differences between experimental groups were insignificant, they had to be pooled to show a statistically significant power calculation. None of the three studies demonstrated a significant progesterone deficiency, each employed a different progestogen, and each had different inclusion criteria recruiting patients only after they had reached at least 8 weeks of gestation. In addition, only a total of 50 treated and 45 control patients were identified. In the study by Levine,[23] patients were allocated alternately, not randomly, and the series published by Swyer and Daley[24] was not 'blind', as treated patients were administered an implant while some controls were offered a placebo tablet. A Cochrane meta-analysis looking at the same data also showed a statistically significant reduction in miscarriage in favor of those randomized to the progestogen group (OR 0.37; 95% CI 0.17–0.91).[25] Patients with primary recurrent spontaneous abortion (RSA) were not differentiated from those with secondary RSA. The recommendations from the American College of Obstetricians and Gynecologists[26] conclude that it has not been shown conclusively that progesterone treatment or corpus luteum support influence outcome in women with RPL, and that luteal phase progesterone support is of unproven efficacy.

In a more recent trial,[27] a significant reduction in the miscarriage rate was observed in women receiving dydrogesterone (10 mg orally) in early pregnancy compared with those who remained untreated ($p<0.05$). In this trial, women with an average of 3.3 previous unexplained recurrent abortions were randomized to receive either no treatment ($n=30$), dydrogesterone ($n=48$), or human chorionic gonadotropin (hCG; 5000 IU intramuscularly every 4 days; $n=36$) from as soon as pregnancy was confirmed until the 12th week of gestation. This trial does not, however, conform to the standards cited in Table 6b.1.

CONCLUSIONS

In the UK, three progestogenic products are licensed for use in early pregnancy: intramuscular progesterone, vaginal progesterone, and oral dydrogesterone, and have been authorized for between 10 and 20 years. However, the number of studies examining the efficacy of progesterone supplementation in early pregnancy remains small, and they do not fulfil the criteria required for meaningful results. In addition, the diversity of biological and pharmacological properties does not allow extrapolation of results across studies. Although there are no obvious adverse effects to mother or fetus, a low level of risk may as yet be unidentified. The observed frequency of another miscarriage after three is over 50%, and the wish to prescribe an apparently safe and well-tolerated treatment is appealing, especially in light of the emerging scientific understanding of early pregnancy failure. As yet, however, the evidence for 'tender loving care' shows a similar improvement in outcomes. The need 'to do something' for a group of unfortunate patients often seems to over-ride the use of an evidence base. While treatment does not appear to do harm, the evidence for the use of progesterone supplementation in recurrent pregnancy loss is contentious at best, dated, and poor at worst.

REFERENCES

1. Csapo AI, Pulkkinen MO, Ruttner B, et al. The significance of the human corpus luteum in pregnancy maintenance. I. Preliminary studies. Am J Obstet Gynecol 1972; 112:1061–7.
2. Jones GS. The luteal phase defect. Fertil Steril 1976; 27:351–6.

3. Daya S, Ward S. Diagnostic test properties of serum progesterone in the evaluation of luteal phase defects. Fertil Steril 1988; 49:168–70.

4. Davis OK, Berkeley AS, Naus GJ, et al. The incidence of luteal phase defect in normal, fertile women, determined by serial endometrial biopsies. Fertil Steril 1989; 51:582–6.

5. Peters AJ, Lloyd RP, Coulam CB. Prevalence of out-of-phase endometrial biopsy specimens. Am J Obstet Gynecol 1992; 166:1738–45; discussion 1745–6.

6. Klopper A, Michie EA. The excretion of urinary pregnanediol after the administration of progesterone. J Endocrinol 1956; 13:360–4.

7. Quenby SM, Farquharson RG. Predicting recurring miscarriage: What is important? Obstet Gynecol 1993; 82:132–8.

8. Ogasawara M, Kajiura S, Katano K, et al. Are serum progesterone levels predictive of recurrent miscarriage in future pregnancies? Fertil Steril 1997; 68:806–9.

9. Roussev RG, Higgins NG, McIntyre JA. Phenotypic characterization of normal human placental mononuclear cells. J Reprod Immunol 1993; 25:15–29.

10. Szekeres-Bartho J, Barakonyi A, Polgar B, et al. The role of γ/δ T cells in progesterone-mediated immunomodulation during pregnancy: a review. Am J Reprod Immunol 1999; 42:44–8.

11. Szekeres-Bartho J, Faust Z, Varga P. The expression of a progesterone-induced immunomodulatory protein in pregnancy lymphocytes. Am J Reprod Immunol 1995; 34:342–8.

12. Druckmann R, Druckmann MA. Progesterone and the immunology of pregnancy. J Steroid Biochem Mol Biol 2005;97:389–96.

13. Raghupathy R, Makhseed M, Azizieh F, et al. Cytokine production by maternal lymphocytes during normal human pregnancy and in unexplained recurrent spontaneous abortion. Hum Reprod 2000; 15:713–18.

14. Chernyshov VP, Vodyanik MA, Pisareva SP. Lack of soluble TNF-receptors in women with recurrent spontaneous abortion and possibility for its correction. Am J Reprod Immunol 2005; 54:284–91.

15. Szekeres-Bartho J, Barakonyi A, Miko E, et al, The role of γ/δ T cells in the feto–maternal relationship. Semin Immunol 2001; 13:229–33.

16. Check JH, Ostrzenski A, Klimek R. Expression of an immunomodulatory protein known as progesterone induced blocking factor (PIBF) does not correlate with first trimester spontaneous abortions in progesterone supplemented women. Am J Reprod Immunol 1997; 37:330–4.

17. Clark DA, Chaouat G, Gorczynski RM. Thinking outside the box: mechanisms of environmental selective pressures on the outcome of the materno–fetal relationship. Am J Reprod Immunol 2002; 47:275–82.

18. Laird SM, Tuckerman EM, Cork BA, et al. A review of immune cells and molecules in women with recurrent miscarriage. Hum Reprod Update 2003; 9:163–74.

19. Azuma K, Calderon I, Besanko M, et al. Is the luteo-placental shift a myth? Analysis of low progesterone levels in successful ART pregnancies. J Clin Endocrinol Metab 1993; 77:195–8.

20. Hill JA. Immunotherapy for recurrent pregnancy loss: 'standard of care or buyer beware'. J Soc Gynecol Investig 1997; 4:267–73.

21. Goldstein P, Berrier J, Rosen S, et al. A meta-analysis of randomized control trials of progestational agents in pregnancy. Br J Obstet Gynaecol 1989; 96:265–74.

22. Daya S. Efficacy of progesterone support for pregnancy in women with recurrent miscarriage. A meta-analysis of controlled trials. Br J Obstet Gynaecol 1989; 96:275–80.

23. Levine L. Habitual abortion. A controlled study of progestational therapy. West J Surg Obstet Gynecol 1964; 72:30–6.

24. Swyer GI, Daley D. Progesterone implantation in habitual abortion. BMJ 1953; i:1073–7.

25. Oates-Whitehead RM, Haas DM, Carrier JA. Progestogen for preventing miscarriage. Cochrane Database Syst Rev 2003; (4):CD003511.

26. American College of Obstetricians and Gynecologists. ACOG Practice Bulletin. Management of recurrent pregnancy loss. Number 24, February 2001. Int J Gynaecol Obstet 2002; 78:179–90.

27. El-Zibdeh MY. Dydrogesterone in the reduction of recurrent spontaneous abortion. J Steroid Biochem Mol Biol 2005; 97:431–4.

DEBATE

6c. Should hCG supplementation be used? – For

James Walker

INTRODUCTION

In the late 1920s, Willard Allen and colleagues[1] carried out experimental work demonstrating that preparations made from corpus luteum extracts could successfully support pregnancies in animals where the ovaries had been ablated. Further work demonstrated that these preparations contained progesterone. However, initial work on the use of progesterone in maintaining early pregnancy in castrated rabbits failed. It was not until a study in 1938[2] that the maintenance of pregnancy in castrated animals was achieved using progesterone. This was achieved when the castration was carried out after the 11th day following mating, when implantation of the embryos had occurred. Other work suggested a role for estrogen in supporting the early pregnancy.[3] However, unlike in small animals, which almost inevitably abort after ovariectomy, the results in pregnancies in larger animals and humans was mixed, with many case being cited in which abortion was seen to follow removal of the corpus luteum, while in others pregnancy appeared to continue successfully after ovariectomy in midpregnancy without hormonal support. It became clear that the effect was gestation-dependent.[4] In human pregnancy, exogenous progesterone support was required only until around 8 weeks' gestation, after which it was not required. The explanation of this became obvious with the realization that the corpus luteum is critical in early pregnancy, after which time the trophoblast takes over the hormonal support. This 'handover' time appeared to be between 7 and 8 weeks' gestation.

Because progesterone was thought to be important for the maintenance of normal pregnancy, the concept that a deficiency in progesterone might lead to miscarriage was a natural follow-on. By the late 1940s, it had been shown that functional reproductive deficits sufficient to cause infertility or recurrent abortion were present in women who appeared to be having regular menstrual cycles.[5] These abnormalities were due to a deficit in progesterone secretion during the luteal phase of the cycle (luteal phase deficiency, LPD). This disorder was characterized by inadequate endometrial maturation, and was reported in up to 60% of women with recurrent miscarriage. However, these early studies are open to question, since there was no reliable method of dating the cycle. Since many of these studies presumed that the patient's menstrual pattern is a normal 28-day cycle, these endometrial abnormalities could be related to prolonged cycles. However, more recent studies on the hormonal cycle have confirmed abnormalities of corpus luteal function, with deficiency in progesterone levels in the luteal phase and early pregnancy of those with a history of miscarriage, but in a lower percentage.[6] In one of the few prospective studies evaluating women with three or more consecutive miscarriages, LPD was believed to be the cause in 17%.[7] Those found to have LPD are more likely to have early losses (prior to the detection of fetal heart activity) than later loss.[8]

INTERVENTION – ESTROGEN

If hormonal lack is associated with miscarriage, hormonal support might be a possible therapy. The problem with steroid hormones is that they cannot be taken by mouth, and synthetic substitutes are required. Because of the early work showing the benefit of an estrogen,[3] the first therapeutic trials were with diethylstilbestrol, a non-steroidal estrogenic substance. This was given in large doses. None of these studies showed benefit, and by the 1970s there was evidence of the effect of this medication on the female offspring.[9–11] Therefore, not only did hormonal support not appear to be beneficial, it had major side-effects in the female offspring. These included abnormalities of the cervix, recurrent pregnancy loss and, in extreme cases, clear cell carcinoma of the vagina. These studies had a major effect on the role of hormonal support in pregnancy, with the fear that hormones could have a significant effect on the unborn child.

INTERVENTION – PROGESTERONE

Progesterone is the main supportive hormone of early pregnancy, and in recent years there has been an increased interest in its use in in vitro fertilization (IVF). This treatment is given early to support the luteal phase. The reasoning is as much for endometrial maturation as for pregnancy support, even though the early animal work did not show any benefit of progesterone prior to implantation. In assisted conception, the randomized trials of progesterone support in the luteal phase demonstrate an increased successful pregnancy rate.[12] However, in studies on the use of progesterone purely to prevent miscarriage, there was no benefit for this therapy, irrespective of the route of administration or type of progesterone used.[13] It is only in those with a history of recurrent miscarriage that there was a trend towards an improved live birth rate. In all studies, there appear to be no obvious side-effects. Therefore, there does appear to be some possible benefit of the use of progesterone in a targeted population to improve the live birth rate.

INTERVENTION – hCG

Human chorionic gonadotropin (hCG) is the hormone responsible for the corpus luteal support in early pregnancy. If the pregnancy is failing, levels of hCG may well be low, resulting in low progesterone. Rather than giving exogenous progesterone, hCG could be used directly, since this would stimulate the natural hormone and reduce the risks of abnormal effects on the fetus. Again, much work has been done in the area of assisted conception. Here, hCG does appear to be of benefit in increasing birth rates, but may not be any better than progesterone on its own.[12] In recurrent miscarriage, two early small studies were supportive of benefit,[14,15] and this led to larger trials. From these, a meta-analysis of four studies[14–17] showed a reduced risk of miscarriage for women with a history of recurrent miscarriage (odds ratio 0.26, 95% confidence interval 0.14–0.52) (Figure 6c.1).[18] However, the authors cautioned readers, as they felt that there was some weakness in the larger trials. One of the studies in the analysis found particular benefit in women with oligomenorrhea (Figure 6c.2).[17,18]

THE PROBLEMS

The problems with all of these trials are the methods of recruitment and timing of intervention. Most studies require the presence of an ultrasound-proven fetal heart rate, even though, once this is present, it is unlikely that hormonal support will be beneficial, since successful implantation has occurred and the gestation is probably in advance of the time when most benefit would be achieved. All of the studies in human pregnancy have not shown any benefit after 8 weeks' gestation. Also by this time, the levels of endogenous hCG are so high that it is unlikely that any exogenous therapy will increase them. If an earlier recruitment is used, trialists worry that they will

Study	Experiment: n/N	Control: n/N	Peto OR (95% CI)	Weight (%)	Peto OR (95% CI)
Harrison et al[15]	0/10	7/10		13.8	0.05 [0.01–0.32]
Harrison et al[16]	6/36	8/31		32.2	0.58 [0.18–1.87]
Quenby and Farquharson[17]	6/36	10/29		34.9	0.39 [0.13–1.20]
Svigos[14]	1/13	9/15		19.1	0.11 [0.02–0.51]
Total (95% CI) $\chi^2=6.46$ (df=3), $z=3.91$	13/95	34/85		100.0	0.26 [0.14–0.52]

0.1 0.2   1   5 10

Figure 6c.1 Meta-analysis of four trials of the use of hCG in the management of recurrent miscarriage.[18] OR, odds ratio; CI, confidence interval. Reproduced from Scott JR, Pattison N. Cochrane Database Syst Rev 2000(2): CD000101 with permission from John Wiley & Sons, Ltd, UK.

include those who will inevitably miscarry. A recent medium-sized study, using early recruitment, demonstrated a significant benefit from both an oral progesten and, less so, hCG, in recurrent miscarriage.[19] Therefore, all the early work and recent trials suggest a potential benefit of hormonal support in a targeted population. The problem is what that target group is. Studies suggest that up to 30% of women may benefit from therapy,[19] and these would be those with a history of early loss[20] and/or oligomenorrhea.[17]

CONCLUSIONS

hCG therapy is not a panacea for all cases of recurrent miscarriage, but it appears to be beneficial in a particular targeted group. The problem is how to diagnose these women. Certainly, those with a proven cause, such as antiphospholipid syndrome and chromosomal abnormalities, will not benefit. Those with repeated early loss (prior to a positive fetal heartbeat) and those with an irregular cycle would appear to be more likely to benefit.

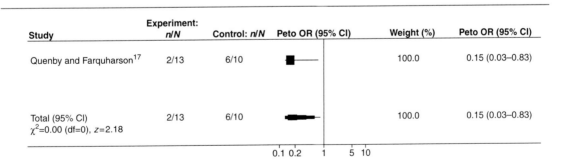

Study	Experiment: n/N	Control: n/N	Peto OR (95% CI)	Weight (%)	Peto OR (95% CI)
Quenby and Farquharson[17]	2/13	6/10		100.0	0.15 (0.03–0.83)
Total (95% CI) $\chi^2=0.00$ (df=0), $z=2.18$	2/13	6/10		100.0	0.15 (0.03–0.83)

0.1 0.2   1   5 10

Figure 6c.2 Meta-analysis of four trials of the use of hCG in the management of recurrent miscarriage showing a subanalysis of those with oligomenorrhea.[18] OR, odds ratio; CI, confidence interval. Reproduced from Scott JR, Pattison N. Cochrane Database Syst Rev 2000(2): CD000101 with permission from John Wiley & Sons, Ltd, UK.

Using these criteria, around 30% of cases of recurrent miscarriage could be offered hormonal support, with a success rate of around 85%.[19] Whether to use a progestogen or hCG is a more difficult argument. However, with the concerns over in utero effects, hCG has the advantage of being more 'natural', with evidence of similar benefits.

I therefore support the use of hCG in the treatment of recurrent miscarriage in an appropriately assessed population.

REFERENCES

1. Allen WM, Corner GW. Physiology of the corpus luteum: III. Normal growth and implantation of embryos after very early ablation of the ovaries, under the influence of extracts of the corpus luteum. Am J Physiol 1929; 88:340–6.
2. Allen WM, Heckel GP. Maintenance of pregnancy by progesterone in rabbits castrated on the 11th day. Am J Physiol 1938; 125:31–5.
3. Heckel GP, Allen WM. Maintenance of the corpus luteum and inhibition of parturition in the rabbit by injection of estrogenic hormone. Endocrinology 1939; 24:137–9.
4. Russ W. The maintenance of pregnancy in the human after removal of both ovaries – case report. Ann Surg 1940; 111:871–3.
5. Jones GES. Some newer aspects of the management of infertility. JAMA 1949; 141:1123–9.
6. Miller H, Durant JA, Ross DM, et al. Corpus luteum deficiency as a cause of early recurrent abortion: a case history. Fertil Steril 1969; 20:433–8.
7. Tulppala M, Bjorses UM, Stenman UH, et al. Luteal phase defect in habitual abortion: progesterone in saliva. Fertil Steril 1991; 56:41–4.
8. Li TC, Iqbal T, Anstie B, et al. An analysis of the pattern of pregnancy loss in women with recurrent miscarriage. Fertil Steril 2002; 78:1100–6.
9. Vessey MP, Fairweather DV, Norman-Smith B, et al. A randomized double-blind controlled trial of the value of stilboestrol therapy in pregnancy: long-term follow-up of mothers and their offspring. Br J Obstet Gynaecol 1983; 90:1007–17.
10. Lanier AP, Noller KL, Decker DG, et al. Cancer and stilbestrol. A follow-up of 1,719 persons exposed to estrogens in utero and born 1943–1959. Mayo Clin Proc 1973; 48:793–9.
11. Bamigboye AA, Morris J. Oestrogen supplementation, mainly diethylstilbestrol, for preventing miscarriages and other adverse pregnancy outcomes. Cochrane Database Syst Rev 2003; (3):CD004271.
12. Daya S, Gunby J. Luteal phase support in assisted reproduction cycles. Cochrane Database Syst Rev 2004; (3):CD004830.
13. Oates-Whitehead RM, Haas DM, Carrier JA. Progestogen for preventing miscarriage. Cochrane Database Syst Rev 2003; (4):CD003511.
14. Svigos J. Preliminary experience with the use of human chorionic gonadotrophin therapy in women with repeated abortion. Clin Reprod Fertil 1982; 1:131–5.
15. Harrison RF. Treatment of habitual abortion with human chorionic gonadotrophin: results of open and placebo-controlled studies. Eur J Obstet Gynecol Reprod Biol 1985; 20:159–68.
16. Harrison RF. Human chorionic gonadotrophin (hCG) in the management of recurrent abortion; results of a multi-centre placebo-controlled study. Eur J Obstet Gynecol Reprod Biol 1992; 47:175–9.
17. Quenby S, Farquharson RG. Human chorionic gonadotropin supplementation in recurring pregnancy loss: a controlled trial. Fertil Steril 1994; 62:708–10.
18. Scott JR, Pattison N. Human chorionic gonadotrophin for recurrent miscarriage. Cochrane Database Syst Rev 2000; (2):CD000101.
19. El-Zibdeh MY. Dydrogesterone in the reduction of recurrent spontaneous abortion. J Steroid Biochem Mol Biol 2005; 97:431–4.
20. Quenby SM, Farquharson RG. Predicting recurring miscarriage: What is important? Obstet Gynecol 1993; 82:132–8.

DEBATE

6d. Should hCG supplementation be used? – Against

Siobhan M Quenby and Roy G Farquharson

INTRODUCTION

Human chorionic gonadotropin (hCG) is a glycoprotein composed of two dissimilar subunits: α and β. The α subunit is similar to pituitary gonadotropins, while the β-hCG is very similar to luteinizing hormone (LH). hCG and LH bind to the same receptor in the corpus luteum. Therefore, both maternal LH and embryonic hCG can regulate hormone secretion from the corpus luteum. During the luteal phase of the menstrual cycle, either the corpus luteum undergoes spontaneous regression within about 14 days or, if pregnancy occurs, hCG binds to the LH/hCG receptor and extends its viability. hCG stimulates the corpus luteum to produce a number of different hormones, including estrogens, progestins, relaxins, and inhibin.[1,2] These hormones in turn maintain early pregnancy until the placenta can produce sufficient levels of steroids to support the conceptus. Increasing levels of hCG are secreted by the syncytiotrophoblast of the early placenta, and appear in serum. The rapidly increasing serum levels of hCG are sufficient to maintain the corpus luteum until its functional capacity diminishes at about the 7th week of gestation, after which the corpus luteum regresses. The decline in corpus luteum function is coincident with the shift in progesterone production from the corpus luteum to the placenta, which then produces sufficient steroids to maintain the rest of the pregnancy.[3]

In the human, several sources of evidence demonstrate that hCG is necessary for the maintenance of the corpus luteum. Firstly, the administration of exogenous hCG in the absence of pregnancy has been shown to prolong corpus luteum function, provided that exposure to hCG occurs before the onset of luteal regression, which begins on about the 10th postovulatory day. Secondly, ovariectomy or removal of the corpus luteum before the 8th week of pregnancy causes miscarriage, whereas pregnancy continues independently of corpus luteum function after the 9th week of gestation.[3]

Early pregnancy failure is associated with low serum levels of hCG. Low serum hCG may be due to the death of trophoblast several weeks before expulsion of the conceptus. Robust observational evidence indicates that hCG is critical to early pregnancy and that a lack of hCG is related to miscarriage. Understandably, the attractive theory emerges that there may be a beneficial effect of hCG supplementation in idiopathic recurring pregnancy loss (RPL) and in those women with an 'endocrine cause' for their recurring pregnancy loss. Clearer attention to the type of pregnancy loss is needed, as historical studies contain poor descriptive information, which in turn can lead to ascertainment and reporting bias.[4]

The exogenous administration of hCG is strategically aimed at stimulating progesterone production from the corpus luteum and thereafter the fetoplacental unit. In recurring miscarriage patients, a preconceptual, whole-cycle study of the progesterone profile fails to provide proof that such patients have a suboptimal progesterone rise in the luteal phase. Interestingly, a suboptimal luteal estradiol rise was evident[5] in the oligomenorrheic group.

THE USE OF hCG SUPPLEMENTATION DURING EARLY PREGNANCY

THREATENED MISCARRIAGE

Recent evidence is available from a randomized controlled trial in which hCG supplementation has been used to treat threatened miscarriage and prevent pregnancy loss in 183 women.[6] The study design was robust, based on a prospective, double-blind, placebo-controlled trial. Compared with placebo, the authors clearly demonstrated no benefit from the use of hCG in early pregnancy, with similar miscarriage rates in both treatment groups (11% vs 12%, risk ratio (RR) 1.1, 95% confidence interval (CI) 0.63–1.6).

PREGNANCY FOLLOWING OVULATION INDUCTION

Single-center non-randomized observational studies have reported improved pregnancy outcome when hCG has been used in very early pregnancy.[7] However, in the absence of a prospective randomized controlled trial design, there are clear concerns regarding selection and ascertainment bias that are inherent in all studies of this nature. The authors have focused on the possibility of 'luteal dysfunction' as a primary cause, but fail to define or measure this entity prior to conception.

As with many studies in this area, the mechanism of hCG action in improving outcome or correcting luteal dysfunction is not clearly identified.

RECURRING MISCARRIAGE

In the absence of evidence-based practice, several authors have examined the role of hCG supplementation during early pregnancy in differing clinical scenarios. A well-recognized review has suggested that hCG is not recommended in women with recurring miscarriage, as it is of no proven value,[8] but the same author states that an exception to this rule applies when oligomenorrhea is present prior to conception. A Cochrane review[9] suggested that evidence for the use of hCG treatment in the

prevention of recurrent miscarriage remains inconclusive and that there was insufficient support for its routine use in clinical practice.

A double-blind, placebo-controlled trial examining hCG supplementation has been reported with cases of idiopathic recurring miscarriage.[10] Eighty-one patients were recruited before 6 weeks' gestation, proven by ultrasonography, following their referral. All patients were given supportive therapy, which consisted of review and a reassurance ultrasound scan fortnightly between 6 and 14 weeks in their pregnancy. Patient characteristics showed little difference in the age or number of previous miscarriages between each group of patients in the trial. Unsuccessful pregnancies (total = 15) included ectopic pregnancy (2) and first-trimester (12) and second-trimester (1) miscarriage, and there were no third-trimester intrauterine deaths. In the regular menstrual cycle group, hCG had no beneficial effect on the success rate above that obtained by reassurance and placebo injections (86% vs 86%)(Table 6d.1). The high success rate in the placebo group (86%) reflects the reported benefits of studies of supportive therapy.[11,12] In the subgroup of patients with oligomenorrhea, there was a statistically significant advantage conferred by hCG. Of 13 patients treated with hCG, 11 had a favorable outcome (85%). However, of 10 patients treated with placebo, only 4 had a favorable outcome (40%) (Table 6d.1). A two-tailed Fisher exact test was used to give a p-value of 0.039. hCG elevated the success rate of the oligomenorrheic group to that established in the regular menstrual cycle group (85% vs 86%).

Table 6d.1 Results of a randomized controlled trial of hCG in women with recurrent miscarriage and regular menstrual cycles or oligomenorrhea

	Oligomenorrhea		Regular cycle	
	Placebo	hCG	Placebo	hCG
Miscarriages	6	2	4	4
Live births	4	11	25	25
Success rate	40%	85%	86%	86%
p-value		<0.039		

PLACEBO EFFECT

Prediction of success following idiopathic recurring miscarriage has concentrated the minds of clinicians and empowered patients who have suffered pregnancy loss.[12,13] Previous studies of supportive therapy alone for RPL have observed success rates ranging from 33% to 77%.[11,14] Subsequent pregnancy success is driven mainly by maternal age and number of losses. The average patient is approximately 32 years old and has suffered three consecutive losses. Given these parameters, there is a 75% chance of success in the next pregnancy, irrespective of treatment intervention and relying exclusively on supportive care and ultrasound reassurance every 2 weeks until 12 weeks. However, the figure decreases to 42% for a patient with five miscarriages, aged 45 (see Chapter 19).[12] For any given treatment intervention, this baseline success rate would need to be bettered, which in turn would require a power calculation invoving the largest patient recruitment so far and which would need to outperform existing reported randomized controlled trials.

OTHER hCG TRIALS AND META-ANALYSIS

The efficacy of hCG in early pregnancy had historically been examined in three trials.[15–17] Two found hCG to improve pregnancy outcome[15,16] and one showed no statistically significant benefit.[17] All trials had methodological difficulties. Svigos' series[15] did not use placebo for the control group and gave no details of randomization procedures.

The first Dublin trial[16] consisted of only 20 patients and did not report on the method of blinding or randomization, and the difference in outcome between the two groups was large so as to seem implausible (100% vs 30% success rate). The second Dublin trial[17] stated that some data was lost, as it was controlled by a drug company.

Meta-analysis is a methodological tool that applies statistical methods and scientific strategies to limit bias and to allow appraisal and synthesis of results from relevant studies on a specific topic. The results of the first meta-analysis are held in the electronic Cochrane database of perinatal trials, and this trial has been entered into that database.[9] Table 6d.2 shows the data from the original reports in the Cochrane database.[9] Hence, the figures are slightly different to those in the opposing debate in favor of hCG supplementation. Both versions of the meta-analysis results indicate that hCG may have a beneficial effect upon the risk of miscarriage for all women with a history of recurrent miscarriage, as the confidence interval for the total result does not cross 1 (Table 6d.2). However the overall analysis is greatly influenced by the two earliest studies,[15,16] both of which had significant methodological weaknesses. The confidence intervals for the later two studies[10,17] do cross 1, implying that any improvement could have occurred by chance.

OLIGOMENORRHEA AND RECURRENT MISCARRIAGE

When oligomenorrheic women with recurrent miscarriage are considered independently, hCG does

Table 6d.2 hCG versus placebo for recurrent miscarriage[a]

| Study | Miscarriages per treated pregnancy | | Odds ratio (95% confidence interval) |
	Treatment	Control	
Quenby and Farquharson[10]	6/41	10/39	0.39 (0.13–1.20)
Svigos[15]	1/13	9/15	0.11 (0.02–0.51)
Harrison[16]	0/10	7/10	0.05 (0.01–0.32)
Harrison[17]	6/36	8/31	0.58 (0.18–1.87)
Total	13/95	34/85	0.26 (0.14–0.52)

Between-trial test for heterogeneity; χ^2 (df =3) = 6.46.
[a] Figures quoted are the original figures of the papers in the Cochrane database.[9]

confer a statistically significant reduced risk of miscarriage. However, the Liverpool study is the only trial to differentiate between regular cycles and oligomenorrhea, and the patient numbers (13 in the treatment arm and 10 in the placebo arm) are too small to draw significant conclusions. This observation is underpinned by the Cochrane review.[9]

Further observational data (1994–2000) from the same unit (Figure 6d.1), based on a quasirandomized patient preference basis, shows continued benefit for women with recurrent miscarriage and oligomenorrhea who receive hCG in early pregnancy. The data fail to show significant improvement, but do indicate that some level of benefit may be present for this specific patient group.

We have performed a prospective cohort study investigating the possibility of using elements of the medical history and investigation of women with recurrent miscarriage to predict future pregnancy outcome.[5] We found that oligomenorrhea (infrequent periods more than 35 days apart) was an important risk factor for predicting subsequent miscarriage in this population of women suffering recurrent miscarriage. Further investigation of women

with recurrent miscarriage and oligomenorrhea detected a difference in the hormone profile of these women compared with those with regular menstrual cycles.[5] Hasegawa et al[18] demonstrated that, in a population of 119 consecutive women with spontaneous first-trimester miscarriage, the incidence of oligomenorrhea was over-represented at 11% (compared with 0.9% in the general female population[19]). In the oligomenorrheic women, a normal fetal karyotype was shown in 34%, versus 12.5% ($p < 0.01$) in the women with normal menstrual cycles. Further analysis revealed that, for those women with anembryonic pregnancy and normal karyotype, the incidence of oligomenorrhea was 57%. These results suggest that oligomenorrhea is associated with loss of normal rather than abnormal pregnancies.

OVERVIEW AND CONCLUSIONS

At present, hCG support should not be offered to those women with recurring miscarriage unless oligomenorrhea is present. In the latter group, there is a need for a large prospective randomized

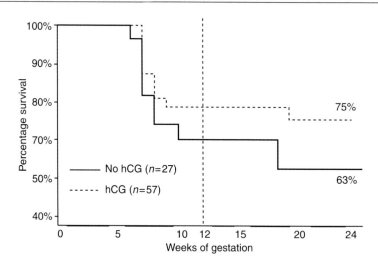

Figure 6d.1 Quasirandomized study of hCG supplementation on pregnancy outcome in 84 patients with oligomenorrhea.

controlled trial of hCG versus placebo in early pregnancy support. A power calculation demands recruitment of 300 women with oligomenorrhea and recurrent miscarriage (150 in each arm) to have an 80% chance of reaching statistical significance at the 5% level. As a result, the trial would need to be multicentered, and is logistically possible, but financially demanding. The use of hCG supplementation should be confined exclusively to the realms of a randomized controlled trial before advocating a potentially beneficial treatment in the early anxious stages of a subsequent pregnancy. Within the parameters of such a trial, adherence to standardized nomenclature[4] and exclusion of abnormal karyotypes are essential.[20,21]

REFERENCES

1. Illingworth PJ, Reddi K, Smith K, et al. Pharmacologic rescue of the corpus luteum results in increased inhibin production. Clin Endocrinol 1990; 33:323–32.
2. Duncan WC, McNeilly AS, Fraser HM, et al. Luteinising hormone receptor in the human corpus luteum: lack of down-regulation during maternal recognition of pregnancy. Hum Reprod 1996; 11:2291–7.
3. Csapo AI, Pulkkinen MO, Rutner B, et al. The significance of human corpus luteum function in pregnancy maintenance. Am J Obstet Gynecol 1972; 112:1061–7.
4. Farquharson RG, Jauniaux E, Exalto N. Updated and revised nomenclature for description of early pregnancy events. Hum Reprod 2005; 20:3008–11.
5. Quenby SM, Farquharson RG. Predicting recurring miscarriage: What is important? Obstet Gynecol 1993; 82:132–8.
6. Qureshi NS, Edi-osagie EC, Ogbo V, et al. First trimester threatened miscarriage treatment with human chorionic gonadotrophins: a randomised controlled trial. Br J Obstet Gynaecol 2005; 112:1536–41.
7. Blumenfeld Z, Ruach M. Early pregnancy wastage: the role of repetitive human chorionic gonadotrophin supplementation during the first 8 weeks of pregnancy. Fertil Steril 1992; 58:19–23.
8. Li TC. Guide for practitioners: recurrent miscarriage: principles of management. Hum Reprod 1998; 13: 478–82.
9. Scott JR, Pattison N. Human chorionic gonadotrophin for recurrent miscarriage. Cochrane Database Syst Rev 2000; (2):CD000101.
10. Quenby SM, Farquharson RG. Human chorionic gonadotrophin supplementation in recurring pregnancy loss: a controlled trial. Fertil Steril 1994; 62:708–10.
11. Liddell HS, Pattison NS, Zanderigo A. Recurrent miscarriage outcome after supportive care in early pregnancy. Aust NZ J Obstet Gynaecol 1991; 31:3202.
12. Brigham SA, Conlon C, Farquharson RG. A longitudinal study of pregnancy outcome following idiopathic recurring miscarriage. Hum Reprod 1999; 14:2868–71.
13. Kavalier F. Investigation of recurrent miscarriages. BMJ 2005; 331:121–2.
14. Stray Pedersen B, Stray Pedersen S. Etiological factors and subsequent obstetric performance in 195 couples with a prior history of habitual abortion. Am J Obstet Gynecol 1983; 148:140–6.
15. Svigos J. Preliminary experience with the use of human chorionic gonadotrophin therapy in women with repeated abortion. Clin Reprod Fertil 1982; 1:131–5.
16. Harrison RF. Treatment of habitual abortion with human chorionic gonadotropin: results of open and placebo-controlled studies. Eur J Obstet Gynecol Reprod Biol 1985; 20:159–68.
17. Harrison RF. Human chorionic gonadotrophin (hCG) in the management of recurrent abortion: results of a multi-centre placebo controlled study. Eur J Obstet Gynaecol 1992; 47:175–9.
18. Hasegawa I, Takakuwa K, Tanaka K. The roles of oligomenorrhoea and fetal chromosomal abnormalities in spontaneous abortion. Hum Reprod 1996; 11:2304–5.
19. Munster K, Schmidt L, Helm P. Length and variation in the menstrual cycle: a cross-sectional study from a Danish county. Br J Obstet Gynaecol 1992; 99:422–9.
20. Morikawa M, Yamada H, Kato EH, et al. Embryo loss pattern is predominant in miscarriages with normal chromosome karyotype among women with repeated miscarriage. Hum Reprod 2004; 19:2644–7.
21. Stephenson MD, Awartini KA, Robinson WP. Cytogenetic analysis of miscarriages from couples with recurring miscarriage: a case–control study. Hum Reprod 2002; 17: 446–51.

7. Antiphospholipid syndrome – pathophysiology

Gilad Twig, Yaniv Sherer, Miri Blank, and Yehuda Shoenfeld

INTRODUCTION

Antiphospholipid syndrome (APS) was first defined as a syndrome in 1983,[1] consisting of a triad of manifestations involving arterial and/or venous thrombosis, recurrent fetal loss, accompanied by mild to moderate thrombocytopenia and elevated titers of antiphospholipid (aPL) antibodies: lupus anticoagulant (LA) and/or anticardiolipin antibodies (aCL). Today, this syndrome is known to be systemic and may affect almost every organ and tissue in the body. The cause of APS is still considered a mystery – yet, as in many other autoimmune diseases, a combination of environmental and genetic factors has been proposed. Recent data indicate that infectious agents may play a major role in the etiology of APS. The pathophysiology of APS includes all arms of the coagulation system, as well as other mechanisms not related to hypercoagulability. In fact, aPL have been shown to be directly toxic to the developing fetus, as these antibodies can be passively transferred from humans to naive mice and will induce pregnancy loss in those mice[2] (Figure 7.1). Active immunization with human pathogenic monoclonal anticardiolipin antibody induces clinical manifestations of APS in BALB/c mice.[3] Additionally, the serum from women with APS is highly teratogenic to rat embryos in culture and also affects embryonic growth.[4] Moreover, purification of the immunoglobulin G (IgG) fraction of the sera of women with APS directly affects the embryo and yolk sac, reducing their growth.[5] This chapter discusses the etiology and pathophysiology of APS, with special emphasis on the reproductive system.

ETIOLOGY OF APS

aPL have long been known to require a cofactor in order to have their effects. Today this co-factor (apolipoprotein H or β_2-glycoprotein I (β_2GPI)) is thought to be the antigen to which aPL bind. Binding of aPL to β_2GPI forms divalent IgG–β_2GPI complexes that have increased affinity for membrane phospholipids.[6] The physiological function of β_2GPI is unknown. β_2GPI deficiency is not associated with disease; homozygous β_2GPI-null mice also appear to suffer no pathological effects.[7] The binding of aPL–β_2GPI to cell membranes, including trophoblasts, results in injury and/or activation. Like many other autoimmune diseases, APS may have a multifactorial etiology in which genetic susceptibility is made apparent by environmental factors.

One environmental factor that has been intensively investigated in recent years is infection. In a series of 100 APS patients,[8] various infections were shown to precede the development of APS, including skin infections (18%), human immunodeficiency virus (HIV) (17%), pneumonia (14%), hepatitis C virus (13%), and urinary tract infection (10%). *Helicobacter pylori*, a common bacterial pathogen that colonizes the gastric mucosa and induces chronic gastric inflammation, has been associated with APS. In pregnant women, *H. pylori* infection can cause intrauterine fetal growth retardation,[9] and increases the risk of reproductive disorders.[10] Molecular mimicry between (β_2GPI) and bacterial and viral epitopes is the principal mechanism that links infections to APS. In the case of *H. pylori*, 34% of patients were positive for anti-β_2GPI antibodies that showed high homology to the

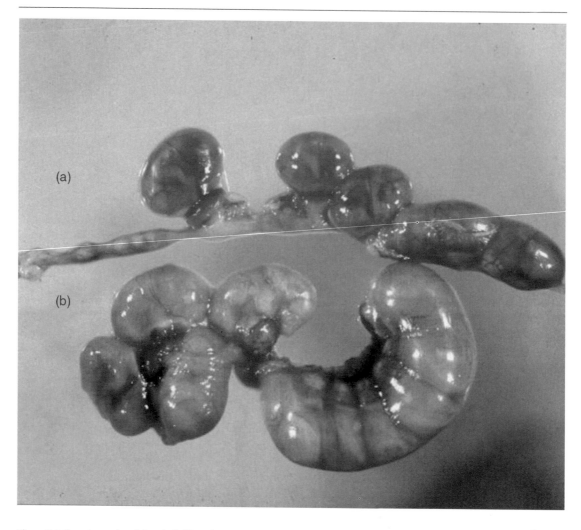

Figure 7.1 Experimental antiphospholipid syndrome (APS). (a) APS uterine horn showing resorbed pregnancies and live fetuses at day 14 of pregnancy. (b) Control uterine horn showing developing pregnancies with no resorptions at day 14.

target epitopes of *H. pylori* structures.[11,12] Indeed, β_2GPI has been found to be immunogenic in vivo. Immunization of BALB/c or PL/J mice or New Zealand white rabbits with β_2GPI resulted in generation of anti-β_2GPI antibodies.[13] The high titers of mouse anti-β_2GPI antibodies has been associated with an increased proportion of fetal resorptions (the equivalent of fetal loss in humans), thrombocytopenia, and prolonged activated partial thromboplastin time (aPTT), indicating the presence of LA, a presentation characteristic of experimental APS.[13]

Direct experimental evidence for molecular mimicry of bacterial pathogens has emerged from the effect of immunization with certain microbial pathogens that share epitope homology with the β_2GPI molecule. Pathogenic anti-β_2GPI auto-antibodies directed against the TLRVYK epitope were formed in mice immunized with *Haemophilus influenzae* or *Neisseria gonorrhoeae* that exhibit the TLRVYK sequence, or with tetanus toxoid that does not present linearly the sequence TLRVYK but can still serve as a mimotope. The formed anti-β_2GPI autoantibodies have been shown to be pathogenic and capable of inducing the clinical picture of experimental APS, manifested by a high percentage of fetal loss, thrombocytopenia, and a prolonged aPTT.[14] Moreover, the pathogenic effect of monoclonal antibodies to β_2GPI is inhibited by the addition of synthetic peptides including the TLRVYK sequence. The latter prevented the development of APS in mice injected with monoclonal antibodies to β_2GPI, or decreased the degree of endothelial cell activation, monocyte adhesion, and expression of adhesion molecules in vitro.[15] Infection may be one of the mechanisms giving rise to APS. In humans, infection with varicella zoster virus (VZV) has been associated with APS.[16] Although HIV, hepatitis A, hepatitis B, and hepatitis C are also associated with an increased prevalence of aCL antibodies, most of these are not β_2GPI-dependent.[17] The difference between APS and the mere presence of aPL may be due to diseases such as syphilis and Lyme disease raising antibodies that recognize phospholipids directly, whereas in APS the infections raise antibodies that recognize epitopes on phospholipid-binding proteins such as β_2GPI.

MECHANISMS OF REPRODUCTIVE FAILURE IN APS

THROMBOSIS

As mentioned above, systemic thromboembolism is the principal manifestation of APS. Evidence for thrombi in the placental circulation and the beneficial effect of antithrombotic therapy in APS patients suffering from recurrent pregnancy loss (RPL) suggest a central role for this mechanism in reproductive failure. The underlying basis for the hypercoagulable state in APS is complex, and involves altered activity of all three major components that govern hemostasis: platelets, fibrinolysis, and the coagulation cascade. The coagulation system in APS

was shown to be altered at different levels. aPL inhibit both protein C activation and the function of activated protein C (APC), thereby preventing the inactivation of activated factors V and VIII.[18] This inhibition is conditional upon the presence of β_2GPI which is a pre-requisite for the binding of aPL to protein C. In addition, autoantibodies directed against protein C, protein S, and thrombomodulin have been detected in some APS patients.[19]

Tissue factor (TF), an initiator of the extrinsic coagulation cascade, which is not normally expressed by intravascular cells, has been shown to be altered in APS patients. It has been shown that TF-related procoagulant activity and TF mRNA levels in monocytes are increased in primary APS patients with thrombosis when compared with those without thrombosis.[20] Injection of purified IgG aCL from APS patients with previous thrombotic episodes induced a significant increase in both monocyte procoagulant activity and TF expression, as compared with purified IgG or IgM aCL from two systemic lupus erythematosus (SLE) patients without thrombosis.[21] In addition, functional anti-TF pathway inhibitor activity has been detected in the sera of a subset of APS patients, showing a correlation between the degree of inhibition and associated occurrence of arterial thrombosis and stroke.[22]

Endothelial cells are affected by aPL autoantibodies. Potentiation of human umbilical vein endothelial cells (HUVEC) procoagulant activity by aPL contained in sera from SLE patients is strongly decreased after depleting IgG from the sera.[23] Human anti-β_2GPI IgM monoclonal antibodies and polyclonal anti-β_2GPI antibodies have been shown to induce tissue factor at both protein and mRNA level in HUVEC monolayers in vitro.[24] aPL can further up-regulate adhesion molecules (E-selectin, intercellular adhesion molecule 1 (ICAM-1) and vascular cell adhesion molecule 1 (VCAM-1)) expression and secretion of the proinflammatory cytokines interleukin-1b (IL-1b) and IL-6.[25] Increased plasma levels of soluble VCAM-1 have been found in primary APS patients with recurrent thrombotic events, and elevated levels of tissue plasminogen activator and von Willebrand factor (vWF) (as endothelial perturbation markers) have been associated with aPL in SLE.

Decreased endothelial cell prostacyclin (PGI$_2$), the principal inhibitor of platelet aggregation, and increased thromboxane A$_2$ (TXA$_2$) production by platelets have both been implicated as mechanisms predisposing to thrombosis in patients with APS. aPL enhance platelet TXA$_2$ production, and allow platelet activation to occur without a compensatory increment in the vascular biosynthesis of PGI$_2$.[26]

Hypofibrinolysis can further aggravate the prothrombotic state in APS. Endothelial cell dysfunction can increase plasma levels of plasminogen activator inhibitor type-1 (PAI-1) and tissue-type plasminogen activator (tPA) antigens.[27] In addition the hypofibrinolytic state can be further aggravated by the presence of autoantibodies against components of the fibrinolytic system such as as anti-plasmin/plasminogen[28] and anti-tPA.[29]

Platelets play a central role in primary hemostasis and are involved in the prothrombotic state of APS patients. Monoclonal aCL obtained from patients with APS increased platelet interaction with the subendothelium.[21] It has been proposed that a minor degree of platelet activation can lead to exposure of phospholipids, which can potentially be amplified to a much larger degree in the serum of APS patient than in controls.[21] β$_2$GPI initially binds to these phospholipids, then binds aPL to form β$_2$GPI–phospholipid complexes. The latter can further activate platelet aggregation by allowing the interaction between the Fc portion and the platelet surface FcγRII receptors (the only FcγR molecules present on platelets).[21,30] In addition to activation of the FcγRII receptors, the β$_2$GPI–phospholipid complexes can also exert their action through complement activation, as complement generated in the presence of aPL binds to negatively charged phospholipids and activates platelets.[31]

In addition to the systemic prothrombotic effects, APS autoantibodies may alter the placental circulation by attacking certain placental epitopes. Annexin A5, a potent anticoagulant protein that has a thrombomodulatory role in the placental circulation, is such a target.[32] Annexin V is found on the apical surface of placental syncytiotrophoblasts, and forms clusters on exposed phospholipids, thereby forming a protective shield on the phospholipid surface. Annexin V blocks phospholipids from becoming available for coagulation reactions. The annexin V protective shield could be damaged by either binding to anti-annexin V or preventing its binding to the phospholipid membrane, or by blocking autoantibodies against annexin V/phospholipids.[33] Anti-annexin V autoantibodies have been detected in patients with SLE and APS associated with pregnancy loss, while reduced levels of annexin V have been observed on the placental villi of women having aPL and RPL and a thrombogenic background.[34]

Recently, complement activation was reported as essential and causative of APL-induced fetal injury. Treatment with heparin prevented this activation both in-vivo and in-vitro.[35]

ARACHIDONIC ACID AND PROSTACYCLIN

aPL inhibit arachidonic acid release.[36] Arachidonic acid is an essential prerequisite for PGI$_2$ production (PGI$_2$ is a physiological inhibitor of thrombocyte aggregation, and a potent vasodilatator). aPL have been shown to increase the concentration of TXA$_2$, thus altering the PGI$_2$/ TXA$_2$ balance.[37] The alteration in the PGI$_2$/TXA$_2$ balance has two effects: vasoconstriction, which impedes the blood supply to the fetus, and platelet activation, with the procoagulant effects described above.

In a mouse model of experimental APS, Shoenfeld and Blank[38] infused aCL into pregnant mice in order to induce APS. Mice that were cotreated with a thromboxane receptor antagonist had a significant reduction in the fetal resorption rate from 45% to 19.8% and an increase in mean placental and embryo weights. There was also an increased platelet count (from 597 100 to 1 075 000 platelets/mm^3) in treated mice, indicating the effect of thrombocyte aggegation in APS.

ANTICYTOKINE EFFECT

The anti-inflammatory cytokine IL-3 is important for the maintenance of normal pregnancy. IL-3 enhances placental and fetal development while increasing the number of megakaryoctes. The serum level of IL-3 in pregnant patients with primary APS or APS secondary to SLE was found to be lower than in controls.[39] In vitro studies have revealed that low-dose aspirin (10 mg/μl) stimulates IL-3 production through its ability to raise leukotriene production, while higher doses of aspirin failed to induce IL-3 generation.[39,40] Furthermore, ciprofloxacin treatment significantly decreased the rate of pregnancy loss in BALB/c mice with experimental APS. This effect correlated with an increases in the serum IL-3 level and in bone marrow megakaryocytes.[41] Other cytokines may also be involved. The level of the proinflammatory and prothrombotic cytokine tumor necrosis factor α (TNF-α), has been shown to be significantly higher in patients with APS than in healthy controls.[42]

INDUCTION OF PLACENTAL CELL APOPTOSIS

Most the literature describes placental pathology in terms of aPL being directed against negatively charged phospholipids, leading to placental infarction and eventually pregnancy loss. aPL may affect the adhesion molecules between the elements of the syncytiotrophoblast. Cellular activation increases the expression of cell adhesion molecules,[43,44] which may promote leukocyte adhesion to the endothelial surface. Although the thrombogenic effects of aPL are mediated by ICAM-1, VCAM-1, and P-selectin,[45] aPL may damage the trophoblast in a manner unrelated to thrombosis, as the cytotrophoblast cells express phospholipid on their surface. This concept is supported by histological evidence from patients with aPL and fetal death. Women with aPL have decreased vasculosyncitial membranes, increased syncytial knots, and substantially more fibrosis, hypovascular villi, and infarcts than women without APS.[46] The changes in syncytial membranes may be secondary to thrombosis, but thrombosis could also be secondary to placental damage that allows free transplacental passage of maternal aPL. Addition of IgG purified from women with SLE/APS, positive for aCL/anti-DNA antibodies, reduced yolk sac and embryonic growth more than sera negative for aPL but positive for anti-phosphatidylserine and anti-laminin.[47] The sera of SLE/APS patients has

also been shown to inhibit the rate of trophoblastic cell growth and to accelerate the rate of apoptosis of cultured human placental cells.[47,48]

aPL can alter the secretion of human chorionic gonadotropin (hCG). Our team has shown that the addition of human polyclonal purified aCL, which were shown to induce experimental APS, suppressed the pulsatile secretion of hCG.[49] In vitro, monoclonal aPL halved trophoblastic hCG and human phospholipid production.[50] These results may be secondary to the effect of aPL on trophoblast differentiation and invasion.

aPL do not seem to be teratogenic to the embryo, however. The offspring of SLE/APS patients do not have a higher rate of anomalies, although the pregnancies are often complicated by intrauterine growth retardation.[51]

CONCLUSIONS

APS is a systemic syndrome whose etiology involves both environmental and genetic factors. Infections may be highly important in the etiology of this syndrome, and molecular mimicry is probably the mechanism by which infectious agents induce aPL. aPL exert their pathogenic effects via various mechanisms, including the induction of a hypercoagulable state. Indeed, therapy of APS is usually directed towards eliminating the enhanced thrombosis. In RPL, the combination of low-molecular-weight heparin and low-dose aspirin is considered to be the treatment of choice. However, when therapy fails, other interventions aimed at controlling the levels of autoantibodies rather than their effects should be considered, as other mechanisms involving autoantibodies are also important in APS. Hence, immunomodulation might theoretically block some of the more detrimental effects of aPL rather than anticoagulant therapy alone.

ACKNOWLEDGMENTS

This study was supported in part by the Federico Foundation Ernesto Hecht Research Grant (to Y Sherer).

REFERENCES

1. Hughes GR. Thrombosis, abortion, cerebral disease, and the lupus anticoagulant. BMJ 1983; 287:1088–9.

2. Blank M, Cohen J, Toder V, et al, Induction of anti-phospholipid syndrome in naive mice with mouse lupus monoclonal and human polyclonal anti-cardiolipin antibodies. Proc Natl Acad Sci USA. 1991; 88:3069–73.

3. Bakimer R, Fishman P, Blank M, et al. Induction of primary anti-phospholipid syndrome in mice by immunization with a human monoclonal anticardiolipin antibody (H-3). J Clin Invest 1992; 89:1558–63.

4. Ornoy A, Yacobi S, Avraham S, et al. The effect of sera from women with SLE and/or antiphospholipid syndrome on rat embryos in culture. Reprod Toxicol 1998; 12:185–91.

5. Ornoy A, Yacobi S, Tartakover Matalon S, et al. The effects of antiphospholipid antibodies obtained from women with SLE APS and associated pregnancy loss on rat embryos and placental explants in culture. Lupus 2003; 12:573–8.

6. Rand JH. The antiphospholipid syndrome. Annu Rev Med 2003; 54:409–24.

7. Sheng Y, Reddel SW, Herzog H, et al. Impaired thrombin generation in β_2-glycoprotein I null mice. J Biol Chem 2001; 276:13817–21.

8. Cervera R, Asherson RA, Acevedo ML, et al. Antiphospholipid syndrome associated with infections: clinical and microbiological characteristics of 100 patients. Ann Rheum Dis 2004: 63:1312–17.

9. Eslick GD, Yan P, Xia HH, et al. Foetal intrauterine growth restrictions with *Helicobacter pylori* infection. Aliment Pharmacol Ther 2002: 16:1677–82.

10. Figura N, Piomboni P, Ponzetto A, et al. *Helicobacter pylori* infection and infertility. Eur J Gastroenterol Hepatol 2002: 14:663–9.

11. Sorice M, Pittoni V, Griggi T, et al. Specificity of anti-phospholipid antibodies in infectious mononucleosis: a role for anti-cofactor protein antibodies. Clin Exp Immunol 2000; 120:301–6.

12. Blank M, Shoenfeld Y. β_2-Glycoprotein-I, infections, antiphospholipid syndrome and therapeutic considerations. Clin Immunol 2004; 112:190–9.

13. Blank M, Faden D, Tincani A, et al. Immunization with anticardiolipin cofactor (β_2-glycoprotein I) induces experimental antiphospholipid syndrome in naive mice. J Autoimmun 1994; 7:441–55.

14. Blank M, Krause I, Fridkin M, et al. Bacterial induction of autoantibodies to β_2-glycoprotein-I accounts for the infectious etiology of antiphospholipid syndrome. J Clin Invest 2002; 109:797–804.

15. Blank M, Shoenfeld Y, Cabilly S, et al. Prevention of experimental antiphospholipid syndrome and endothelial cell activation by synthetic peptides. Proc Natl Acad Sci USA 1999; 96:5164–8.

16. Manco Johnson MJ, Nuss R, Key N, et al. Lupus anticoagulant and protein S deficiency in children with postvaricella purpura fulminans or thrombosis. J Pediatr 1996; 128:319–23.

17. Guglielmone H, Vitozzi S, Elbarcha O, et al. Cofactor dependence and isotype distribution of anticardiolipin antibodies in viral infections. Ann Rheum Dis 2001; 60:500–4.

18. de Groot PG, Horbach DA, Derksen RH. Protein C and other cofactors involved in the binding of antiphospholipid antibodies: relation to the pathogenesis of thrombosis. Lupus 1996; 5:488–93.

19. Pengo V, Biasiolo A, Brocco T, et al. Autoantibodies to phospholipid-binding plasma proteins in patients with thrombosis and phospholipid-reactive antibodies. Thromb Haemost 1996; 75:721–4.

20. Cuadrado MJ, Lopez-Pedrera C, Khamashta MA, et al. Thrombosis in primary antiphospholipid syndrome: a pivotal role for monocyte tissue factor expression. Arthritis Rheum 1997; 40:834–41.

21. Reverter JC, Tassies D, Font J, et al. Effects of human monoclonal anticardiolipin antibodies on platelet function and on tissue factor expression on monocytes. Arthritis Rheum 1998; 41:1420–7.

22. Forastiero RR, Martinuzzo ME, Broze GJ. High titers of autoantibodies to tissue factor pathway inhibitor are associated with the antiphospholipid syndrome. J Thromb Haemost 2003: 1:718–24.

23. Oosting JD, Derksen RH, Blokzijl L, et al. Antiphospholipid antibody positive sera enhance endothelial cell procoagulant activity – studies in a thrombosis model. Thromb Haemost 1992; 68:278–84.

24. Kornberg A, Renaudineau Y, Blank M, et al. Anti-β_2-glycoprotein I antibodies and anti-endothelial cell antibodies induce tissue factor in endothelial cells. Isr Med Assoc J 2000; 2(Suppl):27–31.

25. Meroni PL, Raschi E, Camera M, et al. Endothelial activation by aPL: a potential pathogenetic mechanism for the clinical manifestations of the syndrome. J Autoimmun 2000: 15:237–40.

26. Lellouche F, Martinuzzo M, Said P, et al. Imbalance of thromboxane/prostacyclin biosynthesis in patients with lupus anticoagulant. Blood 1991; 78:2894–9.

27. Jurado M, Paramo JA, Gutierrez-Pimentel M, et al. Fibrinolytic potential and antiphospholipid antibodies in systemic lupus erythematosus and other connective tissue disorders. Thromb Haemost 1992; 68:516–20.

28. Yang CD, Hwang KK, Yan W, et al. Identification of anti-plasmin antibodies in the antiphospholipid syndrome that inhibit degradation of fibrin. J Immunol 2004; 172:5765–73.

29. Cugno M, Cabibbe M, Galli M, et al. Antibodies to tissue-type plasminogen activator (tPA) in patients with antiphospholipid syndrome: evidence of interaction between the antibodies and the catalytic domain of tPA in 2 patients. Blood 2004; 103:2121–4.

30. Font J, Espinosa G, Tassies D, et al. Effects of β_2-glycoprotein I and monoclonal anticardiolipin antibodies in platelet interaction with subendothelium under flow conditions. Arthritis Rheum 2002; 46:3283–9.

31. Shibata S, Sasaki T, Hirabayashi Y, et al. Risk factors in the pregnancy of patients with systemic lupus erythematosus: association of hypocomplementaemia with poor prognosis. Ann Rheum Dis 1992; 51:619–23.

32. Wang X, Campos B, Kaetzel MA, et al. Annexin V is critical in the maintenance of murine placental integrity. Am J Obstet Gynecol 1999: 180:1008–16.

33. Rand JH, Wu XX, Andree HA, et al. Pregnancy loss in the antiphospholipid-antibody syndrome – a possible thrombogenic mechanism. N Engl J Med 1997; 337:154–60.

34. Matsubayashi H, Arai T, Izumi S, et al. Anti-annexin V antibodies in patients with early pregnancy loss or implantation failures. Fertil Steril 2001; 76:694–9.

35. Girardi G, Redecha P, Salmon JE. Heparin prevents antiphospholipid antibody-induced fetal loss by inhibiting complement activation. Nat Med 2004; 10:1222–6.

36. Carreras LO, Vermylen JG. 'Lupus' anticoagulant and thrombosis – possible role of inhibition of prostacyclin formation. Thromb Haemost 1982; 48:38–40.

37. Robbins DL, Leung S, Miller-Blair DJ, et al. Effect of anticardiolipin/β_2-glycoprotein I complexes on production of thromboxane A2 by platelets from patients with the antiphospholipid syndrome. J Rheumatol 1998; 25:51–6.

38 Shoenfeld Y, Blank M. Effect of long-acting thromboxane receptor antagonist (BMS 180,291) on experimental antiphospholipid syndrome. Lupus 1994; 3:397–400.

39. Fishman P, Falach-Vaknin E, Sredni B, et al. Aspirin–interleukin-3 interrelationships in patients with anti-phospholipid syndrome. Am J Reprod Immunol 1996; 35:80–4.

40. Fishman P, Falach-Vaknin E, Sredni B, et al. Aspirin modulates inter-leukin-3 production: additional explanation for the preventive effects of aspirin in antiphospholipid antibody syndrome. J Rheumatol 1995; 22:1086–90.

41. Blank M, George J, Fishman P, et al. Ciprofloxacin immunomo-dulation of experimental antiphospholipid syndrome associated with elevation of interleukin-3 and granulocyte–macrophage colony-stimulating factor expression. Arthritis Rheum 1998; 41:224–32.

42. Bertolaccini ML, Atsumi T, Lanchbury JS, et al. Plasma tumor necrosis factor α levels and the 238A promoter polymorphism in patients with antiphospholipid syndrome. Thromb Haemost 2001; 85:198–203.

43. Simantov R, LaSala JM, Lo SK, et al. Activation of cultured vascular endothelial cells by antiphospholipid antibodies. J Clin Invest 1995; 96:2211–19.

44. Meroni PL, Raschi E, Camera M, et al. Endothelial activation by aPL: a potential pathogenetic mechanism for the clinical manifestations of the syndrome. J Autoimmun 2000; 15:237–40.

45. Pierangeli SS, Espinola RG, Liu X, et al. Thrombogenic effects of antiphospholipid antibodies are mediated by intercellular cell adhe-sion molecule-1, vascular cell adhesion molecule-1, and P-selectin. Circ Res 2001; 88:245–50.

46. Out HJ, Kooijman CD, Bruinse HW, et al. Histo-pathological findings from patients with intrauterine fetal death and antiphospholipid antibodies. Eur J Obstet Gynecol 1991; 41:179–86.

47. Ornoy A, Yacobi S, Matalon ST, et al. The effects of antiphospholipid antibodies obtained from women with SLE/APS and associated preg-nancy loss on rat embryos and placental explants in culture. Lupus 2003; 12:573–8.

48. Matalon ST, Shoenfeld Y, Blank M, et al. Antiphosphatidylserine antibodies affect rat yolk sacs in culture: a mechanism for fetal loss in antiphospholipid syndrome. Am J Reprod Immunol 2004; 51:144–51.

49. Shurtz-Swirski R, Inbar O, Blank M, et al. In vitro effect of anti-cardiolipin autoantibodies upon total and pulsatile placental hCG secretion during early pregnancy. Am J Reprod Immunol 1993; 29:206–10.

50. Katsuragawa H, Kanzaki H, Inoue T, et al. Monoclonal antibody against phosphatidylserine inhibits in vitro human trophoblastic hormone production and invasion. Biol Reprod 1997; 56:50–8.

51. Bernstein PS, Divon MY. Etiologies of fetal growth restriction. Clin Obstet Gynecol 1997; 40:723–9.

8. Diagnosis of aPL-associated abortions

Marighoula Varla-Leftherioti

Antiphospholipid antibodies (aPL) are a heterogeneous group of autoantibodies directed against different antigens, predominantly anionic phospholipids or phospholipid-containing structures. aPL have been associated with pregnancy disorders, including spontaneous miscarriage, recurrent miscarriage, pregnancy-induced hypertension, preeclampsia, and intrauterine growth retardation. aPL can be detected using sensitive solid-phase immunoassays or coagulation tests. Both assays are easy to perform, but care is required in the selection of the appropriate tests and in interpretation of the results. In order to distinguish between those women at risk of abortion and those not at risk, it is important to consider the following parameters: (a) the assays to be used, (b) the type and (c) the isotype of aPL to be identified, (d) the antibody level to be evaluated, (e) the interpretation of the results in relation to the heterogeneity of aPL and clinical data, and (f) the timing for testing.

ASSAYS FOR THE DETECTION OF aPL

aPL that do not prolong phospholipid-dependent clotting assays can be detected by immunoassays using phospholipid-coated surfaces. Hence, antibodies against cardiolipin (aCL), phosphatidylethanolamine (aPE), phosphatidylserine (aPS), phosphatodylcholine (aPC), phosphatidylglycerol (aPG), phosphatidylinositol (aPI), phosphatidic acid (aPA), and β_2-glycoprotein I (aβ_2GPI) must be identified by standardized enzyme-linked immunosorbent assays (ELISA) using surfaces coated with the relevant phospholipid (usually complexed with cofactor proteins). The results are expressed in aPL units, with 1 unit being equivalent to the binding capacity of 1 μg/ml pure phospholipid. Depending on their immunoglobulin isotype (IgG, IgM, or IgA), aPL units are defined as GPL, MPL, and APL units. For the results to be reliable, the assays must be properly standardized, standard calibrators must be used, and the range of normal values must derive from measurements of aPL levels in a large number of normal individuals.[1]

For the detection of aPL that prolong phospholipid-dependent clotting assays (lupus anticoagulant, LA) clotting time prolongation assays are used, in which prolongation of clotting is not corrected with normal plasma, but with the addition of phospholipids. These tests include the activated partial thromboplastin time (aPTT), the diluted Russell's viper venom time (dRVVT), and the kaolin clotting time (KCT).[2]

TYPE OF aPL

Classically, the workup for the diagnosis of aPL-associated abortions was limited to the detection of LA (prolongation of at least one phospholipid-dependent clotting assay) and the detection of β_2GPI-dependent IgG and IgM aCL antibodies in the serum (aCL-IgG >20 GPL units/ml or/and aCL-IgM >20 MPL units/ml). LA and increased aCL-IgG antibodies are independently associated with recurrent first- and second-trimester fetal loss and can be used as prognostic and diagnostic markers.[3] It has been reported that women positive for LA or aCL have a 16% and 38% rate of pregnancy loss, respectively.[4,5]

It has recently become apparent that, although extremely useful, the diagnostic tests for LA and aCL may not be sufficient for diagnosing all patients with aPL-associated pregnancy loss or to elucidate the underlying pathology. A percentage of women experiencing recurrent miscarriages may be negative for aCL but positive for other aPL.

Several studies have shown that if only aCL are measured, 10–63% of positive APL are detected and 37–90% of women with reproductive autoimmune failure syndrome (RAFS) will have the diagnosis missed.[6–8] Although aPL other than LA and aCL have not been shown to be causative of pregnancy loss,[9] it has been suggested that, at least for the diagnosis of RAFS-related abortions, a full aPL panel should be measured (LA, aCL, aPE, aPS, aPC, aPG, aPI, aPA, and aβ_2GPI).[10] The diagnostic and prognostic value of some of these antibodies has been well documented. It has been shown that the trophoblastic layer directly in contact with the maternal circulation is more reactive with aPS than aCL,[11] and that the aPS assay is more sensitive than the aCL assay for identifying women with autoimmune abortions.[12] The presence of IgG and IgM aPE antibodies also appears to be a risk factor for early fetal losses (because of their effect on trophoblast formation) as well as for mid-to-late pregnancy loss (due to binding to PE–kininogen complexes, which results in thrombin-induced platelet aggregation).[13]

Studies in women with recurrent miscarriage, not receiving anticoagulation, have shown that LA is mainly associated with second- rather than first-trimester abortions.[14] Moreover, the presence of aCL in the absence of LA most likely reduces the chance of live birth by 36–48% compared with the absence of both aCL and LA,[15] while the detection of aCL before gestation or an increase during pregnancy are considered as bad prognostic markers for the outcome of pregnancy.[16] Measurement of aPS and aPE is indicated in women with early recurrent pregnancy loss (RPL), since they represent those aPL that affect cell division during embryogenesis and the normal function of the trophoblast.[17] The roles of other aPL (e.g., aPC, aPG, aPA, and aPI) and antibodies against cofactor proteins are less clear, but they have been reported to have diagnostic significance. Some studies have shown a predominance of aPC, aPG, aPA, and aPI in women with recurrent spontaneous abortion (RSA),[18–20] while antibodies against cofactor proteins (prothrombin and annexin V) have also been reported to be more significant in reproductive failure than aCL alone.[21] Anti-β_2GPI testing does not seem to identify additional patients with RSA who had initial negative tests for aCL (possibly because of the strong correlation between the two autoantibodies).[22] Finally, the presence of more than one aPL appears to be a more accurate variable than the presence of one aPL in predicting pregnancy loss.[23]

ISOTYPE OF aPL

Most aPL are of the IgG or IgM class, but a small proportion (10%) may be IgA. Some studies report a predominance of IgG antibodies in women with repeated miscarriages,[18] while others have found that the majority of aPL are of the IgM isotype.[24] In a recent study, positivity for IgM aCL was found to show a stronger correlation to pregnancy outcome than IgG aCL positivity.[15] Abortion occurs more often in the presence of both IgG and IgM antibodies than in the presence of one isotype alone. Hence, in order to avoid misdiagnosis and obtain helpful information, testing should include at least the detection of both IgG and IgM antibodies.

TITER OF aPL

Since low levels of aPL may be found in otherwise-normal women, low titers detected in women with repeated miscarriages cannot be considered as risk factors for aPL-associated abortions (above the risk conferred by their medical history), and are of doubtful clinical significance.[25] In contrast, medium and high titers of aCL and/or other aPL antibodies (>40 GPL units) identify the women who would benefit from pharmacological prophylaxis in the next pregnancy. Eighty percent of women with very high levels of aCL (>80 GPL) and a history of previous miscarriage(s) are expected to have fetal death in their next pregnancy.[26]

HETEROGENEITY OF aPL

Depending on their type, aPL group members affect pregnancy by acting through different pathways.

aCL, aPE, and aPS target relevant phospholipids on endothelial cells and lead to thrombosis in placental vessels. However, aPE and aPS also target relevant phospholipids on the trophoblast and affect the formation of the syncytium. Furthermore, these antibodies and the aPC, aPG, and aPI target relevant phospholipids in pre-embryonic tissues.[27] The above data must be taken into account in the workup. In second-trimester abortions where thromboses have been found in the placental material of previously missed abortions, it is advisable to test for antibodies with anticoagulant effect on the endothelium (aCL, aPS, and aPE), as there may be classical antiphospholipid syndrome (APS), while in women with early pregnancy and pre-embryonic losses, the work up should include aPL inhibiting trophoblastic cell function (aPS and aPE) and possibly those affecting implantation (aPS, aPE, aPC, aPI, aPG, and aPA).

TIME OF TESTING

Finally, since aPL may appear transiently in normal individuals,[28] it is recommended that in order to establish the diagnosis of aPL-associated abortions, increased titers of aPL must be present in the serum in two measurements with an interval of 6 weeks between the assays.[29] Furthermore, it is important to note that aPL that are increased during an unsuccessful pregnancy may decrease afterwards. Hence, aPL assays are of diagnostic value if performed during pregnancy or at a time close to pregnancy loss. Occasionally, aCL seem to remain high outside pregnancy.[30]

REFERENCES

1. Tincani A, Allegri F, Balestrieri G, et al. Minimal requirements for antiphospholipid antibodies ELISAs proposed by the European Forum on antiphospholipid antibodies. Thromb Res 2004; 114:553–8.
2. Jennings I, Kitchen S, Woods TA, et al. Potentially clinically important inaccuracies in testing for the lupus anticoagulant: an analysis of results from three surveys of the UK National External Quality Assessment Scheme (NEQAS) for Blood Coagulation. Thromb Haemost 1997; 77:934–7.
3. Creagh MD, Malia RG, Cooper SM, et al. Screening for lupus anticoagulant and anticardiolipin antibodies in women with fetal loss. J Clin Pathol 1991; 44:45–7.
4. Pattison NS, Chamley LW, McKay EJ, et al. Antiphospholipid antibodies in pregnancy: prevalence and clinical associations. Br J Obstet Gynaecol 1993; 100:909–13.
5. Lockwood CJ, Romero R, Feinberg RF, et al. The prevalence and biologic significance of lupus anticoagulant and anticardiolipin antibodies in a general obstetric population. Am J Obstet Gynecol 1989; 161:369–73.
6. Yetman DL, Kutteh WH. Antiphospholipid antibody panels and recurrent pregnancy loss: prevalence of anticardiolipin antibodies compared with other antiphospholipid antibodies. Fertil Steril 1996; 66:540–6.
7. Rote NS. Antiphospholipid antibodies other than lupus anticoagulant and anticardiolipin antibodies in women with recurrent pregnancy loss, fertile controls, and antiphospholipid syndrome. Obstet Gynecol 1997; 90:642–4.
8. Coulam CB, Stern JJ, Kaider BD, et al. Comparison of frequency of anticardiolipin and other antiphospholipid antibodies among women with reproductive autoimmune failure syndrome. Am J Reprod Immunol 1997; 37:353–4.
9. Branch DW, Silver R, Pierangeli S, et al. Antiphospholipid antibodies other than lupus anticoagulant and anticardiolipin antibodies in women with recurrent pregnancy loss, fertile controls, and antiphospholipid syndrome. Obstet Gynecol 1997; 89:549–55.
10. Coulam CB. The role of antiphospholipid antibodies in reproduction: questions answered and raised at the 18th Annual Meeting of the American Society of Reproductive Immunology. Am J Reprod Immunol 1999; 41:1–4.
11. Lyden TW, Vogt E, Ng AK, et al. Monoclonal antiphospholipid antibody reactivity against human placental trophoblast. J Reprod Immunol 1992; 22:1–14.
12. Rote NS, Dostal-Johnson D, Branch DW. Antiphospholipid antibodies and recurrent pregnancy loss: correlation between the activated partial thromboplastin time and antibodies against phosphatidylserine and cardiolipin. Am J Obstet Gynecol 1990; 163:575–84.
13. Sugi T, Matsubayashi H, Inomo A, et al. Antiphosphatidylethanolamine antibodies in recurrent early pregnancy loss and mid-to-late pregnancy loss. J Obstet Gynaecol Res 2004; 30:326–32.
14. Carp HJ, Menashe Y, Frenkel Y, et al. Lupus anticoagulant. Significance in habitual first-trimester abortion. J Reprod Med 1993; 38:549–52.
15. Nielsen HS, Christiansen OB. Prognostic impact of anticardiolipin antibodies in women with recurrent miscarriage negative for the lupus anticoagulant. Hum Reprod 2005; 20:1720–8.
16. Kwak JY, Barini R, Gilman-Sachs A, et al. Down-regulation of maternal antiphospholipid antibodies during early pregnancy and pregnancy outcome. Am J Obstet Gynecol 1994; 171:239–46.
17. McIntyre JA. Antiphospholipid antibodies in implantation failures. Am J Reprod Immunol 2003; 49:221–9.
18. Kaider AS, Kaider BD, Janowicz PB, et al. Immunodiagnostic evaluation in women with reproductive failure. Am J Reprod Immunol 1999; 42:335–46.
19. Ulcova-Gallova Z, Krauz V, Novakova P, et al. Anti-phospholipid antibodies against phosphatidylinositol, and phosphatidylserine are more significant in reproductive failure than antibodies against cardiolipin only. Am J Reprod Immunol 2005; 54:112–17.
20. Franklin RD, Kutteh WH. Antiphospholipid antibodies (APA) and recurrent pregnancy loss: treating a unique APA positive population. Hum Reprod 2002; 17:2981–5.
21. Bizzaro N, Tonutti E, Villalta D, et al. Prevalence and clinical correlation of anti-phospholipid-binding protein antibodies in anticardiolipin-negative patients with systemic lupus erythematosus and women with unexplained recurrent miscarriages. Arch Pathol Lab Med 2005; 129:61–8.

22. Lee RM, Emlen W, Scott JR, et al. Anti-β_2-glycoprotein I antibodies in women with recurrent spontaneous abortion, unexplained fetal death, and antiphospholipid syndrome. Am J Obstet Gynecol 1999; 181:642–8.

23. Aoki K, Hayashi Y, Hirao Y, et al. Specific antiphospholipid antibodies as a predictive variable in patients with recurrent pregnancy loss. Am J Reprod Immunol 1993; 29:82–7.

24. Matzner W, Chong P, Xu G, et al. Characterization of antiphospholipid antibodies in women with recurrent spontaneous abortions. J Reprod Med 1994; 39:27–30.

25. Silver RM, Porter TF, van Leeuween I, et al. Anticardiolipin antibodies: clinical consequences of 'low titers'. Obstet Gynecol 1996; 87:494–500.

26. Reece EA, Garofalo J, Zheng XZ, et al. Pregnancy outcome. Influence of antiphospholipid antibody titer, prior pregnancy losses and treatment. J Reprod Med 1997; 42:49–55.

27. Coulam CB. Antiphospholipid antibody round table report. Am J Reprod Immunol 2002; 48:262–5.

28. Harris EN, Pierangeli S, Birch D. Anticardiolipin Wet Workshop Report. Fifth International Symposium on Antiphospholipid Antibodies. Am J Clin Pathol 1994; 101:616–24.

29. Coulam CB, Branch DW, Clark DA, et al. American Society for Reproductive Immunology. Report of the Committee for Establishing Criteria for Diagnosis of Reproductive Autoimmune Syndrome. Am J Reprod Immunol 1999; 41:121–32.

30. Ruiz JE, Cubillos J, Mendoza JC, et al. Autoantibodies to phospholipids and nuclear antigens in non-pregnant and pregnant Colombian women with recurrent spontaneous abortions. J Reprod Immunol 1995; 28:41–51.

9. Management of antiphospholipid syndrome in pregnancy

Wendell A Wilson and Nigel Harris

INTRODUCTION

Appropriate management can greatly reduce the fetal and maternal morbidity in antiphospholipid syndrome (APS), an autoimmune disease that is now recognized as a leading cause of recurrent pregnancy loss (RPL). RPL occurs in about 1% of women.[1,2] In about 15% of otherwise-healthy women, antiphospholipid antibodies (aPL) appear to be the sole explanation for their pregnancy loss.[3,4] aPL have also been associated with:

- preterm birth, prior to 34 weeks' gestation[5,6]
- placental insufficiency and fetal growth restriction[5,6]
- preeclampsia[5,6]
- venous, arterial, and small-vessel thrombophilia[7,8]

The aims of therapy of APS during pregnancy include the improvement of all these morbidities.

UNFRACTIONATED HEPARIN AND LOW-MOLECULAR-WEIGHT HEPARIN

At present, maternally administered unfractionated heparin (UH) or low-molecular-weight heparin (LMWH) given concurrently with low-dose aspirin are generally considered standard therapy to prevent pregnancy loss in women with APS.[9–12] This treatment has been endorsed by an international panel of experts, and it is usually started pre-pregnancy or as early as possible in the first trimester, after ultrasound demonstration of a live embryo. The live birth rate in APS is improved by about 50% with this therapy to about 80% of treated pregnancies. Notwithstanding the foregoing recommendations,

there is room for debate about some aspects of current therapy, because:

- there have been relatively few controlled studies on which to base recommendations
- APS pregnancy is a somewhat heterogeneous clinical syndrome
- there was no general consensus on the definition of APS pregnancy prior to publication of the Sapporo consensus criteria.[13]

Although there is consensus about the value of heparin given concurrently with low-dose aspirin therapy, it is not clear what benefit, if any, is produced by the aspirin component. Aspirin, given alone, did not improve the live birth rate compared with placebo,[14,15] although the latter study of 'low-risk APS pregnancy' included some pregnancies that fail to satisfy current APS criteria. The study by Pattison et al[14] included aPL-positive women who had three or more prior pregnancy losses (predominantly in the first trimester) and no history of thromboses or systemic lupus erythematosus (SLE); it showed a relatively high live birth rate of about 80% using either aspirin or placebo, suggesting that there may indeed be a subgroup of women with 'low-risk APS pregnancy' who may not need anticoagulant or antiplatelet therapy. Three studies have compared the effect of aspirin alone with the effect of aspirin with the addition of heparin. Two studies[16,17] showed a statistically significant benefit from adding heparin to the aspirin. An 80% live birth rate was seen after heparin and aspirin, compared with 44% after aspirin alone in Kutteh's trial,[16] and a 71% live birth rate after heparin compared with 42% in the trial by Rai et al.[17] However, in the trial by Farquharson et al,[18] the live birth rate was similar whether aspirin was used alone or in combination with heparin. When the three trials were combined in a meta-analysis,[19] there was a common odds ratio of 2.63 in favor of adding heparin to the regimen (95% confidence interval (CI) 1.46–4.75).

The dose of heparin therapy needed for APS pregnancy is also debatable.[9,20] More aggressive, full-dose heparin therapy may be appropriate for women who have a prior history of either venous, arterial, or small-vessel thrombosis or pregnancy loss that occurred later than the 10th week of gestation, because these groups of women appear to have an increased risk of recurrence of thrombosis during pregnancy or the puerperium. However, there is some debate concerning the importance of the second factor.

The action of UH and LMWH in treating APS pregnancy is thought to be mainly due to their potent anticoagulant effects. APS is considered to be essentially an autoimmune thrombophilia that is causally related to the persistent presence of heterogeneous antibodies directed against phospholipids and/or phospholipid-binding proteins.[8,21] However, heparins may also bind directly to aPL[22,23] possibly inhibiting their activity in causing APS. In addition, recent studies in experimental models suggest that aPLs may in part cause APS by activating the complement system and that heparin may prevent fetal loss in APS by inhibiting complement activation, in particular the formation of the activation products C3a and C5a;[24] it is possible that C3a and C5a amplify the procoagulant effects of aPL, thus causing thrombophilia. Detailed studies are needed to assess the relevance of these mechanisms to human pregnancy.

Consensus guidelines for the management of APS pregnancy were published in 2003 by a study group from the International Symposium on aPL.[11] In general, patients with recurrent (three or more) prior early pregnancy loss (before the 10th week of gestation) who have no prior venous, arterial, or small-vessel thrombosis are managed with UH or LMWH in low doses (e.g., enoxaparin 1 mg/kg/day). Outside of the context of APS, this dosage is generally considered prophylactic rather than therapeutic in the prevention and management of venous thrombosis. APS patients with prior venous, arterial, or small-vessel thrombosis are managed with a full therapeutic dose (e.g., enoxaparin 1 mg/kg body weight every 12 hours). Some authorities suggest that women with prior late fetal loss (10 weeks gestation or later) and no prior history of thrombosis should also receive full or almost full therapeutic UH or LMWH doses, because these women may also have a higher risk of thromboembolism during or after pregnancy than women who experience early pregnancy losses.[9,10,12,25] Our experience with APS pregnancy has been in keeping with this approach. It may therefore be useful to separate patients according to whether there is a history of previous thrombosis, or whether the previous pregnancy losses were early or late.

- 1. *APS patients who have a prior history of thrombosis.* Most of these patients will be on long-term or lifelong thromboprophylaxis with warfarin. Before pregnancy is contemplated or attempted, these women should be informed of the teratogenic potential of warfarin during the first 14 weeks of pregnancy. Prior to conception, warfarin should be replaced with a full therapeutic dose of UH or LMWH, supervised by a clinician with expertise in managing APS pregnancy.

- 2. *APS patients who have at least one fetal loss after the 10th week of gestation, no prior thromboses, and no other features of APS.* Although these patients have not had prior thromboses, some studies suggest that they may also be at significantly increased risk of thrombosis during pregnancy or the puerperium, and should be managed similarly to group 1 (see above) patients during pregnancy and the puerperium.[9,10,12,25]

- 3. *APS patients with three or more prior early pregnancy losses only (prior to 10 weeks' gestation) and no other features of APS.* RPL that occurs prior to the 10th week of gestation is frequently due to other causes than APS and is less specific for APS than pregnancy loss that occurs after 10 weeks. There is a paucity of controlled studies that address the management of recurrent pregnancy loss prior to 10 weeks' gestation. However, if other causes of fetal loss have been excluded, these patients should be managed with LMWH in lower doses (1 mg/kg/day) and low-dose aspirin, begun prior to conception.[9,10]

RISKS OF THERAPY

The risks of heparin therapy appear to be significantly reduced with LMWH. Hemorrhage, osteoporosis, and heparin-induced thrombocytopenia in particular appear to be substantially less frequent with LMWH than with UH. The increased bioavailability and longer therapeutic half-life of LMWH also allow less frequent injections. Additionally, there is no overlap between the anticoagulant effect and the antithrombotic effect – hence, there is no bleeding with LMWH, and little need for monitoring. Because of these factors and recent studies that suggest LMWH to be as effective in preventing pregnancy loss in APS,[26–29] LMWH has to a large extent supplanted UH.

MONITORING OF UH AND LMWH IN APS PREGNANCY

Full-dose UH therapy requires monitoring of partial thromboplastin time (PTT) or factor Xa level. Patients in whom the baseline PTT is prolonged due to the presence of lupus anticoagulant in APS should be monitored by factor Xa level. Full anticoagulation with LMWH may require monitoring by Xa level, since LMWH does not prolong the PTT. Further studies are needed to address the potential value of monitoring factor Xa level in APS pregnancy.

OTHER THERAPIES

In meta-analyses of APS pregnancy,[12,25] heparin given concurrently with aspirin improved the live birth rate from about 25% to 75%. These and other studies have shown that pregnancy losses continue in 20–30% of women, in spite of therapy. Alternate therapies have included glucocorticoids or intravenous immunoglobulin (IVIG).

GLUCOCORTICOIDS

Glucocorticoid therapy predated the use of heparin in treating APS pregnancy. Early enthusiasm for glucocorticoids waned after a small randomized trial showed heparin to be as effective as high-dose prednisone.[30] In addition, most subsequent controlled studies have not confirmed a beneficial effect for glucocorticoids in APS pregnancy.[31–33] Well-known prednisone toxicities such as gestational diabetes, hypertension, preeclampsia, infections, and osteoporosis contributed to the abandonment of prednisone therapy for APS pregnancy.[12,25,29] Prednisone therapy does have a place in treating the SLE in those women who have APS that is secondary to SLE. Among such women with SLE requiring prednisone therapy, the lowest dose of prednisone should be used that produces satisfactory SLE control. Recent studies in experimental models of APS pregnancy, mentioned above, point to a role for complement activation in causing fetal loss. If this mechanism, which is potentially both proinflammatory and procoagulant, is validated in human pregnancy, it may provide novel therapeutic targets in APS pregnancy.

HYDROXYCHLOROQUINE

In the past, it was customary to discontinue hydroxychloroquine during SLE pregnancy because of its presumed potential for fetal toxicity.[34] However, women with SLE who are taking hydroxychloroquine (Plaquenil) have been shown to be at increased risk of SLE flare if the hydroxychloroquine is discontinued.[34] The treating physician may not recognize the true cause of such flares, because the flare may be delayed for weeks to months after the hydroxychloroquine is stopped. In addition, recent studies have shown that, contrary to previous dogma, hydroxychloroquine is not associated with fetal toxicity when used in conventional doses[35,36] (≤6.5 mg/kg lean body weight). Most authorities therefore now consider it preferable to continue hydroxychloroquine throughout SLE pregnancy, to reduce the risk of an SLE flare. Such flares may have adverse effects on fetal and maternal morbidity and increase prednisone requirements.[34–37] In APS patients who also have SLE, this approach is additionally supported by studies showing that hydroxychloroquine reduces the thrombogenic potential of aPL in a mouse model, possibly because of its antiplatelet effects.[38] Although there have been no trials of hydroxychloroquine in APS pregnancy, there is evidence that hydroxychloroquine may reduce the thrombosis risk associated with aPL in non-pregnant SLE patients.[39]

'PROBABLE APS' PREGNANCY

The live birth rate does not appear to be improved by heparin therapy in women who do not fulfil clinical criteria for APS.[14,15] In particular, heparin therapy does not improve the live birth rate in women who have only one or two prior early pregnancy losses (<10 weeks' gestation) with a low titer of aPL and no other features of APS.[14,15]

INTRAVENOUS IMMUNOGLOBULIN

IVIG therapy has been of interest because of its efficacy in treating other autoimmune syndromes, and recent experimental studies that suggest it may improve thrombogenicity in experimental APS. However, clinical trials have found that it is no more effective in preventing pregnancy loss than heparin with aspirin in unselected APS pregnancy.[40–42] The value of IVIG in the subgroup of women miscarrying despite conventional therapy needs to be adequately addressed by future studies.

Some preliminary observational data have reported that IVIG may lower the incidence of the late obstetric complications described above compared with heparin and low-dose aspirin. These complications include preeclampsia,[41–44] intrauterine growth restriction (IUGR),[40,43–45] and premature births,[43,44] leading to fewer admissions to the neonatal intensive care unit (14% of seven patients in the IVIG group compared with 44% of nine in the placebo group) in the trial by Branch et al.[40] Kwak et al[45] used IVIG in six patients who were refractory to other forms of treatment and had complications in late pregnancy. Three pregnancies were complicated by IUGR, another three had twin

pregnancies. aPL titers of both immunoglobulin G (IgG) and IgM were significantly decreased after each infusion. The development of IUGR correlated with rising antibody titers. Again, future trials are necessary in order to confirm these results, and to determine whether the possible improvement in obstetric complications is real and justifies using IVIG, with its prohibitive cost. At present, it seems that IVIG may have a place as a second line of treatment in patients who are refractory to heparin or who continue to suffer the late obstetric complications of APS.

TREATMENT OF REFRACTORY APS

As stated above, pregnancy losses continue in 20–30% of women, despite conventional therapy with heparin and aspirin. There are few definitive answers regarding therapy in these patients. The clinical features of the subsequent pregnancy loss may give some insight into appropriate management. If the treated pregnancy terminates in a first-trimester missed abortion, there may be a confounding factor such as unrelated structural malformations[46] or chromosome aberrations in the embryo. Ogasawara et al[47] have reported that 40% of abortuses had chromosomal aberrations in their series of 10 patients with recurrent miscarriage and APS. Takakuwa et al[48] found 20% of abortuses to be chromosomally abnormal in their series of 10 patients with APS. If the patient aborts a chromosomally aberrant fetus, it may be a chance event unrelated to APS. In these circumstances, the patient should be given the same regimen of LMWH again with or without aspirin.

If the treated pregnancy terminates in a further midtrimester fetal death, the likelihood of chromosomal aberrations is far less, and there may be a true failure of treatment. In these cases, it must be remembered that the optimal doses of heparins are still to be worked out, and a higher dose may be necessary. However, the use of higher doses of LMWH should be weighed against the risk of side-effects. If the pregnancy loss was accompanied by other autoimmune phenomena, including complications of SLE, or vasculitis, steroids should be added to the regimen. Another alternative is IVIG. The addition of either of these two drugs should be considered if artificial termination of pregnancy was required due to other autoimmune phenomena. However, if the pregnancy required artificial termination for a maternal indication, the patient should be carefully counselled as to whether another pregnancy is warranted. The past obstetric history will help the patient and physician arrive at an optimal decision. If the pregnancy loss is due to obstetric complications such as preeclampsia or abruption, IVIG may be the appropriate choice for use in the next pregnancy.[49] Plasmapheresis has also been described as a method for washing out the antibodies.[50,51] However, plasmapheresis is considered to be a salvage therapy for pregnant women with secondary APS or catastrophic APS.

It is against this background of uncertainty that the results of treatment should be interpreted. There are no clear guidelines regarding optimal therapy in failure of treatment; however, skill and clinical judgment will be necessary to manage the following pregnancy.

LABOR AND POSTPARTUM

It has been reported that LMWH should be stopped at 36 weeks' gestation to avoid the risk of epidural hematoma in patients needing epidural block, and UH should be substituted.[25,52] However, LMWH is often continued until 1 day before labor begins. If the patient has been free of LMWH, epidural analgesia is probably quite safe. After labor has begun, UH is stopped.[29,52] Aspirin therapy is usually stopped at 34 weeks' gestation to allow ductus arteriosus closure.

MONITORING OF PREGNANCY

Prompt management of potential problems is facilitated by patient education and monitoring as for high risk pregnancies. The American College of

Obstetricians and Gynecologists (ACOG) guidelines[29, 52] include the following:

- kidney and liver function baseline studies (e.g., creatinine clearance, urine protein, and hepatic enzymes)
- education about thrombosis, preeclampsia, and heparin therapy
- monitoring of the platelet count in patients on heparin
- monitoring for preeclampsia
- after the late second trimester, sonograms every 3–4 weeks
- consideration of umbilical Doppler flow evaluations or more frequent fetal heart monitoring if IUGR is suspected
- early delivery for fetal or maternal compromise

CONCLUSIONS

It is clear from the above that the current management of APS pregnancy improves the pregnancy outcome, especially with regard to the live birth rate. However, treatment is not uniformly effective, and heparin injections are inconvenient, expensive, and generally painful. Occasional internal bleeding remains a problem that has been reduced, but not eliminated, by using LMWH. However, it is gratifying that although the infants of APS mothers treated by current methods have an increased risk of prematurity, they appear to grow and develop quite normally when followed for up to 5 years of age.[53]

REFERENCES

1. Alberman E. The epidemiology of repeated abortion. In: Beard RW, Sharp F, eds. Early Pregnancy Loss: Mechanisms and Treatment. London: Springer-Verlag; 1988: 9–17.
2. Salat-Baroux J. Recurrent spontaneous abortions. Reprod Nutr Dev 1988; 28:1555–68. [in French]
3. Stephenson MD. Frequency of factors associated with habitual abortion in 197 couples. Fertil Steril 1996; 66:24–9.
4. Yettman DL, Kutteh WH. Antiphospholipid antibody panels and recurrent pregnancy loss: prevalence of anticardiolipin antibodies compared with other antiphospholipid antibodies. Fertil Steril 1996; 66: 540–6.

5. Branch WD, Silver RM, Blackwell JL, et al. Outcome of treated pregnancies in women with antiphospholipid syndrome: an update of the Utah experience. Obstet Gynecol 1992; 80:614–20.

6. Lima F, Khamashta MA, Buchanan NM, et al. A study of sixty pregnancies in patients with the antiphospholipid syndrome. Clin Exp Rheumatol 1996; 14:131–6.

7. Cervera R, Piette JC, Font J, et al. Antiphospholipid syndrome: clinical and immunologic manifestations and patterns of disease expression in a cohort of 1000 patients. Arthritis Rheum 2002; 46:1019–27.

8. Levine JS, Branch DW, Rauch J. The antiphospholipid syndrome. N Engl J Med 2002; 346:752–63.

9. Branch DW, Khamashta MA. Antiphospholipid syndrome: obstetric diagnosis, management, and controversies. Obstet Gynecol 2003; 101:1333–44.

10. Derksen RH, Khamashta MA, Branch DW. Management of the obstetric antiphospholipid syndrome. Arthritis Rheum 2004; 50:1028–39.

11. Tincani A, Branch W, Levy RA, et al. Treatment of pregnant patients with antiphospholipid syndrome. Lupus 2003; 12:524–9.

12. Lassere M, Empson M. Treatment of antiphospholipid syndrome in pregnancy – a systematic review of randomized therapeutic trials. Thromb Res 2004; 114:419–26.

13. Wilson WA, Gharavi AE, Koike T, et al. International consensus statement on preliminary classification for definite antiphospholipid syndrome. Arthritis Rheum 1999; 42:1309–11.

14. Pattison NS, Chamley LW, Birdsall M, et al. Does aspirin have a role in improving pregnancy outcome for women with the antiphospholipid syndrome? A randomized controlled trial. Am J Obstet Gynecol 2000; 183:1008–12.

15. Cowchock S, Reece EA, Balaban D, et al. Do low risk pregnant women with antiphospholipid antiboidies need to be treated? Organising Group of the Antiphospholipid Treatment Trial. Am J Obstet Gynecol 1997; 176:1099–100.

16. Kutteh WH. Antiphospholipid antibody-associated recurrent pregnancy loss: treatment with heparin and low-dose aspirin is superior to low-dose aspirin alone. Am J Obstet Gynecol 1996; 174:1584–9.

17. Rai R, Cohen H, Dave M, et al. Randomised controlled trial of aspirin and aspirin plus heparin in pregnant women with recurrent miscarriage associated with phospholipid antibodies (or antiphospholipid antibodies). BMJ 1997; 314:253–7.

18. Farquharson RG, Quenby S, Greaves M. Antiphospholipid syndrome in pregnancy: a randomized, controlled trial of treatment. Lupus 2002; 100:408–13.

19. Carp HJA. Antiphospholipid syndrome in pregnancy. Curr Opin Obstet Gynaecol 2004; 16:129–35.

20. Erkan D, Merrill JT, Yazici Y, et al. High thrombosis rate after fetal loss in antiphospholipid syndrome. Arthritis Rheum 2001; 44:1466–7.

21. Gharavi AE, Pierangeli S, Wilson WA. The molecular basis of antiphospholipid syndrome. Lupus 2003; 12:579–83.

22. Ermel LD, Marshburn PB, Kutteh WH. Interaction of heparin with antiphospholipid antibodies (APA) from the sera of women with recurrent pregnancy loss (RPL). Am J Reprod Immunol 1995; 33:14–20.

23. Franklin RD, Kutteh WH. Effects of unfractionated and low molecular weight heparin on antiphospholipid antibody binding in vitro. Obstet Gynecol 2003; 101:455–62.

24. Girardi G, Redecha P, Salmon JE. Heparin prevents antiphospholipid antibody-induced fetal loss by inhibiting complement system activation. Nat Med 2004; 10:1222–6.

25. Empson M, Lassere M, Craig JC, et al. Recurrent pregnancy loss with antiphospholipid antibody: a systematic review of therapeutic trials. Obstet Gynecol 2002; 99:135–44.

26. Triolo G, Ferrante A, Ciccia F, et al. Randomized study of subcutaneous low molecular weight heparin plus aspirin versus intravenous immunoglobulin in the treatment of recurrent fetal loss associated with antiphospholipid antibodies. Arthritis Rheum 2003; 48:728–31.

27. Stephenson MD, Ballem PJ, Tsang P, et al. Treatment of antiphospholipid antibody syndrome (APS) in pregnancy: a randomized pilot trial comparing low molecular weight heparin to unfractionated heparin. J Obstet Gynaecol Can 2004; 26:729–34.

28. Gris JC, Balducchi JP, Quere I, et al. Enoxaparin sodium improves pregnancy outcome in aspirin-resistant antiphospholipid/antiprotein antibody syndromes. Thromb Haemost 2002; 87:536–7.

29. American College of Obstetricians and Gynecologists. Anticoagulation with low-molecular-weight heparin during pregnancy. ACOG Committee Opinion 211. Washington, DC: ACOG, 1998.

30. Cowchock FS, Reece EA, Balaban D, et al. Repeated fetal losses associated with antiphospholipid antibodies: a collaborative randomized trial comparing prednisone with low-dose heparin treatment. Am J Obstet Gynecol 1992; 166:1318–23.

31. Lockshin MD, Druzin ML, Qamar T. Prednisone does not prevent recurrent fetal death in women with antiphospholipid antibody. Am J Obstet Gynecol 1989; 160:439–43.

32. Laskin CA, Bombardier C, Hannah ME, et al. Prednisone and aspirin in women with autoantibodies and unexplained recurrent fetal loss. N Engl J Med 1997; 337:148–53.

33. Silver RK, MacGregor Sholl, JS, et al. Comparative trial of prednisone plus aspirin versus aspirin alone in the treatment of anticardiolipin antibody-positive obstetric patients. Am J Obstet Gynecol 1993; 169:1411–17.

34. Canadian Consensus Conference on Hydroxychloroquine. J Rheumatol 2000; 27:2919–21.

35. Motta M, Tincani A, Faden D, et al. Follow-up of infants exposed to hydroxychloroquine given to mothers during pregnancy and lactation. J Perinatol 2005; 25:86–9.

36. Khamashta MA, Buchanan NMM, Hughes GRV. The use of hydroxychloroquine in lupus pregnancy the British experience. Lupus 1996; S1:65–6.

37. Parke A, West B. Hydroxychloroquine in pregnant patients with systemic lupus erythematosus. J Rheumatol 1996; 23:1715–18.

38. Espinola RG, Pierangeli SS, Ghara AE, et al. Hydroxychloroquine reverses platelet activation induced by human IgG antiphospholipid antibodies. Thromb Haemost 2002; 87:518–22.

39. Petri M. Thrombosis and systemic lupus erythematosus: the Hopkins Lupus Cohort perspective. Scand J Rheumatol 1996; 25: 191–3.

40. Branch DW, Peaceman AM, Druzin M, et al. A multicenter, placebo-controlled pilot study of intravenous immune globulin treatment of antiphospholipid syndrome during pregnancy. Am J Obstet Gynecol 2000; 182:122–7.

41. Vaquero E, Lazzarin N, Valensise H, et al. Pregnancy outcome in recurrent spontaneous abortion associated with antiphospholipid antibodies: a comparative study of intravenous immunoglobulin versus prednisone plus low-dose aspirin. Am J Reprod Immunol 2001; 45:174–9.

42. Spinnato JA, Clark AL, Pierangeli SS, et al. Intravenous immunoglobulin therapy for the antiphospholipid syndrome in pregnancy. Am J Obstet Gynecol 1995; 172:690–4.

43. Harris EN, Pierangeli SS. Utilization of intravenous immunoglobulin therapy to treat recurrent pregnancy loss in the antiphospholipid syndrome: a review. Scand J Rheumatol 1998; 107(Suppl):97–102.

44. Valensie H, Vaquero E, De Carolis C. Normal fetal growth in women with antiphospholipid syndrome treated with high dose intravenous immunoglobulin (IVIG). Prenat Diagn 1995; 15:509–17.

45. Kwak JY, Quilty EA, Gilman-Sachs A, et al. Intravenous immunoglobulin infusion therapy in women with recurrent spontaneous abortions of immune etiologies. J Reprod Immunol 1995; 28:175–88.

46. Philipp T, Kalousek DK. Transcervical embryoscopy in missed abortion. J Assist Reprod Genet 2001; 18:285–90.

47. Ogasawara M, Aoki K, Okada S, et al. Embryonic karyotype of abortuses in relation to the number of previous miscarriages. Fertil Steril 2000; 73:300–4.

48. Takakuwa K, Asano K, Arakawa M, et al. Chromosome analysis of aborted conceptuses of recurrent aborters positive for anticardiolipin antibody. Fertil Steril 1997; 68:54–8.

49. Galli M, Barbui T. Antiphospholipid antibodies and pregnancy. Best Pract Res Clin Haematol 2003; 16:211–25.

50. Takeshita Y, Tsurumi Y, Touma S, et al. Successful delivery in a pregnant woman with lupus anticoagulant positive systemic lupus erythematosus treated with double filtration plasmapheresis. Therap Apher 2001; 5:22–4.

51. Von Baeyer H. Plasmapheresis in immune hematology: review of clinical outcome data with respect to evidence-based medicine and clinical experience. Therap Apher Dial 2003; 7:127–40.

52. ACOG Practice Bulletin No. 68: Antiphospholipid Syndrome. Obstet Gynecol 2005; 106:1113–21.

53. Ruffatti A, Dalla Barba B, Del Ross T, et al. Outcome of fifty-five newborns of antiphospholipid antibody-positive mothers treated with calcium heparin during pregnancy. Clin Exp Rheumatol 1998; 16:605–10.

10. Defects in coagulation factors leading to recurrent pregnancy loss

Aida Inbal and Howard JA Carp

INTRODUCTION

The etiology of pregnancy loss often remains an enigma, even after exclusion of uterine abnormalities and of genetic, immunological, infectious, or endocrine disorders. Recently, thrombophilias, whether hereditary or acquired, have been found in a significant number of women with recurrent abortions without apparent cause. The evidence for pregnancy loss having a thrombotic basis is due to the widely reported association between antiphospholipid antibodies (aPL) and recurrent pregnancy loss (RPL). aPL are thought to cause pregnancy loss by thrombosis in decidual vessels, impairing the blood supply to the fetus and leading to fetal death. Due to the assumption that aPL induce thrombosis causing pregnancy loss, it has been assumed that any prothrombotic state may also increase the chance of pregnancy loss due to a thrombotic mechanism, and that if this process recurs three or more times, there is recurrent miscarriage. Hereditary thrombophilias that have been reported to be associated with recurrent pregnancy loss include antithrombin, protein C, and protein S deficiencies, factor V Leiden (FVL), the G20210A mutation in the factor II (FII) gene, and homozygosity for the thermolabile variant of methylenetetrahydrofolate reductase (MTHFR C677T), which leads to hyperhomocysteinemia specifically in the presence of low folate levels. In addition, deficiencies of factor XIII (FXIII) and fibrinogen are associated with pregnancy loss. Both of these are bleeding diatheses that become apparent in childhood, and are associated with impaired wound repair in addition to pregnancy loss and excessive bleeding. This chapter deals with the association between decreased or increased levels of coagulation factors and pregnancy loss. The various factors and their association with the trophoblast are shown in Figure 10.1.

BLEEDING DIATHESES LEADING TO PREGNANCY LOSS

HEREDITARY FACTOR XIII DEFICIENCY

Coagulation factor XIII (FXIII) is a plasma transglutaminase that participates in the final step of the coagulation cascade. Following activation by thrombin, the active form (FXIIIa) crosslinks fibrin chains through γ-glutamyl–ε-lysine bonds, creating a stable clot resistant to fibrinolysis.[1] In plasma, FXIII circulates as a heterotetramer (A2B2) composed of two catalytic A subunits (FXIII-A) and two carrier B subunits (FXIII-B).[2] FXIIIa is synthesized by megakaryocytes, monocytes, and monocyte-derived macrophages, whereas FXIII-B is synthesized by hepatocytes. Platelets, monocytes, and macrophages contain only the A subunits of FXIII dimers.[2]

In contrast to factors FVII, FVIII, FIX, FX, and fibrinogen, which increase during normal pregnancy, the concentration of plasma FXIII decreases during pregnancy, reaching 50% of normal at term. Likewise, the activity of FXIIIA is significantly decreased at the time of abortion.[3]

FXIII deficiency is a hereditary bleeding disorder, characterized by severe bleeding manifestations, delay in wound healing, and recurrent abortions in homozygous women.[2] Women who are homozygous for FXIII deficiency will not carry the pregnancy until term unless treated with FXIII concentrate throughout pregnancy.[4] The minimal

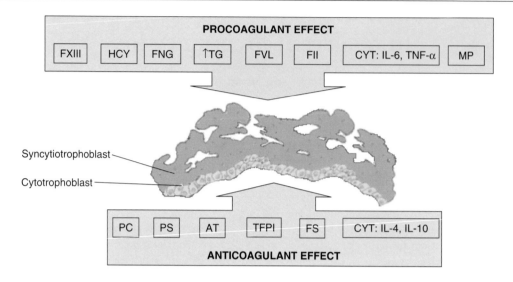

Figure 10.1   Procoagulant and anticoagulant balance of the trophoblast. FXIII, factor XIII; HCY, homocysteine; FNG, fibrinogen; ↑TG, increased thrombin generation; FVL, factor V Leiden; FII, prothrombin gene mutation (G20210A); CYT, cytokines; IL-6/4/10, interleukin-6/4/10; TNF-α, tumor necrosis factor α; MP, microparticles; PC, protein C; PS, protein S; AT, antithrombin; TFPI, tissue factor pathway inhibitor; FS, fibrinolytic system.

level of FXIII-A required for normal pregnancy is unknown; however, only 0.5–2% of FXIII-A is required for normal hemostasis.[2]

The mechanism by which FXIII supports normal pregnancy is unknown. FXIII is essential for implantation, placental attachment, and further placental development by crosslinking not only between fibrin chains but also between fibronectin and collagen, the major components of connective tissue matrix.[2,5] Hence, FXIII seems to play an essential role in the interaction between the blastocyst and the endometrium at implantation. FXIIIa also crosslinks fibrin(ogen) and fibronectin, both of which are important for maintaining the attachment of the placenta to the uterus.[6] FXIII deficiency may result in periplacental hemorrhage and subsequent spontaneous fetal loss. This hypothesis is supported by evidence from a mouse model of FXIII deficiency: pregnant FXIII-A-subunit knockout mice suffer excessive uterine bleeding followed by embryonic demise.[7] Kobayashi et al[8] have reported that FXIII-A is present in the extracellular

space of the extravillous cytotrophoblast shell adjacent to Nitabuch's layer. FXIII-A has also been co-localized with fibrinogen and fibronectin at Nitabuch's layer.[9] FXIII-A has been reported to be absent from the placental bed in women with FXIII deficiency, leading to deficient cytotrophoblastic shell formation.[9] Thus, deficiency of FXIII-A at the site of implantation will adversely affect fibrin–fibronectin crosslinking, resulting in detachment of the placenta from the uterus and subsequent miscarriage.[7,9] Recent studies have shown FXIII-A to have proangiogenic activity both in vitro and in vivo.[10] Since embryo implantation requires adequate angiogenesis, the supportive role of FXIII in implantation may be partly due to its proangiogenic activity.

Whatever the cause of pregnancy loss in FXIII-deficient women, administration of FXIII throughout pregnancy results in successful outcomes.[2,4,5] A plasma-derived concentrate has been available since 1980. The FXIII concentrate seems to have a half-life of 10–12 days.[11] Recently, a recombinant

FXIII-A-subunit protein has become available, with a half-life similar to that of the plasma-derived concentrate.[12]

The timing and dose of FXIII replacement for pregnant women and the optimal level of FXIII remain unknown. The level of plasma FXIII generally achieved for successful pregnancy is 10% in women with FXIII deficiency.[11] We treat pregnant women prophylactically with 20 IU/kg of FXIII concentrate every 4 weeks to achieve a FXIII level of above 3%. A booster dose of 1000 IU is also given before amniocentesis or labor.

OTHER ALTERATIONS IN FXIII

It is unknown if there is an association between normal or decreased levels of FXIII and RPL. Whereas plasma FXIII-B concentrations increase during pregnancy, FXIII-A tends to decrease, resulting in an overall steady reduction in plasma FXIII, reaching approximately 50% of normal at term.[13] The A subunit rises with the onset of labor and falls postpartum.[13] This is in contrast to the progressive increase in levels of fibrinogen, FVII, FVIII, FIX, and FX during pregnancy.[14] Whether the reduction of plasma FXIII during pregnancy represents decreased synthesis of FXIII-A, increased utilization or destruction, or simple dilution by the expanded plasma volume is not clear. In a cohort of non-FXIII-deficient women with a history of two or more first-trimester miscarriages, plasma FXIII levels were not found to be predictive for subsequent pregnancy loss.[15] A substitution of tyrosine by phenylalanine at position 204 in exon 5 of the FXIII-A gene was found in one study to be more prevalent in women suffering three or more miscarriages.[16] The Phe204 FXIII-A variant has been associated with lower specific activity. However, in subsequent studies, this association has not been confirmed.

FIBRINOGEN DEFICIENCY

Fibrinogen, a major blood glycoprotein, is a dimer of three polypeptide chains: Aα, Bβ, and γ. It is synthesized by hepatic parenchymal cells and its half-life is 3–4.5 days.[17] Thrombin cleaves fibrinogen to fibrin monomer, which then polymerizes and is stabilized by FXIII. Fibrin(ogen) is also a target for fibrinolytic factors that dissolve excess fibrin to maintain vascular patency and integrity. Fibrinogen is also a primary bridging molecule, linking activated platelets together via their glycoproteins (GP) IIb/IIIa.[18]

The three overlapping hereditary abnormalities of fibrinogen – afibrinogenemia, dysfibrinogenemia, and hypofibrinogenemia – have been associated with recurrent pregnancy loss. Afibrinogenemia – a defect in hepatic fibrinogen secretion or release – is inherited as an autosomal recessive trait and is associated with bleeding diathesis, impaired wound repair, and recurrent pregnancy loss. A related form of this disorder is hypofibrinogenemia. Hereditary dysfibrinogenemias are characterized by the biosynthesis of structurally and functionally abnormal fibrinogen.

Brenner[19] has reported that women with dysfibrinogenemia are candidates for miscarriage. Of 64 pregnancies in women with dysfibrinogenemia, 39% terminated in miscarriage. The mechanisms whereby dysfibrinigenemias are associated with a tendency to thrombosis have been reviewed by Mosesson.[20]

Hypofibrinogenemic women[21] and experimental afibrinogenemic mice[22] show similar features with regard to bleeding tendency, miscarriage, and abnormal scar formation. Based on the mouse model, absence or a significant decrease in maternal fibrinogen is sufficient to cause rupture of the maternal vasculature, thereby affecting embryonic trophoblast infiltration leading to hemorrhage and subsequent miscarriage.

Cryoprecipitate, fresh-frozen plasma and fibrinogen concentrate are the sources of fibrinogen that are commercially available. Replacement therapy throughout pregnancy is feasible for patients with pregnancy losses.[23] It has been suggested that the minimal level of normal fibrinogen to maintain pregnancy is about 60 mg/100 ml.[24] A cryoprecipitate infusion of 0.2 bags/kg body weight (approximately 250 mg/bag) will raise the fibrinogen concentration to 100 mg/dl. Since the half-life of fibrinogen is approximately 4 days, two weekly infusions of cryoprecipitate during the gestational period should be sufficient to keep the fibrinogen level above 60 mg/dl and prevent pregnancy loss.

The benefits of substitution therapy should be weighed against the possibility of inducing thrombosis. Catastrophic thrombosis has been reported during fibrinogen replacement therapy in patients with afibrinogenemia and dysfibrinogenemia.[25] Prophylactic heparin or low-molecular-weight heparin (LMWH) has been advocated for the peripartum period in these patients.[26]

THROMBOPHILIAS

The evidence for pregnancy loss having a thrombotic mechanism rests on three pillars: increased prevalence of thrombophilias in RPL, a higher incidence of pregnancy loss in the presence of thrombophilias, and the demonstration of thrombosis in decidual vessels. The hereditary thrombophilias cause an increased tendency to venous thrombosis and comprise a number of conditions, such as antithrombin, protein C, and protein S deficiencies, FVL, prothrombin gene (FII) mutation G20210A, homozygosity for the MTHFR mutation C677T, and increased FVIII. There are also various acquired hypercoagulable states, the most common of which is antiphospholipid syndrome (APS), which is discussed elsewhere in this book. Proteins C and S and antithrombin are physiological anticoagulants. Deficiencies of these anticoagulants are uncommon.[27] FVL is the most common cause of inherited thrombophilia.[27] It results from the substitution of adenine for guanine at nucleotide 1691 of the factor V gene (G1691A), which causes the arginine in residue 506 of the factor V protein to be replaced by glutamine (Arg506Gln). The resulting protein is called factor V Leiden. This mutation slows down the proteolytic inactivation of FVa, by activated protein C (termed activated protein C resistance, APCR), which in turn leads to augmented generation of thrombin. In the G20210A mutation of the prothrombin gene, adenine is substituted for guanine at the 3′ untranslated part of the prothrombin gene.

This mutation leads to more efficient mRNA processing of the prothrombin gene, which in turn is associated with an increased level of prothrombin and generation of thrombin. FVL and the G20210A mutation in the prothrombin gene are common among healthy whites (with prevalences of 5% and 1.5%, respectively), but are rare in Asians and Africans. Homozygosity for MTHFR (C677T) may lead to hyperhomocysteinemia, mainly when folate storage is decreased, which may also predispose to thrombosis. The mechanism is multifactorial.

THROMBOSIS IN DECIDUAL VESSELS

Thrombophilia has been suggested to be a cause for microembolism in the placenta resulting in abortion or adverse outcome of pregnancy.[28] However, it remains an assumption that hereditary thrombophilias lead to thrombosis in placental vessels in RPL, as no group has assessed the placenta in recurrent miscarriage with hereditary thrombophilias. Genetic polymorphisms of the thrombophilic genes of the parents have a 50% likelihood of transmission to the fetus, potentially affecting trophoblast function. Thus, to determine the true risk for adverse pregnancy outcome associated with genetic thrombophilias, it is necessary to test the offspring for these thrombophilias. In 1978, Rushton[29] reported histological findings in 1486 abortuses. Thrombosis was found in the placenta of 12.1% of abortuses examined. However, at that time, there was no possibility of examining hereditary thrombophilias. Many et al[28] have compared the placental findings in women with severe pregnancy complications with and without thrombophilias. The number of women with villous and multiple infarcts was significantly higher in women with thrombophilias. The number of placentas with fibrinoid necrosis of the decidual vessels was also significantly higher in women with thrombophilias. However, a study by Mousa and Alfirevic[30] could not confirm these results, but found a high incidence of placental infarcts (50%) and thrombosis in both women with and women without thrombophilias. Arias et al[31] evaluated 13 placentas of women with preeclampsia, preterm labor, intrauterine growth restriction (IUGR), or stillbirth. Of 13 women, 10 (77%) had thrombophilias, including aPL, protein C, protein S, and antithrombin deficiencies, APCR, and FVL. However, rather than decidual thrombosis, a fetal thrombotic vasculopathy was found with fibrotic villi, or stem villi obliterated by fibrous tissue. It is important to note that these histological changes are on the fetal side of the placenta, not the maternal side. There was also fetal stem vessel thrombosis, infarcts, hypoplasia, spiral artery thrombosis, and perivillous fibrin deposition. The fact that no specific placental lesion has been found in thrombophilia could have a number of explanations. There may be other thrombophilias as yet unknown, which could explain the high incidence of placental pathology, or the lesions may be the result of inflammatory changes in the placenta associated with the underlying pathology, and unrelated to thrombophilia. Even in APS, thrombosis has not been convincingly demonstrated in decidual vessels. On the contrary, after treatment with monoclonal aPL, stained placental sections have shown most reactivity to be localized to the cytotrophoblast, suggesting that the trophoblast may be directly damaged by mechanisms unrelated to thrombosis.[32] As in hereditary thrombophilias, these histological changes were on the fetal, rather than maternal, side of the placenta. It seems that cell surface-associated membrane receptors rather than soluble factors (e.g., thrombophilic factors) are most relevant candidates to affect pregnancy outcome.[33]

The maternal spiral arteries become remodeled by pregnancy hormones and the trophoblast into uteroplacental arteries toward the end of the first trimester. In the uteroplacental arteries, the lumen is larger, and the media is replaced by endovascular trophoblast cells. If there is thrombosis of the maternal uteroplacental arteries, it is by no means certain that thrombosis can also occur in first-trimester arteries. It is possible that first-trimester miscarriage may be due to failure in the mechanisms governing implantation or due to chromosomal or other abnormalities in the fetus, whereas second-trimester losses may be a consequence of thrombotic events in the placenta. Prothrombotic

polymorphisms may contribute to thrombotic events in the placenta rather than to failure of implantation. However, no study has assessed the placenta in first-trimester pregnancy loss in the presence of thrombophilia, compared with second-trimester losses, nor has any study assessed the placenta in the presence of genetic pregnancy loss compared with pregnancy losses with a normal karyotype.

PREVALENCE OF THROMBOPHILIAS IN FIRST-TRIMESTER MISCARRIAGE

Opinions are divided whether thrombophilias are more prevalent in women with any pregnancy loss or RPL. Prevalences have been reported to range between 3% and 42%. Part of the confusion may stem from the fact that there are studies comparing the prevalence of thrombophilias in all forms of pregnancy loss with parous patients. Other studies have sought differences in prevalences of thrombophilias in recurrent first-trimester losses compared with late losses. Others have sought the prevalence in patients with late obstetric complications. Some papers have found an increased prevalence of certain thrombophilias, but not others.

The papers describing the prevalences in different forms of RPL and pregnancy complications have been described by Kupferminc.[34] When pregnancy loss is not broken down into subgroups, thrombophilias seem to be more prevalent. Brenner et al[35] tested women with three or more first-trimester losses, two or more second-trimester losses, or one or more third-trimester loss. FVL was more prevalent in the pregnancy loss group than in controls; however, neither the MTHFR C677T nor prothrombin mutations were more common in women with pregnancy loss than controls. Forty-nine percent of women with pregnancy loss had a thrombophilia, compared with 22% of controls. Thrombophilias were more common in second- and third-trimester losses, but first-trimester recurrent miscarriage was not associated with thrombophilia. Due to the controversy over the prevalence of thrombophilia and pregnancy loss, Rey et al[36] carried out a meta-analysis of

31 studies in the literature. There was a significant association between hereditary thrombophilias and pregnancy loss.

Similar disagreement is found in the literature with regard to recurrent miscarriage. The disagreements in the literature have prompted the need for meta-analyses to determine whether the prevalence is increased in recurrent miscarriage. Krabbendam et al[37] have reported a meta-analysis of 11 studies regarding the association between thrombophilias and recurrent miscarriage. There were significantly higher serum homocysteine levels among women with a history of recurrent miscarriage, but no increased prevalence of the MTHFR C677T mutation. No relation was observed for the levels of antithrombin, protein C, or protein S. Nelen et al[38] have performed a meta-analysis to assess the relationship between recurrent early pregnancy loss and hyperhomocysteinemia. Overall, the pooled odds ratio (OR) for elevated homocysteine was 2.7 (95% confidence interval (CI) 1.5–5.2), for afterload homocysteine it was 4.2 (95% CI 2.0–8.8), and for MTHFR it was 1.4 (95% CI 1.0–2.0). These data support hyperhomocysteinemia as a risk factor for recurrent early pregnancy loss.

There are some publications separating early and late pregnancy losses and the prevalence of thrombophilias. Preston et al[39] reported on hereditary thrombophilias and fetal loss in a cohort of women with FVL or deficiencies of antithrombin, protein C, or protein S. Of 843 women with thrombophilia, 571 had 1524 pregnancies; of 541 control women, 395 had 1019 pregnancies. The incidences of miscarriage (fetal loss at or before 28 weeks of gestation) and stillbirth (fetal loss after 28 weeks of gestation) were assessed jointly and separately. The risk of fetal loss was increased in women with thrombophilia (OR 1.35; 95% CI 1.01–1.82). The OR was higher for stillbirth than for miscarriage: 3.6 (95% CI 1.4–9.4) versus 1.27 (95% CI 0.94–1.71), respectively. The highest OR for stillbirth was in women with combined defects, 14.3 (95% CI 2.4–86.0), compared with 5.2 (95% CI 1.5–18.1) in antithrombin deficiency, 2.3 (95% CI 0.6–8.3) in protein C deficiency, 3.3 (95% CI 1.0–11.3) in protein S

deficiency, and 2.0 (95% CI 0.5–7.7) in FVL mutation. Sarig et al[40] evaluated 145 patients with recurrent miscarriage and 145 matched controls. At least one thrombophilic defect was found in 66% of study group patients, compared with 28% in controls. Late pregnancy wastage occurred more frequently in women with thrombophilia compared with women without thrombophilia. Grandone et al[41] investigated the FVL mutation in 43 women with two or more unexplained fetal losses and 118 controls. The FVL mutation was more frequent in women with second-trimester loss, but the prevalence of the mutation in women with first-trimester loss and controls was similar.

PREVALENCE OF THROMBOPHILIAS IN LATE OBSTETRIC COMPLICATIONS

Kupferminc et al[42] and a systematic review of 25 studies by Alfirevic et al[43] have reported that various hereditary thrombophilias are more prevalent in pregnant women with IUGR, preeclampsia, abruptio placentae, or stillbirth. In a case–control study of 232 women with a history of one or more second- or third-trimester losses by Gris et al,[44] 21.1% of patients and 3.9% of controls had at least one thrombophilia ($p < 0.00001$). The OR for stillbirth associated with any positive thrombophilia was 5.5 (95% CI 3.4–9.0). Logistic regression analysis showed four risk factors for stillbirth: protein S deficiency, positive anti-β_2-glycoprotein I (β_2GPI) IgG antibodies, positive anticardiolipin IgG antibodies, and the FVL mutation. The conclusion was that late fetal loss, through placenta thrombosis, might sometimes be the consequence of a maternal multifactorial prothrombotic state. Many et al[45] investigated women with intrauterine fetal death (IUFD) at 27 weeks of gestation or more. In 40 women with unexplained IUFD, the prevalence of inherited thrombophilias was 42.5% in the study group, compared with 15% in controls (OR 2.8; 95% CI 1.5–5.3; $p = 0.001$). However, this increased prevalence has been disputed by Infante-Rivarde et al.[46] A systematic review by Alfirevic et al[43] has shown that placental abruption was more often associated with homozygous and heterozygous

FVL, heterozygous G20210A, and hyperhomocysteinaemia. Women with preeclampsia/eclampsia were more likely to have heterozygous FVL mutation, heterozygous G20210A prothrombin gene mutation, homozygous MTHFR C677T, protein C deficiency, protein S deficiency, or APCR. Stillbirth was more often associated with FVL, protein S deficiency, and activated protein C resistance. Women with IUGR had a higher prevalence of G20210A, MTHFR C677T, or protein S deficiency. However, Alfirevic et al[43] concluded that 'Women with adverse pregnancy outcome are more likely to have a positive thrombophilia screen but studies published so far are too small to adequately assess the true size of this association.'

COHORT STUDIES

Case–control studies can only show associations between thrombophilias and pregnancy losses. In order to infer cause and to come to conclusions about treatment, cohort studies are necessary. There are few cohort studies of patients with thrombophilias, in whom longitudinal studies have been performed to assess the true incidence of pregnancy loss. Two studies have examined the subsequent live birth rate in women with recurrent miscarriage and hereditary thrombophilias. In the report by Ogasawara et al,[15] the subsequent miscarriage rate was not different for patients with decreased protein C or S activity, or antithrombin deficiency. Carp et al[47] found the live birth rate to be similar to that expected in recurrent miscarriage, whether the patient had FVL, G20210A, MTHFR C677T, protein C, protein S, or antithrombin deficiencies. Salomon et al[48] have followed up 191 thrombophilic patients who attended an ultrasound clinic to prospectively assess obstetric complications. The blood flow to the fetus was not compromised. No association was found between thrombophilias and preeclampsia or IUGR. Lindqvist et al[49] assessed pregnancy complications in 270 patients with APCR. This subgroup did not differ significantly from the non-APCR patients in terms of pregnancy complications, but was characterized by an eight-fold higher risk of VTE. In our series of 21 pregnancies

with FVL that were followed up prospectively, there was one case of HELLP syndrome (hemolysis, elevated liver enzymes, and low platelet count), but no other obstetric complications, and no deep vein thrombosis or pulmonary embolus (unpublished data). However, Sanson et al[50] investigated women with deficiencies of antithrombin, protein S, and protein C. In the 60 deficient subjects, 22.3% of the 188 pregnancies resulted in miscarriage or stillbirth, as compared with 11.4% of the 202 pregnancies in the 69 non-deficient subjects. The relative risk of abortion and stillbirth per pregnancy for deficient women as compared with non-deficient women was 2.0 (95% CI 1.2–3.3). A longitudinal follow-up study is sorely needed to compare the incidence of miscarriage, stillbirth, IUGR, and preeclampsia in women with hereditary thrombophilias.

TREATMENT

This chapter only gives an outline of the treatment options, as it is followed by a debate on the place of treatment. Suffice it to say here that there are isolated reports that the presence of hereditary thrombophilias warrants thromboprophylaxis. However, the role of treatment can only be determined in well-designed randomized trials where the effect of treatment is compared with untreated or placebo-treated patients. As yet, there are no randomized placebo-controlled trials assessing prophylactic treatment with anticoagulants in hereditary thrombophilias.

In hereditary thrombophilias, a recent prospective study by Gris et al[51] has compared enoxaparin with aspirin in patients with thrombophilia and one pregnancy loss. Enoxaparin was found to be superior to low-dose aspirin. However, this study did not distinguish between early and late pregnancy losses, nor did it correct for early losses due to genetic or other factors known to affect the subsequent live birth rate. Carp et al[52] have reported a comparative cohort study comparing enoxaparin with no treatment in women with hereditary thrombophilias and recurrent miscarriage. The primary outcome measure was the incidence of subsequent live births. Of the 37 pregnancies in treated patients 26 (70.2%) terminated in live births, compared with 21 of 48 (43.8%) in untreated patients (OR 3.03; 95% CI 1.12–8.36). The beneficial effect was mainly seen in primary aborters, i.e., women with no previous live births (OR 9.75; 95% CI 1.59–52.48). This benefit was also found in patients with a poor prognosis for a live birth (five or more miscarriages), where the live birth rate was increased from 18.2% to 61.6%. Although this trial was not randomized or blinded, it is the only trial in the literature comparing the effect of treatment with a cohort of untreated patients with hereditary thrombophilias. There has been no trial of anticoagulants comparing the effects of treatment with untreated patients regarding late obstetric complications. The optimal dose of anticoagulants has not yet been determined. In a randomized prospective study, no difference was found between 40 mg and 80 mg of enoxaparin (Clexane, Sanofi Aventis Ltd, France) in women with thrombophilia and pregnancy losses.[53]

The mode of action of treatment also requires clarification. It has been assumed that thrombophilias act via thrombosis. However, anticoagulants also have anti-inflammatory effects. Heparin increases serum tumor necrosis factor (TNF)-binding protein, protecting against systemic harmful manifestations of TNF.[54] Low-molecular-weight heparins (LMWH) inhibit TNF-α production.[55] Thrombosis results in an inflammatory response in the vein wall. Both heparin and LMWH limit the anti-inflammatory response,[56] including neutrophil extravasation and decreasing vein wall permeability. Heparin also has direct effects on the trophoblast. It has been reported to restore the invasive properties of the trophoblast in APS,[57] and to enhance placental human chorionic gonadotropin (hCG) production. The anti-inflammatory effects of heparins and the direct placental effects may be as relevant, if not more so, than the anticoagulant effects.

OTHER PROTHROMBOTIC MECHANISMS OF
PREGNANCY LOSS

There are other mechanisms that may induce thrombosis, or may allow thrombosis to become apparent in patients with genetic predispositions to thrombosis.

CYTOKINES

Cytokines are low-molecular-weight peptides or glycopeptides, produced by lymphocytes, monocytes/macrophages, mast cells, eosinophils, and blood vessel endothelial cells. Two cytokines have been associated with initiation of coagulation in infections: TNF-α and interleukin-6 (IL-6) upregulate the expression of tissue factor (TF), which initiates the extrinsic phase of the coagulation cascade and subsequent thrombin generation.

Cytokine imbalances have been described in RPL,[58] APS,[59] preeclampsia,[60] preterm births,[61] and IUGR.[62] The predominance of prothrombotic cytokines may well lead to placental thrombosis in genetically susceptible individuals.

MICROPARTICLES

Placental apoptosis has been described as a salient feature of pregnancy loss.[63] Following apoptosis and cell activation, the cell membrane is remodeled, with the release of microparticles. The microparticles express procoagulant phospholipids, such as phosphotidylserine, on their external surface. These phospholipids are normally found inside the cell membrane. Microparticles lead to increased expression of adhesion molecules, thus amplifying the procoagulant and/or inflammatory response on the endothelial cell surface. Microparticles have been found in increased numbers in normal pregnancy, when there is constant deportation of trophoblast into the maternal circulation. Both Laude et al[64] and Carp et al[65] have found increased levels of circulating microparticles in women with RPL. However, it has not been determined whether endothelial microparticles may cause pregnancy loss through subsequent thrombotic mechanisms, or may be a consequence of embryonic death. Between 29% and 60% of recurrent first-trimester miscarriages are due to chromosomal aberrations that are incompatible with life and lead to miscarriage irrespective of other associations or causes of pregnancy loss, including the presence of microparticles. Even in missed abortion due to chromosomal aberrations, the trophoblast undergoes apoptosis with subsequent microparticle formation and thrombosis. However, in some patients, circulating endothelial microrparticles may themselves possibly induce thrombosis and subsequent loss of a normal pregnancy.

HORMONES AND THROMBOSIS

The hormones of pregnancy – estrogen, progesterone, and hCG – all affect thrombosis. Estrogen may alter the concentrations of clotting factors to a prothrombotic profile, for example raising FVII[66] and plasminogen activator inhibitor 1 (PAI-1)[67] and reducing antithrombin III.[67] In mice, estrogen sulfotransferase (a cytosolic enzyme that catalyzes the sulfoconjugation of estrogens) plays a critical role in modulating estrogen activity in the mouse placenta during midgestation.[68] Inactivation of estrogen sulfotransferase caused local and systemic estrogen excess and an increase in TF, leading to placental thrombosis and fetal loss. Additionally, estrogen can either stimulate or inhibit the production of IL-1 and TNF.[67]

Progesterone, however, seems to have opposing effects. It has prothrombotic effects, including upregulation of TF expression,[70] but also induces the production of cytokines such as IL-4, which upregulates protein S, which inhibits coagulation.[71] The progestogen dydrogesterone inhibits production of TNF-α (prothrombotic), but increases the levels of IL-4 (antithrombotic) and IL-6 (prothrombotic).[72]

In addition to its endocrine luteotrophic role, hCG could also have a local role within the uterine environment. Specific binding sites for hCG have been shown in various cells of the endometrium and decidua. The local role of hCG in the endometrium has not been fully elucidated. Uzumcu et al[73] have assessed endometrial production of cytokines when stimulated by hCG. Increasing doses of hCG caused a dose-dependent increase in TNF-α and IL-6 secretion, both of which have been reported to be thrombogenic.

FETAL THROMBOPHILIA

As placental histology usually shows a fetal vasculopathy rather than maternal thrombosis, fetal thrombophilia may explain the pathological changes. The hemostatic balance in the placenta may be determined by both maternal and fetal factors cooperatively regulating coagulation at the fetomaternal interface.[74] Humans have an almost unique placentation in which trophoblast cells line the maternal blood lakes rather than endothelial cells. Using genomewide expression analysis, Sood et al[33] identified a panel of genes that determine the ability of fetal trophoblast cells to regulate hemostasis at the fetomaternal interface. Additionally, the trophoblast was shown to sense the presence of activated coagulation factors via the expression of protease-activated receptors. Engagement of these receptors was reported to result in specific changes in gene expression. Hence, fetal genes might modify the risks associated with maternal thrombophilia. Additionally, coagulation activation at the fetomaternal interface might affect trophoblast physiology and alter placental function in the absence of frank thrombosis. We have seen fetal deaths in utero in which sonograms have shown complete occlusion of the umbilical blood vessels. However, it is impossible to say whether the thromboses caused fetal death or whether the changes occurred postmortem.

REFERENCES

1. Lorand L, Losowsky MS, Miloszewski KJ. Human factor XIII fibrin stabilizing factor. Progr Thromb Haemost 1980; 5:245–90.
2. Muszbek L, Adany R, Mikkola H. Novel aspects of blood coagulation factor XIII. I. Structure, distribution, activation, and function. Crit Rev Clin Lab Sci 1996; 33:357–421.
3. Schubring C, Grulich-Henn J, Burkhard PAT, et al. Fibrinolysis and factor XIII in women with spontaneous abortion. Eur J Obstet Gynecol Reprod Biol 1990; 35:215–21.
4. Burrows RF, Ray JG, Burrows EA. Bleeding risk and reproductive capacity among patients with factor XIII deficiency: a case presentation and review of the literature. Obstet Gynecol Surv 2000; 55:103–7.
5. Mosher DF, Schad PE, Kleinman HK. Cross-linking of fibronectin to collagen by blood coagulation factor XIII. J Clin Invest 1979; 64:781–7.
6. Wartiovaara J, Leivo I, Virtanen I, et al. Cell surface and extracellular matrix glycoprotein fibronectin. Expression in embryogenesis and in teratocarcinoma differentiation. Ann NY Acad Sci 1978; 312:132–41.

7. Koseki-Kuno S, Yamakawa M, Dickneite G, et al. Factor XIII A subunit deficient mice developed severe uterine bleeding events and subsequent spontaneous miscarriages. Blood 2003; 102:4410–12.

8. Kobayashi T, Asahina T, Okada Y, et al. Studies on the localization of adhesive proteins associated with the development of extravillous cytotrophoblast. Trophoblast Res 1999; 13:35–53.

9. Asahina T, Kobayashi T, Okada Y, et al. Maternal blood coagulation factor XIII is associated with the development of cytotrophoblastic shell. Placenta 2000; 21:388–93.

10. Dardik R, Loscalzo J, Inbal A. Factor XIII (FXIII) and angiogenesis. J Thromb Haemost 2005; 4:19–25.

11. Anwar T, Miloszewski K. Factor XIII deficiency. Br J Haematol 1999; 107:468–84.

12. Reynolds TC, Butine MD, Visich JE, et al. Safety, pharmacokinetics, and immunogenicity of single-dose rFXIII administration J Thromb Haemost 2005; 3:922–8.

13. Hayano Y, Ima N, Kasaraura T. Studies on the physiologic changes of blood coagulation factor XIII during pregnancy and their significance. Acta Obstet Gynaecol Jpn 1982; 34:469–77.

14. Stirling Y, Woolf L, North WRS, et al. Haemostasis in normal pregnancy. Thromb Haemost 1984; 52:176.

15. Ogasawara MS, Aoki K, Katano K, et al. Factor XII but not protein C, protein S, antithrombin III, or factor XIII is a predictor of recurrent miscarriage. Fertil Steril 2001; 75:916–19.

16. Anwar R, Gallivan L, Edmonds SD, et al. Genotype/phenotype correlations for coagulation factor XIII: specific normal polymorphisms are associated with high or low factor XIII specific activity. Blood 1999; 93:897–905.

17. Galanakis DK. Fibrinogen anomalies and disease. A clinical update. Hematol Oncol Clin North Am 1992; 6:1171–87.

18. Doolittle RF. The molecular biology of fibrin. In: Stamatoyannopoulos GS, Nienhuis AW, Majerus PW, Harmus H, eds. The Molecular Basis of Blood Diseases. Philadelphia: WB Saunders, 1994:701–23.

19. Brenner B. Inherited thrombophilia and fetal loss. Curr Opin Hematol 2000; 7:290–5.

20. Mosesson MW. Dysfibrinogenemia and thrombosis. Semin Thromb Hemost 1999; 25:311–19.

21. Ridgway HJ, Brennan SO, Faed JM, et al. Fibrinogen Otago: a major α chain truncation associated with severe hypofibrinogenaemia and recurrent miscarriage. Br J Haematol 1997; 98:632–9.

22. Suh TT, Holmback K, Jensen N, et al. Resolution of spontaneous bleeding events but failure of pregnancy in fibrinogen-deficient mice. Genes Dev 1995; 9:2020–33.

23. Inamoto Y, Terao T. First report of a case of congenital afibrinogenemia with successful delivery. Am J Obstet Gynecol 1985; 153:803–4.

24. Gilabert J, Reganon E, Vila V, et al. Congenital hypofibrinogenemia and pregnancy: obstetric and hematological management. Gynecol Obstet Invest 1987; 24:271–6.

25. MacKinnon HH, Fekete JF. Congenital afibrinogenemia: vascular changes and multiple thromboses induced by fibrinogen infusions and contraceptive medication. CMAJ 1971; 140:597–9.

26. Beck EA. Congenital abnormalities of fibrinogen. Clin Haematol 1979; 8:169–81.

27. Seligsohn U, Lubetsky A. Genetic susceptibility to venous thrombosis. N Engl J Med 2001; 344:1222–31.

28. Many A, Schreiber L, Rosner S, et al. Pathologic features of the placenta in women with severe pregnancy complications and thrombophilia. Obstet Gynecol 2001; 98:1041–4.

29. Rushton DI. Simplified classification of spontaneous abortions. J Med Genet 1978; 15:1–9.

30. Mousa HA, Alfirevic Z. Do placental lesions reflect thrombophilia state in women with adverse pregnancy outcome? Hum Reprod 2000; 15:1830–3.

31. Arias F, Romero R, Joist H, et al. Thrombophilia: a mechanism of disease in women with adverse pregnancy outcome and thrombotic lesions in the placenta. J Matern Fetal Med 1998; 7:277–86.

32. Lyden TW, Vogt E, Ng AK, et al. Monoclonal antiphospholipid antibody reactivity against human placental trophoblast. J Reprod Immunol 1992; 22:1–14.

33. Sood R, Kalloway S, Mast AE, et al. Fetomaternal cross talk in the placental vascular bed: control of coagulation by trophoblast cells. Blood 2006; 107:3173–80.

34. Kupferminc MJ. Thrombophilia and pregnancy. Reprod Biol Endocrinol 2003; 1:111.

35. Brenner B, Sarig G, Weiner Z, et al. Thrombophilic polymorphisms are common in women with fetal loss without apparent cause. Thromb Haemost 1999; 82:6–9.

36. Rey E, Kahn SR, David M, et al. Thrombophilic disorders and fetal loss: a meta-analysis. Lancet 2003; 361:901–8.

37. Krabbendam I, Franx A, Bots ML, et al. Thrombophilias and recurrent pregnancy loss: a critical appraisal of the literature. Eur J Obstet Gynecol Reprod Biol 2005; 118:143–53.

38. Nelen WL, Blom HJ, Steegers EA, et al. Hyperhomocysteinemia and recurrent early pregnancy loss: a meta-analysis. Fertil Steril 2000; 74:1196–9.

39. Preston FE, Rosendaal FR, Walker ID, et al. Increased fetal loss in women with heritable thrombophilia. Lancet 1996; 348:913–16.

40. Sarig G, Younis JS, Hoffman R, et al. Thrombophilia is common in women with idiopathic pregnancy loss and is associated with late pregnancy wastage. Fertil Steril 2002; 77:342–7.

41. Grandone E, Margaglione M, Colaizzo D, et al. Factor V Leiden is associated with repeated and recurrent unexplained fetal losses. Thromb Haemost 1997; 77:822–4.

42. Kupferminc MJ, Eldor A, Steinman N, et al. Increased frequency of genetic thrombophilias in women with complications of pregnancy. N Engl J Med 1999; 340:9–13.

43. Alfirevic Z, Roberts D, Martlew V. How strong is the association between maternal thrombophilia and adverse pregnancy outcome? A systematic review. Eur J Obstet Gynecol Reprod Biol 2002; 101:6–14.

44. Gris JC, Quere I, Monpeyroux F, et al. Case–control study of the frequency of thrombophilic disorders in couples with late fetal loss and no thrombotic antecedent. The Nimes Obstetricians and Haematologists Study (NOHA). Thromb Haemost 1999; 81:891–9.

45. Many A, Elad R, Yaron Y, et al. Third-trimester unexplained intrauterine fetal death is associated with inherited thrombophilia. Obstet Gynecol 2002; 99:684–7.

46. Infante-Rivard C, Rivard GE, Yotov WV, et al. Absence of association of thrombophilia polymorphisms with intrauterine growth restriction. N Engl J Med 2002; 347:19–25.

47. Carp HJA, Dolitzky M, Inbal A. Hereditary thrombophilias are not associated with a decreased live birth rate in women with recurrent miscarriage. Fertil Steril 2002; 78:58–62.

48. Salomon O, Seligsohn U, Steinberg DM, et al. The common prothrombotic factors in nulliparous women do not compromise blood flow in the feto–maternal circulation and are not associated with preeclampsia or intrauterine growth restriction. Am J Obstet Gynecol 2004; 191:2002–9.

49. Lindqvist PG, Svensson PJ, Marsá K, et al. Activated protein C resistance (FV:Q506) and pregnancy. Thromb Haemost 1999; 81:532–7.

50. Sanson BJ, Friederich PW, Simioni P, et al. The risk of abortion and stillbirth in antithrombin-, protein C-, and protein S-deficient women. Thromb Haemost 1996; 75:387–8.

51. Gris JC, Mercier E, Quere I, et al. Low-molecular-weight heparin versus low-dose aspirin in women with one fetal loss and a constitutional thrombophilic disorder. Blood 2004; 103:3695–9.

52. Carp HJA, Dolitzky M, Inbal A. Thromboprophylaxis improves the live birth rate in women with consecutive recurrent miscarriages and hereditary thrombophilia. J Thromb Hemost 2003; 1:433–8.

53. Brenner B, Hoffman R, Carp HJA, et al. The LIVE–ENOX Investigators. Efficacy and safety of two doses of enoxaparin in women with thrombophilia and recurrent pregnancy loss: the LIVE-ENOX study. J Thromb Haemost 2005; 3:227–9.

54. Lantz M, Thysell H, Nilsson E, et al. On the binding of tumor necrosis factor (TNF) to heparin and the release in vivo of the TNF-binding protein I by heparin. J Clin Invest 1991; 88:2026–31.

55. Baram D, Rashkovsky M, Hershkoviz R, et al. Inhibitory effects of low molecular weight heparin on mediator release by mast cells: preferential inhibition of cytokine production and mast cell-dependent cutaneous inflammation. Clin Exp Immunol 1997; 110:485–91.

56. Downing LJ, Strieter RM, Kadell AM, et al. Low-dose low-molecular-weight heparin is anti-inflammatory during venous thrombosis. J Vasc Surg 1998; 28:848–54.

57. Bose P, Black S, Kadyrov M, et al. Adverse effects of lupus anticoagulant positive blood sera on placental viability can be prevented by heparin in vitro. Am J Obstet Gynecol 2004; 191:2125–31.

58. Carp HJA, Torchinsky A, Fein A, et al. Hormones, cytokines and fetal anomalies in habitual abortion. J Gynecol Endocrinol 2002; 15:472–83.

59. Krause I, Blank M, Levi Y, et al. Anti-idiotype mmunomodulation of experimental antiphospholipid syndrome via effect on Th1/Th2 expression. Clin Exp Immunol 1999; 117:190–7.

60. Darmochwal-Kolarz D, Rolinski J, Leszczynska-Goarzelak B, et al. The expressions of intracellular cytokines in the lymphocytes of preeclamptic patients. Am J Reprod Immunol 2002; 48:381–6.

61. Maymon E, Ghezzi F, Edwin SS, et al. The tumor necrosis factor alpha and its soluble receptor profile in term and preterm parturition. Am J Obstet Gynecol 1999; 181:1142–8.

62. Hahn-Zoric M, Hagberg H, Kjellmer I, et al. Aberrations in placental cytokine mRNA related to intrauterine growth retardation. Pediatr Res 2002; 51:201–6.

63. Brill A, Torchinsky A., Carp HJA, et al. The role of apoptosis in normal and abnormal embryonic development. J Assist Reprod Genet 1999; 16:512–19.

64. Laude I, Rongieres-Bertrand C, Boyer-Neumann C, et al. Circulating procoagulant microparticles in women with unexplained pregnancy loss: a new insight. Thromb Haemost 2001; 85:18–21.

65. Carp HJA, Dardik R, Lubetsky A, et al. Prevalence of circulating procoagulant microparticles in women with recurrent miscarriage: a case controlled study. Hum Reprod 2004; 19:191–5.

66. Meilahn EN, Kuller LH, Matthews KA, et al. Hemostatic factors according to menopausal status and use of hormone replacement therapy. Ann Epidemiol 1992; 2:445–55.

67. Cosman F, Baz-Hecht M, Cushman M, et al. Short-term effects of estrogen, tamoxifen and raloxifene on hemostasis: a randomized-controlled study and review of the literature. Thromb Res 2005; 116:1–13.

68. Tong MH, Jiang H, Liu P, et al. Spontaneous fetal loss caused by placental thrombosis in estrogen sulfotransferase-deficient mice. Nat Med 2005; 11:153–9.

79. Polan ML, Daniele A, Kuo A. Gonadal steroids modulate human monocyte interleukin-1 (IL-1) activity. Fertil Steril 1988; 49:964–8.

70. Schatz F, Krikun G, Caze R, et al. Progestin-regulated expression of tissue factor in decidual cells: implications in endometrial hemostasis, menstruation and angiogenesis. Steroids 2003; 68:849–60.

71. Smiley ST, Boyer SN, Heeb MJ, et al. Protein S is inducible by interleukin 4 in T cells and inhibits lymphoid cell procoagulant activity. Proc Natl Acad Sci USA 1997; 94:11484–9.

72. Raghupathy R, Al Mutawa E, Makhseed M, et al. Modulation of cytokine prouction by dydrogesterone in lymphocytes from women with recurrent miscarriage. Br J Obset Gynaecol 2005; 112:1096–101.

73. Uzumcu M, Coskun S, Jaroudi K, et al. Effect of human chorionic gonadotropin on cytokine production from human endometrial cells in vitro. Am J Reprod Immunol 1998; 40:83–8.

74. Rosing J. Mechanisms of OC related thrombosis. Thromb Res 2005; 115(Suppl 1):81–3.

DEBATE

10a. Should thromboprophylaxis be used in hereditary thrombophilias with RPL? – For

Benjamin Brenner

THROMBOPHILIA AND FETAL LOSS

Thrombophilic risk factors are common and can be found in 15–25% of Caucasian populations. Since pregnancy is an acquired hypercoagulable state, women harboring thrombophilia may present with clinical symptoms of vascular complications for the first time during gestation.[1] Recurrent pregnancy loss affects 1–5% of women of reproductive age and bears a significant emotional, social, and economical impact. A number of case–control and cohort studies have suggested an association between inherited thrombophilia and recurrent pregnancy loss (RPL).[2–4] Several recently reported meta-analyses support an association between pregnancy loss and maternal factor V Leiden (FVL) and factor II (FII) G20210A genotypes.[5–7] Recently, Lissalde-Lavigne et al[8] reported findings from the 'NOHA first' study, a large carefully designed case–control study nested in a cohort of nearly 32 700 women of whom 18% had pregnancy loss in the first gestation. The findings of the multivariate analysis clearly demonstrate an overall association between unexplained first pregnancy loss after 10 weeks of gestation and the two thrombophilic risks factors (odds ratio (OR) 3.46 and 2.60, respectively).

Documentation of thrombophilic risk factors in women with pregnancy complications may have significant therapeutic implications, since recent clinical studies have demonstrated the potential efficacy of prophylaxis with low-molecular-weight heparin (LMWH) in these settings.[9,10] While interpretation of the results of these studies has given rise to intensive debate,[11] it is clear that the field of thrombophilia and pregnancy complications continues to be at the focus of medical research and clinical practice.

LMWH THERAPY IN PREGNANCY

Until recently, studies on the treatment of women with inherited thrombophilia and pregnancy loss were predominantly uncontrolled, and included small series of patients treated mostly with LMWH. A collaborative study demonstrated the safety of using LMWH during 486 gestations.[12] A successful outcome was reported in 83 (89%) of 93 gestations in women with a history of RPL and in all 28 gestations in women who had experienced preeclampsia during a previous pregnancy. A retrospective French study on the use of the LMWH enoxaparin during 624 pregnancies revealed a good safety profile.[13] More recently, a review of close to 2800 treated pregnancies evaluated the safety and efficacy of LMWH in pregnancy.[14] The main indications were prophylaxis of venous thromboembolism (VTE) and prevention of pregnancy loss. The rate of bleeding complications was low (<2%) and thrombocytopenia was rare, with no cases of heparin-induced thrombocytopenia. Likewise, clinically significant osteoporosis was extremely rare. The live birth rate was between 85% and 96%, depending on the indication.

LMWH IN WOMEN WITH THROMBOPHILIA AND PREGNANCY LOSS

Our group has treated 61 pregnancies in 50 women with thrombophilia who presented with recurrent fetal loss with enoxaparin throughout gestation and 4–6 weeks into the postpartum period.[15] The dose was 40 mg/day, except for patients with combined thrombophilia or in the case of abnormal Doppler velocimetry suggesting decreased placental perfusion, where the dose was increased to 40 mg twice a day. Of the 61 pregnancies, 46 (75%) resulted in live birth, compared with a success rate of only 20% in these 50 women in prior gestations without antithrombotic therapy. Carp et al[16] have reported a cohort study undertaken to assess the effect of enoxaparin on the subsequent live birth rate in women with three or more consecutive pregnancy losses and hereditary thrombophilia. The live birth rate was higher in women treated with enoxaparin: 26 (70.2%) of 37, compared with 21 (43.8%) of 48 in untreated patients. The beneficial effect was mainly in primary aborters and in those with five or more miscarriages. Gris et al[17] have recently carried out a randomized study to compare the effect of enoxaparin given throughout gestation at a dose of 40 mg daily, compared with low-dose aspirin. The study comprised 160 women with thrombophilia and one previous pregnancy loss after 10 weeks of gestation. The patients treated with enoxaparin had a significantly higher live birth rate than the patients treated with low-dose aspirin (86% vs 29%, respectively). These dramatic differences were found in women with FVL and FII G20210A mutations and in women with protein S deficiency. Moreover, thrombophilic women with the co-presence of protein Z deficiency or antibodies to protein Z had a reduced live birth rate following enoxaparin prophylaxis.[17]

The optimal dosage of LMWH is yet unknown and should be determined by prospective randomized trials. Ideally, large placebo-controlled trials should be advocated. However, logistic and ethical difficulties limit this approach.[11] The LIVE–ENOX study[10] was a multicenter prospective randomized study recently conducted in Israel on women with thrombophilia and pregnancy loss, defined as three or more first-trimester, two or more second-trimester, or at least one third-trimester loss; 180 women were enrolled in the study. The study compared two doses of enoxaparin: 40 mg/day and 40 mg twice daily throughout pregnancy, starting at 5–10 weeks of gestation and for 6 weeks postpartum. The primary endpoint was the delivery of a healthy infant. Secondary endpoints were duration of gestation, birthweight, and incidence of gestational thrombosis and gestational vascular complications. The incidence of preeclampsia in the enoxaparin 40 and 80 mg/day groups was 6.7% and 14.3%, respectively, and the incidence of placental abruption was 13.5% and 8.8%, respectively. Approximately a quarter of the women in both groups had had intrauterine growth restriction (IUGR) in previous gestations (22.5% and 24.2%, respectively). The live birth rate prior to enrollment in the study was only 28%. During the study, the live birth rate was 84% for the 40 mg/day group and 78% for the 80 mg/day group.[9] Late gestational complications decreased after enoxaparin treatment. The incidence of preeclampsia in the enoxaparin 40 and 80 mg/day groups was 3.4% and 4.4%, respectively. Similarly, the incidence of placental abruption in the 40 and 80 mg/day groups was 4.5% and 3.3%, respectively.[10] Both doses of enoxaparin appeared to be safe and well tolerated. The gestation period was longer than 36 weeks in over 80% of patients in each group. However, preterm delivery occurred in 10% and 18.5% of women in the enoxaparin 40 and 80 mg/day groups, respectively. Postpartum bleeding (1.1% of women in each group) and enoxaparin-related allergic local skin reactions at the injection sites were observed in a small number of women (2.2% and 3.3% of those receiving 40 and 80 mg/day, respectively). Thus, prophylaxis with enoxaparin (40 or 80 mg/day) is safe and effective for improving pregnancy outcome and reducing late pregnancy complications in thrombophilic women with a history of pregnancy loss. Prophylaxis with LMWH is indicated in women with thrombophilia and late or recurrent early pregnancy loss. Women with severe thrombophilia (i.e., antithrombin deficiency) or with combined thrombophilic risk factors may require higher doses of LMWH.

MONITORING OF LMWH IN PREGNANCY

The need for monitoring of LMWH therapy in pregnancy is debatable. However, consensus conferences such as the ACCP[18] suggest that changes in pharmacokinetic and pharmacodynamic properties during pregnancy may require monitoring. Indeed, a recent study suggests that monitoring of anti-Xa and free tissue factor pathway inhibitor (TFPI) levels is of value during pregnancy in thrombophilic women treated with enoxaparin.[19] It is debatable whether antithrombotic prophylaxis should be used for unexplained recurrent first- or second-trimester pregnancy loss in women who do not harbor thrombophilia. A recent study by Dolitzky et al[20] found that enoxaparin 40 mg/day and low-dose aspirin were equally effective in this setting. However, selection bias cannot be excluded in the study by Dolitzky et al,[20] since women were enrolled after demonstration of fetal heart beat.

MECHANISM OF ACTION OF LMWH IN PREGNANCY

The mechanisms of action of LMWH in women with placental vascular complications have not been fully elucidated. While the systemic anticoagulant effect in the maternal circulation is important, other mechanisms have been suggested. These include anti-inflammatory effects and modulation of local hemostasis at the placental level. In particular, placental trophoblasts are characterized by a hemostatic balance between TF and TFPI.[21] This balance is hampered in placental vascular complications, as TFPI levels are reduced. Maternal treatment with LMWH restores TFPI levels and improves the TF/TFPI balance in the human placenta.[22]

In about 30–50% of women with pregnancy loss, no specific thrombophilic risk factor can be documented. It is possible that in some of these cases, subtle changes in a number of coagulation proteins can lead to abnormal function of the protein C system that can be detected by global assays.[23] Presentation of membrane hemostatic proteins such as TF, thrombomodulin (TM), and endothelial protein C receptor (EPCR) on trophoblasts may determine a local procoagulant profile of the placenta.[24] Abnormalities in these genes may serve as risk modifiers in thrombophilia-associated gestational vascular complications. Indeed, LMWH therapy improves gestational outcome in obligatory carriers of EPCR knockout mice.[25]

REFERENCES

1. Brenner B. Clinical management of thrombophilia-related placental vascular complications. Blood 2004; 103:4003–9.
2. Grandone E, Margaglione M, Colaizzo D, et al. Factor V Leiden is associated with repeated and recurrent unexplained fetal losses. Thromb Haemost 1997; 77:822–4.
3. Ridker PM, Miletich JP, Buring JE, et al. Factor V Leiden mutation as a risk factor for recurrent pregnancy loss. Ann Intern Med 1998; 15:1000–3.
4. Brenner B, Sarig G, Weiner Z, et al. Thrombophilic polymorphisms are common in women with fetal loss without apparent cause. Thromb Haemost 1999; 82:6–9.
5. Rey E, Kahn SR, David M, et al. Thrombophilic disorders and fetal loss: a meta-analysis. Lancet 2003; 361:901–8.
6. Kovalevsky G, Gracia CR, Berlin JA, et al. Evaluation of the association between hereditary thrombophilias and recurrent pregnancy loss: a meta-analysis. Arch Intern Med 2004; 164:558–63.
7. Dudding TE, Attia J. The association between adverse pregnancy outcomes and maternal factor V Leiden genotype: a meta-analysis. Thromb Haemost 2004; 91:700–11.
8. Lissalde-Lavigne G, Fabbro-Peray P, Cochery-Nouvellon E, et al. Factor V Leiden and prothrombin G20210A polymorphisms as risk factors for miscarriage during a first intended pregnancy: the matched case–control 'NOHA first' study. J Thromb Haemost 2005; 3:2178–84.
9. Brenner B, Bar J, Ellis M, et al. Effects of enoxaparin on late pregnancy complications and neonatal outcome in women with recurrent pregnancy loss and thrombophilia: results from the LIVE–ENOX study. Fertil Steril 2005; 84:770–3.
10. Brenner B, Hoffman R, Carp H, et al. Efficacy and safety of two doses of enoxaparin in women with thrombophilia and recurrent pregnancy loss: the LIVE–ENOX study. J Thromb Haemost 2005; 3:227–9.
11. Walker ID, Kujovich L, Greer IA, et al. The use of LMWH in pregnancies at risk: new evidence or perception? J Thromb Haemost 2005; 3:778–93.
12. Sanson BJ, Lensing AW, Prins MH, et al. Safety of low molecular weight heparin in pregnancy: a systemic review. Thromb Haemost 1999; 81:668–72.

13. Lepercq J, Conard J, Borel-Derlon A, et al. Venous thromboembolism during pregnancy: a retrospective study of enoxaparin safety in 624 pregnancies. Br J Obstet Gynaecol 2001; 108:1134–40.

14. Greer IA, Nelson-Piercy C. Low-molecular-weight heparins for thromboprophylaxis and treatment of venous thromboembolism in pregnancy: a systematic review of safety and efficacy. Blood 2005; 106:401–7.

15. Brenner B, Hoffman R, Blumenfeld Z, et al. Gestational outcome in thrombophilic women with recurrent pregnancy loss treated by enoxaparin. Thromb Haemost 2000; 83:693–7.

16. Carp H, Dolitzky M, Inbal A. Thromboprophylaxis improves the live birth rate in women with consecutive recurrent miscarriages and hereditary thrombophilia. J Thromb Haemost 2003; 1:433–8.

17. Gris JC, Mercier E, Quere I, et al. Low-molecular-weight heparin versus low-dose aspirin in women with one fetal loss and a constitutional thrombophilic disorder. Blood 2004; 103:3695–9.

18. Bates SM, Greer IA, Hirsh J, et al. Use of antithrombotic agents during pregnancy: the Seventh ACCP Conference on Antithrombotic and Thrombolytic Therapy. Chest 2004; 126(3 Suppl):627S-44S.

19. Sarig G, Blumenfeld Z, Leiba R, et al. Modulation of systemic hemostatic parameters by enoxaparin during gestation in women with thrombophilia and pregnancy loss. Thromb Haemost 2005; 94:980–5.

20. Dolitzky M, Inbal A, Weiss A, et al. Randomized study of thromboprophylaxis in women with unexplained consecutive recurrent miscarriages. Fertil Steril 2006: 86:362–6.

21. Aharon A, Brenner B, Katz T, et al. Tissue factor and tissue factor pathway inhibitor levels in trophoblast cells: implications for placental hemostasis. Thromb Haemost 2004; 92:776–86.

22. Aharon A, Lanir N, Drugan A, et al. Placental TFPI is decreased in gestational vascular complications and can be restored by maternal enoxaparin treatment. J Thromb Haemost 2005; 3:2355–7.

23. Sarig G, Lanir N, Hoffman R, et al. Protein C global assay in the evaluation of women with idiopathic pregnancy loss. Thromb Haemost 2002; 88:32–6.

24. Sood R, Kalloway S, Mast AE, et al. Fetomaternal cross talk in the placental vascular bed: control of coagulation by trophoblast cells. Blood 2006; 107:3173–80.

25. Gu JM, Crawley JT, Ferrell G, et al. Disruption of the endothelial cell protein C receptor gene in mice causes placental thrombosis and early embryonic lethality. J Biol Chem 2002; 277:43335–43.

DEBATE

10b. Should thromboprophylaxis be used in hereditary thrombophilias with RPL? – Against

Pelle G Lindqvist

INTRODUCTION

Habitual abortion is usually associated with up to a 75% live birth rate after three consecutive fetal losses.[1,2] Recurrent pregnancy loss (RPL) is often taken to have a broader definition of at least three first-trimester fetal losses and/or two or more second-trimester fetal losses. Factors that are major determinants of the risk of miscarriage are maternal age, the number of prior fetal losses, and whether or not cardiac activity had been detected.[2] The pathogenesis of recurrent fetal loss in the majority of cases is still unclear. Several causes have been suggested: chromosome aberrations, thrombophilias, thyroid abnormality, microparticles, and complement activation.[3]

RELATIONSHIP BETWEEN FIRST-TRIMESTER FETAL LOSS AND THROMBOPHILIA

Treatment of RPL with low-molecular-weight heparin (LMWH) is based on a supposed causative relationship between thrombophilias and recurrent fetal loss. Such a link has not been established and is still disputed. Since the majority of recurrent fetal losses occur in the first trimester and more than 90% of women with heritable thrombophilias in Caucasian populations are carriers of either coagulation factor V Leiden (FVL) or the prothrombin gene mutation G20210A (FII), the analysis below

will focus on these factors. First-trimester fetal loss has not been related to hereditary thrombophilia – either in large cohorts[4,5] or in the largest case–control studies.[6,7] Studies of early RPL show no increased risk in the largest case–control studies.[6,8] Although several meta-analyses and systematic reviews have shown an increased prevalence of thrombophilias in RPL. Meta-analyses may not be a sound method of amassing evidence from these studies, as the majority of studies that have been surveyed are uncontrolled, underpowered, and subject to several types of bias. In addition, the conclusions are mostly drawn from case–control studies, which tend to overestimate risk assessments when compared with cohort studies. With regard to second-trimester (or >10 gestational weeks) or third-trimester fetal loss, there seems to be an increased risk.[7]

SINGLE-GENE MUTATION AND HUMAN EVOLUTION

Both FVL and FII are single-gene mutations that appear to have first occurred some 25 000 years ago.[9,10] A strong relation between these thrombophilias and fetal loss would have had a strong negative impact on the respective gene pool. Instead, the number of carriers of FVL has gone from one person 25 000 years ago to about 50 million carriers of Caucasian descent today.[11] Thus, from an evolutionary perspective, it is unlikely that an increased risk of fetal loss in the general population has been caused by these thrombophilias. However, this does not exclude the possibility of a relationship in small subgroups, i.e., second-trimester fetal losses or habitual abortions. The more prevalent a single-mutation thrombophilia is, the less likely is an increased risk of fetal loss. Thus, a causative link between fetal loss and rare mutations such as antithrombin, protein C, and protein S deficiencies is more likely, as compared with FVL and FII.[12]

TREATMENT STUDIES

There have been some treatment studies published using a 'before and after' design.[13,14] This design lacks a control group, and the result is conditioned by the phenomenon of 'regression toward the mean'.[15] 'Regression toward the mean' is a statistical principle stating that, of related measurements, the expected value of the second is closer to the mean than the observed value of the first.[16] Therefore, in a 'before and after' design, one should expect the group of women with the highest rate of recurrent fetal loss to have a lower rate of RPL by natural

causes, independent of medical intervention (see Chapter 18). Therefore, no conclusions may be drawn from the results.[13,14] The study by Gris et al,[17] comparing enoxaparin treatment with low-dose aspirin in nulliparous carriers of FVL with a single pregnancy loss, has also been criticized for not including untreated controls.[18] The authors write that in the course of their investigation, the creation of a control group 'was tried out, but failed'. Recently, we have compiled data on the magnitude of 'regression toward the mean' (Table 10b.1).[18] In fact, the untreated women with recurrent fetal loss in our prospective cohort have a similar outcome to those treated with enoxaparin.[13,14,18] Moreover, our untreated FVL carriers with a prior fetal loss had similar outcomes to FVL carriers with a single prior fetal loss who were treated with enoxaparin[17,18] (Table 10b.1). A discussion of the optimal dosage of LMWH is not relevant before a relation has been established.[15]

Many of us remember when immunotherapy was considered the optimal treatment for RPL, but immunotherapy was widely introduced before conclusive studies had been performed.[19] There is only

Table 10b.1 Pregnancy outcome in different subgroups of women with prior fetal loss

	Prior live birth rate (%)	Present live birth rate (%)
Recurrent fetal loss[a]		
Enoxaparin 40 or 80 mg/day ($n = 50$)[13,b]	20	75
Enoxaparin 40 mg/day ($n = 89$)[14,b]	28	84
Enoxaparin 80 mg/day ($n = 91$)[14,b]	28	78
No treatment ($n = 37$)[18,c]	28	89
Second-trimester fetal loss		
1 prior ($n = 43$), no treatment[18]	49	98
≥ 2 prior ($n = 10$) prior, no treatment[18]	30	80
Nulliparous women with one prior fetal loss and carriers of		
factor V leiden (FVL)		
Low-dose aspirin ($n = 36$)[17]	0	29
Enoxaparin 40 mg/day ($n = 36$)[17]	0	94
No treatment ($n = 20$)[18,d]	0	95
No treatment ($n = 52$)[18,e]	40	98

[a]Recurrent fetal loss: ≥ 3 first-trimester and/or ≥ 2 second-trimester fetal loss.
[b]Includes or/and ≥ 1 stillbirth.
[c]Includes women with and without thrombophilia.
[d]Nulliparous carriers of FVL with at least 1 prior fetal loss.
[e]FVL carriers with at least 1 prior fetal loss.

one study designed to answer the question of whether it is of value to treat thrombophilic women having habitual abortion[20] with LMWH and no study of women with recurrent second-trimester losses. In 2003, Carp et al[20] raised the possibility that LMWH treatment might be beneficial for women with a history of habitual abortion. Most encouraging were the positive results in the small subgroup of primary aborters. However, the investigation needs to be reproduced in a randomized manner.

Due to the lack of studies designed to address the issue at hand, we have as yet no evidence to recommend LMWH treatment for RPL due to thrombophilia.

REFERENCES

1. Warburton D, Fraser FC. On the probability that a woman who has had a spontaneous abortion will abort in subsequent pregnancies. J Obstet Gynaecol Br Emp 1961; 68:784–8.
2. Brigham SA, Conlon C, Farquharson RG. A longitudinal study of pregnancy outcome following idiopathic recurrent miscarriage. Hum Reprod 1999; 14:2868–71.
3. Carp H, Dardik R, Lubetsky A, et al. Prevalence of circulating procoagulant microparticles in women with recurrent miscarriage: a case-controlled study. Hum Reprod 2004; 19:191–5.
4. Lindqvist PG, Svensson P, Dahlback B. Activated protein C resistance – in the absence of factor V Leiden – and pregnancy. J Thromb Haemost 2006; 4:361–6.
5. Roque H, Paidas MJ, Funai EF, et al. Maternal thrombophilias are not associated with early pregnancy loss. Thromb Haemost 2004; 91:290–5.
6. Rai R, Shlebak A, Cohen H, et al. Factor V Leiden and acquired activated protein C resistance among 1000 women with recurrent miscarriage. Hum Reprod 2001; 16:961–5.
7. Lissalde-Lavigne G, Fabbro-Peray P, Cochery-Nouvellon E, et al. Factor V Leiden and prothrombin G20210A polymorphisms as risk factors for miscarriage during a first intended pregnancy: the matched case–control 'NOHA first' study. J Thromb Haemost 2005; 3:2178–84.
8. Carp H, Salomon O, Seidman D, et al. Prevalence of genetic markers for thrombophilia in recurrent pregnancy loss. Hum Reprod 2002; 17:1633–7.
9. Zivelin A, Griffin JH, Xu X, et al. A single genetic origin for a common Caucasian risk factor for venous thrombosis. Blood 1997; 89:397–402.
10. Zivelin A, Rosenberg N, Faier S, et al. A single genetic origin for the common prothrombotic G20210A polymorphism in the prothrombin gene. Blood 1998; 92:1119–24.
11. Lindqvist PG, Zöller B, Dahlbäck B. Improved hemoglobin status and reduced menstrual blood loss among female carriers of activated protein C resistance (FV Leiden). An evolutionary advantage? Thromb Haemost 2001; 86:1122–3.
12. Preston FE, Rosendaal FR, Walker ID, et al. Increased fetal loss in women with heritable thrombophilia. Lancet 1996; 348:913–16.
13. Brenner B, Hoffman R, Blumenfeld Z, et al. Gestational outcome in thrombophilic women with recurrent pregnancy loss treated by enoxaparin. Thromb Haemost 2000; 83:693–7.
14. Brenner B, Hoffman R, Carp H, et al. Efficacy and safety of two doses of enoxaparin in women with thrombophilia and recurrent pregnancy loss: the LIVE–ENOX study. J Thromb Haemost 2005; 3:227–9.
15. Lindqvist PG, Merlo J. Low molecular weight heparin for repeated pregnancy loss: Is it based on solid evidence? J Thromb Haemost 2005; 3:221–3.
16. Regression toward the mean. Wikipedia, the free encyclopedia, 2006. http://en.wikipedia.org
17. Gris JC, Mercier E, Quere I, et al. Low-molecular-weight heparin versus low-dose aspirin in women with one fetal loss and a constitutional thrombophilic disorder. Blood 2004; 103:3695–9.
18. Lindqvist PG, Merlo J. The natural course of women with recurrent fetal loss. J Thromb Haemost 2006; 4:896–7.
19. Scott JR. Immunotherapy for recurrent miscarriage. Cochrane Database Syst Rev 2003; (1):CD000112.
20. Carp H, Dolitzky M, Inbal A. Thromboprophylaxis improves the live birth rate in women with consecutive recurrent miscarriages and hereditary thrombophilia. J Thromb Haemost 2003; 1:433–8.

11. Uterine anomalies and recurrent pregnancy loss

Daniel S Seidman and Mordechai Goldenberg

INTRODUCTION

Anatomical uterine defects have long been associated with recurrent miscarriage. However, it is frustrating to realize how little is actually known regarding the pathophysiology responsible for the proposed causal association between uterine anomalies and fetal wastage. The lack of a clear understanding of the causative mechanisms may be due to the fact that the prevalence and impact of uterine malformations has so far not been conclusively determined.[1] Even the true incidence of congenital uterine anomalies in the general population is unknown. A review of the available literature reveals a wide range of reported incidences, from 0.2% to 10.0%.[2]

Using newer imaging modalities, it is currently estimated that the incidence of uterine anomalies in the general population is approximately 1%, and is about threefold higher in women with recurrent pregnancy loss (RPL) and poor reproductive outcomes.[2] Below, we will discuss in detail the new modes of imaging that have been introduced over the last two decades and which may modify the previously reported data on the incidence.

In addition to pregnancy loss, uterine malformations predispose women to other reproductive difficulties, including infertility, preterm labor, and abnormal fetal presentation. These poor reproductive outcomes are often attributed to the presence of a uterine septum, intrauterine adhesions, polyps, and fibroids, all of which are amenable to surgical correction. Therefore, an accurate diagnosis is essential in order to offer appropriate treatment.

In this chapter, we will review the common congenital and acquired uterine anomalies associated with RPL, and discuss contemporary diagnosis and treatment options.

DEVELOPMENT AND CLASSIFICATION OF MÜLLERIAN DUCT DEFECTS

Uterine anatomical defects are commonly classified as congenital or acquired. The classification of congenital uterine defects is largely based on the understanding of müllerian duct development.

The two paired müllerian ducts of the embryo ultimately develop into the female reproductive tract. The cephalic ends of the müllerian ducts form the fallopian tubes, and the caudal portions fuse to form the uterus, cervix, and the upper two-thirds of the vagina. The ovaries and lower one-third of the vagina have separate embryological origins. The müllerian ducts grow caudally and become enclosed in peritoneal folds that later develop into the round and ovarian ligaments. In the female embryo, sexual differentiation is marked by degeneration of the wolffian ducts in the absence of fetal testes and testosterone. Absence of müllerian-inhibiting substance allows the müllerian ducts to fully mature. At 9 weeks of gestation, the uterine cervix is recognizable, and by 17 weeks the formation of the myometrium is complete. Vaginal development begins at approximately 9 weeks. The uterovaginal plate forms between the caudal buds of the müllerian ducts and the dorsal wall of the urogenital sinus. These cells will degenerate, thereby increasing the distance between the uterus and urogenital sinus. Hence, the upper two-thirds of the vagina derives from the müllerian ducts while the remainder derives from the urogenital sinus. Complete formation and differentiation of the müllerian ducts into the segments of the female reproductive tract depend on completion of the following three phases of development: organogenesis, fusion both laterally and vertically, and resorption.

In failure of organogenesis, one or both müllerian ducts may not develop fully, resulting in abnormalities such as uterine agenesis or hypoplasia (bilateral) or unicornuate uterus (unilateral). In lateral fusion defects, the process by which the lower segments of the paired müllerian ducts fuse to form the uterus, cervix, and upper vagina fails. Failure of fusion results in anomalies such as bicornuate or didelphys uterus. Vertical fusion refers to fusion of the ascending sinovaginal bulb with the descending müllerian system (i.e., fusion of the lower one-third and upper two-thirds of the vagina). Complete vertical fusion forms a normal patent vagina, while incomplete vertical fusion results in an imperforate hymen.

After the lower müllerian ducts fuse, a central septum is present, which subsequently must be resorbed to form a single uterine cavity and cervix. Failure of resorption results in septate uterus.

Müllerian duct anomalies occur throughout development, although the etiology of these defects remains poorly understood. The most commonly used classification of müllerian duct anomalies is that of the American Fertility Society (now named the American Society for Reproductive Medicine),[3] which is shown in Table 11.1.

SUBSEPTATE UTERUS

Subseptate uterus is considered to be the most common major uterine anomaly in women with RPL[4] and recurrent first-trimester pregnancy loss.[5] Indeed, the subseptate uterus accounted for 70–90% of major anomalies found in low-risk women with uterine anomalies.[6–9]

Table 11.1 Classification of müllerian duct anomalies

---

1. Class I: uterine agenesis or hypoplasia
2. Class II: unicornuate uterus
3. Class III: didelphys uterus
4. Class IV: bicornuate uterus
5. Class V: septate uterus
6. Class VI: arcuate uterus
7. Class VII: diethystilbestrol (DES)-exposed uterus

The association between RPL and subseptate uterus has been attributed to the decreased amount of connective tissue in the relatively avascular septum, resulting in poor decidualization and placentation. In addition, the increased amount of muscle tissue in the septum can cause miscarriage by the production of local uncoordinated myometrial contractility. The view that inadequate blood supply to the developing embryo accounts for the fetal losses is supported by histological evaluation of the septum showing a significantly reduced vascular supply relative to the rest of the uterus.[10,11] If this theory is correct, then the likelihood of miscarriage caused by septal implantation should increase with the severity of the disruption of uterine morphology.[6]

Salim et al[6] showed that the degree of distortion of the uterine cavity in subseptate uterus was higher in women with recurrent miscarriage, compared with low-risk women. The uterine cavity was mainly distorted due to the reduced length of unaffected cavity, rather than increased septum length. The greater degree of uterine cavity distortion in RPL supports the hypothesis of septal implantation as a potential cause of miscarriage, since the likelihood of septal implantation increases with an increasing ratio of septal size to functional cavity.

ARCUATE UTERUS

An arcuate uterus has, by definition, an intrauterine indentation less than 1 cm. Using three-dimensional (3D) ultrasound, it has been found that the prevalence of arcuate uterus was 17% in women with recurrent miscarriage,[6] which is significantly higher than the prevalence of 3.2% in low-risk women.[8] In addition, it has been shown that distortion of the uterine cavity is greater in women with recurrent first-trimester loss, as with the subseptate uterus.

The diagnosis of arcuate uterus is difficult when conventional diagnostic methods such as hysteroscopy or laparoscopy are used, as the diagnostic criteria are far from clear.[12] As a result, little is known about the prevalence and clinical significance. Although many believe that the arcuate uterus has little or no impact on reproduction and obstetric outcomes, some studies have reported an increase in adverse reproductive outcomes, mostly second-trimester loss.[9,13,14] The pathophysiology of fetal loss in women with arcuate uterus remains obscure.

UNICORNUATE UTERUS

A unicornuate uterus is the result of complete, or almost complete, arrest of development of one of the müllerian ducts (Figure 11.1). When the arrest is incomplete (in 90% of patients with unicornuate uterus), a rudimentary horn with or without functioning endometrium is present. If the rudimentary horn is obstructed, it may present as an enlarging pelvic mass, with unilateral cyclical pelvic pain secondary to hematometra. Pregnancies can occur in the rudimentary horn, with an estimated incidence of 2%. These cases may be difficult to diagnose, and may result in rupture of the rudimentary horn.

The incidence of unicornuate uterus has been estimated to be 6.3% of uterine anomalies, and may be associated with urinary tract anomalies, especially renal. Urinary tract anomalies should be suspected in all women with a unicornuate uterus.[15] Unicornuate uterus is associated with the worst reproductive outcome.[16] About one-third of all pregnancies result in miscarriage.[9,17,18] The high miscarriage rate is mostly attributed to abnormal uterine vasculature and decreased muscle mass. Increased cesarean section rates are a result of fetal malpresentation and irregular uterine contractions during labor.

There are no surgical procedures to correct the unicornuate uterus. Prophylactic cervical cerclage has been suggested for the prevention of miscarriage in patients with unicornuate uterus, although there is no clear evidence of cervical incompetence.[19] However, with little data to support the use of cerclage, most clinicians prefer to use careful follow-up, with frequent clinical and sonographic evaluation of cervical length. Resection of the cavitated rudimentary horn is often recommended in symptomatic patients with unicornuate uterus suffering from dysmenorrhea and hematometra. Laparoscopic excision of the rudimentary horn has been shown to be an effective surgical approach.[20]

UTERUS DIDELPHYS

A double uterus results from the complete failure of the two müllerian ducts to fuse (Figures 11.2 and 11.3). Therefore, each duct develops into a separate uterus, each of which is narrower than a

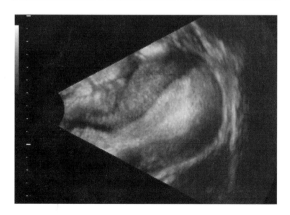

Figure 11.1 Three-dimensional transvaginal ultrasound of a unicornuate uterus using volume contrast imaging. (Courtesy of Professor Yaron Zalael MD, Sheba Medical Center, Tel-Hashomer, Israel.)

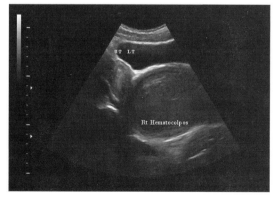

Figure 11.2 Two-dimensional transvaginal ultrasound of a didelphys uterus with obstructed right vagina (hematocolpos). (Courtesy of Professor Yaron Zalael MD, Sheba Medical Center, Tel-Hashomer, Israel.)

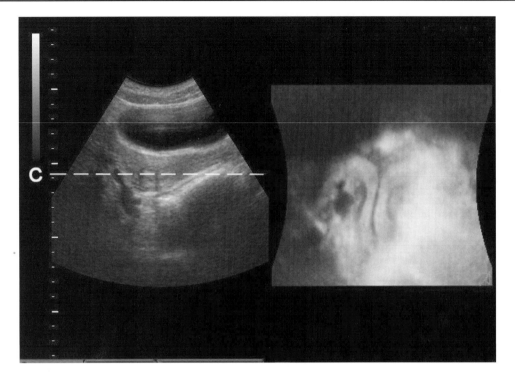

Figure 11.3 Two- and three-dimensional transvaginal ultrasound of a didelphys uterus using volume contrast imaging in plane C. (Courtesy of Professor Yaron Zalael MD, Sheba Medical Center, Tel-Hashomer, Israel.)

normal uterus and has only a single horn. The two uteri may each have a cervix or may share a cervix. In 67% of cases, a uterus didelphys is associated with two vaginas separated by a thin wall. Didelphic uteri are relatively uncommon, with an estimated incidence of 6.3% of uterine anomalies.[6] The two uteri do not always function normally, and are associated with a miscarriage rate of 20.9% and a preterm delivery rate of 24.4%.[6,21] A long-term follow-up of 49 Finnish women with didelphic uterus and a longitudinal vaginal septum reported an obstructed hemivagina in nine women (18%). Eight of these nine women also had ipsilateral renal agenesis.[21] Cesarean section rates are higher, due to uterine dystocia and malpresentation.[22] In addition, didelphic uterus is commonly associated with a patent or obstructed vaginal septum. Fertility in women with didelphic uterus, is not notably impaired.

However, endometriosis is more commonly associated with a didelphic uterus, possibly because of retrograde menstruation.[21]

BICORNUATE UTERUS

A bicornuate uterus results from partial non-fusion of the müllerian ducts (Figure 11.4). The central myometrium may extend to the level of the internal cervical os (bicornuate unicollis) or external cervical os (bicornuate bicollis). The latter is distinguished from uterus didelphys because it demonstrates some degree of fusion between the two horns, while in uterus didelphys the two horns and cervices are separated completely. In addition, the horns of the bicornuate uteri are not fully developed; typically, they are smaller than those of didelphys uteri. Bicornuate uterus is proably the most common

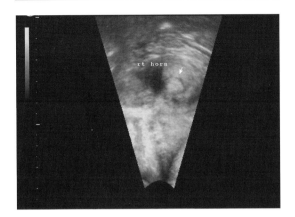

Figure 11.4 Three-dimensional transvaginal ultrasound of a bicornuate uterus. (Courtesy of Professor Yaron Zalael MD, Sheba Medical Center, Tel-Hashomer, Israel.)

uterine anomaly after septate and arcuate uterus.[22] The reproductive outcome seems to be directly correlated with the severity of fundal indentation.[9] It is generally considered that bicornuate uterus does not directly affect infertility, but may be linked with recurrent miscarriages. Bicornuate uterus can be corrected surgically by metroplasty.

T-SHAPED UTERUS AND DIETHYLSTILBESTROL EXPOSURE

Diethylstilbestrol (DES) is a synthetic estrogen that was used from 1948 up to its ban in 1971 to prevent further pregnancy losses in women with RPL. However, approximately two-thirds of embryos exposed in utero developed uterine abnormalities, including a characteristic small, incompletely formed uterus with a T-shaped cavity and a hypoplastic cervix. The spontaneous incidence of T-shaped uterus is unknown in the general population. In addition, approximately half of DES-exposed women have structural cervical defects, including an incompletely formed cervix. The mechanism by which DES disrupts normal uterine development is not known. DES-exposed women are less likely than unexposed women to have a full-term live birth, and are more likely to have premature births,

spontaneous pregnancy losses, or ectopic pregnancies.[23] Women exposed to DES in utero are also at increased risk for breast cancer and clear cell adenocarcinoma of the vagina and cervix.[24]

Goldberg and Falcone,[25] in a meta-analysis study of DES-exposed subjects, found a ninefold increase in ectopic pregnancy, a twofold increase in miscarriage rate, and a twofold increase in preterm delivery compared with a matched control population. Pregnancy rates were similar between DES-exposed women and controls: 72% and 79%, respectively. The poor obstetric outcomes are caused not only by the uterine anomaly, but also by an anti-estrogenic effect at the level of the endometrium.[22] The clinical significance of DES exposure is rapidly diminishing as those affected women pass their reproductive years.[22]

MYOMAS

Myomas are considered the most common acquired anomaly of the uterus. It has been shown[26] that infertile women with fibroids have a lower pregnancy rate when undergoing assisted reproduction than age-matched women with no fibroids. Submucous myomas deform the uterine cavity, and the overlying endometrium is usually thin and inadequate for normal implantation. Submucous fibroids can also be associated with pregnancy loss.[27] The situation is less clear with intramural and subserosal fibroids. In these locations, the size and the number of fibroids may be significant. Significantly lower implantation and pregnancy rates have been found in patients with intramural or submucosal fibroids undergoing in vitro fertilization and intracytoplasmic sperm injection, even when there was no uterine cavity deformation.[28] Furthermore, the pregnancy rate observed within 1 year of myomectomy is higher than that observed in couples with unexplained infertility and no treatment.[29,30]

POLYPS

Polyps are benign hyperplastic endometrial growths that have also been associated with adverse pregnancy outcomes. It is postulated that polyps and fibroids with intracavitary extension may act like foreign bodies within the endometrial cavity.[31] It has also been proposed that polyps and fibroids might induce chronic inflammatory changes in the endometrium that make it unfavorable for pregnancy. Since the presence of polyps has been associated with a worse prognosis for pregnancy, hysteroscopic polypectomy is usually considered if no other explanation for the recurrent loss is found.[32]

INTRAUTERINE ADHESIONS

Intrauterine synechiae may not be a frequent cause of recurrent abortion, but may lead to secondary infertility in these patients. Intrauterine adhesions develop as a result of surgical procedures, typically curettage, or endometritis. Intrauterine scars can probably interfere with the normal implantation process, and may be responsible for pregnancy loss. Intrauterine adhesions are expected to be more common among patients with recurrent abortions, since the formation of adhesions may even follow a simple manual vacuum aspiration for early pregnancy loss.[33] Among 23 patients with an otherwise unexplained history of three or more first- or second-trimester miscarriages and no live births, hysteroscopy showed that 5 (21.8%) had intrauterine adhesions.[34]

INVESTIGATION OF UTERINE INTEGRITY

In patients with RPL, imaging studies are important during the initial workup in order to assess the integrity of the uterus. The guidelines of the Royal College of Obstetricians and Gynaecologists[35] for investigating recurrent miscarriage recommend an ultrasound scan of the pelvis, but this recommendation is based solely on the clinical experience of the guideline development group, rather than on published evidence. Transvaginal sonography (TVS) is usually the initial step, but is now enhanced using 3D-mode ultrasound. TVS allows accurate and rapid characterization of the uterus, including its size and position, as well as the presence of anomalies such

as a duplicated cervix, duplicated uterus, uterine septum, or unicornuate uterus. TVS is also useful in determining the size and location of uterine myomas, as well as the presence of intrauterine polyps and endometrial irregularities that might suggest adhesions.

Recent reports on 2D and 3D TVS, as well as saline contrast sonohysterography, appear promising for diagnosis and classification of congenital uterine anomalies.[36] The ability to visualize both the uterine cavity and the fundal uterine contour on a 3D scan facilitates the diagnosis of uterine anomalies and enables differentiation between septate and bicornuate uteri. The additional use of color Doppler ultrasound may also allow visualization of intraseptal vascularity and may help in distinguishing the avascular from the vascular septum.

Intravenous pyelography is recommended during the workup of congenital anomalies. Defects in the urinary tract are commonly seen when a uterine anomaly is diagnosed.[15]

HYSTEROSALPINGOGRAPHY

Hysterosalpingography (HSG) has long been used to evaluate the contour of the uterine cavity, cervical canal, and fallopian tube.[37] The radio-opaque contrast medium fills the cavity, allowing the accurate identification of filling defects, scarring, or a septum. However, HSG alone cannot differentiate between a septate uterus and a bicornuate uterus. Furthermore, HSG cannot determine the myometrial extension or the size of intrauterine lesions. Therefore, HSG is primarily used to assess tubal patency, and has a limited role in the imaging of uterine malformations.

THREE-DIMENSIONAL ULTRASOUND

3D ultrasound is now accepted as an accurate and reproducible means for the diagnosis of congenital uterine anomalies[38] (Figures 11.1 and 11.5). It has clear advantage over HSG, hysteroscopy, and laparoscopy for the diagnosis of congenital uterine anomalies, since it is a non-invasive method and is currently available in most out patient settings.

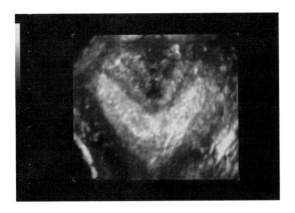

Figure 11.5 Three-dimensional transvaginal ultrasound of a septated uterus (3D rendering). (Courtesy of Professor Yaron Zalael MD, Sheba Medical Center, Tel-Hashomer, Israel.)

The results of 3D ultrasound have been shown to concur with HSG in all cases of arcuate uterus and major congenital anomalies.[8] It has been suggested that the ability to visualize both the uterine cavity and the myometrium on a 3D scan facilitates the diagnosis of uterine anomalies and enables easy differentiation between subseptate and bicornuate uteri.

Salim et al[6] have examined the differences in the morphology of uterine anomalies found in 509 women with a history of unexplained recurrent miscarriage and 1976 low-risk women who were examined for the presence of congenital uterine anomalies by 3D ultrasound. Salim et al[6] detected 121 anomalies in the recurrent miscarriage group and 105 among low-risk women. Surprisingly, there was no significant difference in relative frequency of various anomalies or the depth of fundal distortion between the two groups. However, with both arcuate and subseptate uteri, the length of remaining uterine cavity was significantly shorter and the distortion ratio was significantly higher in the recurrent miscarriage group. Salim et al[6] therefore concluded that the distortion of uterine anatomy is more severe in the congenital uterine anomalies, found in women with a history of recurrent first-trimester miscarriage.

Woelfer et al[14] tried to determine the reproductive outcomes in women with congenital uterine anomalies detected incidentally by 3D ultrasound. In their study, 1089 women with no history of infertility or recurrent miscarriage, undergoing a transvaginal ultrasound scan, were screened for uterine abnormalities: 983 women had a normally shaped uterine cavity, 72 an arcuate, 29 a subseptate, and 5 bicornuate uterus. Women with a subseptate uterus had a significantly higher proportion of first-trimester loss compared with women with a normal uterus. Women with an arcuate uterus had a significantly greater proportion of second-trimester loss and preterm labor. The study by Woelfer et al[14] demonstrated the potential value of 3D ultrasound and contributed evidence to the proposed association between congenital uterine anomalies and adverse pregnancy outcomes.

SONOHYSTEROGRAPHY

Valenzano et al[39] have assessed the diagnostic value and usefulness of transvaginal sonohysterography (SHG) in the detection of uterine anomalies, compared with other diagnostic methods. SHG was able to detect all uterine anomalies found in a study of 54 patients with primary or secondary infertility or repeated spontaneous abortion and with a clinically or sonographically suspected abnormal uterus. SHG was carried out by the intrauterine injection of an isotonic saline solution. The sensitivity and specificity of SHG were the same as for hysteroscopy. However, there was no significant difference between the diagnostic capabilities of the methods analyzed. Valenzano et al[39] therefore concluded that transvaginal SHG with saline solution is a low-cost, easy, and helpful examination method for uterine malformations.

It is now possible to combine 3D ultrasound with SHG. Sylvestre et al[40] carried out a study of 209 infertile patients suspected to have an intrauterine lesion on 3D SHG. Ninety-two patients with a lesion underwent hysteroscopy. In these 92 patients, polyps were found in 48 women, submucous or intramural myomas in 35, both polyps and myomas in 3, müllerian anomalies in 4, thick endometrium in 1, and intrauterine synechiae in 1. It was concluded that 3D SHG allowed precise recognition and localization of lesions. It was further suggested that if 2D and 3D SHG are normal, invasive diagnostic procedures such as hysteroscopy can be avoided.

Alborzi et al[41] performed a prospective study to determine whether SHG can differentiate septate from bicornuate uterus, in 20 patients with a history of RPL and an HSG diagnosis of septate or bicornuate uterus. SHG was found to effectively differentiate septate and bicornuate uterus, and may eliminate the need for laparoscopy in order to differentiate between these uterine anomalies.

The diagnostic accuracy of SHG has been evaluated prospectively compared with HSG and TVS in a study comprising 65 infertile women.[42] Hysteroscopy was used as the gold standard. SHG was found to have the same diagnostic accuracy, and sometimes even to be markedly superior to hysteroscopy with respect to polypoid lesions and endometrial hyperplasia. In the diagnosis of intrauterine adhesions, SHG had limited accuracy, similar to that obtained by HSG, with a high false-positive diagnosis rate.[42]

MAGNETIC RESONANCE IMAGING

Magnetic resonance imaging (MRI) is an accurate non-invasive technique for the evaluation of uterine anomalies. It has been shown to be a valuable tool in the diagnosis of selected cases of müllerian duct anomalies.[43] Although most anomalies will be initially diagnosed with HSG and SHG, further imaging will often be required for definitive diagnosis and elaboration of secondary findings.[44] At this time, MRI is justified only in special cases where its high accuracy and detailed elaboration of uterovaginal anatomy is needed.

The utility of MRI remains limited due to its cost. However, in selected cases, careful use of MRI to delineate the pelvic soft tissues may greatly aid in precise definition of the anomaly and in planning the most appropriate corrective surgery.[45]

DIAGNOSTIC HYSTEROSCOPY

Hysteroscopy offers the best and most direct assessment of the uterine cavity. During the procedure, the intracavitary structures can be directly visualized

and directed biopsies can be obtained when indicated. A retrospective study by Zuppi et al[46] found an association between the hysteroscopic findings in 344 women with recurrent spontaneous abortion and major (and even minor) uterine anomalies. The anomalies were shown to correlate with an increased risk of recurrent miscarriage.[46]

Weiss et al[47] performed hysteroscopy on 165 women referred for RPL: 67 after two and 98 after three or more consecutive miscarriages. The prevalence of uterine anomalies did not differ significantly: 32% and 28%, respectively. Weiss et al[47] concluded that hysteroscopy may be justified following two spontaneous pregnancy losses.

The intramyometrial extension of fibroids cannot be assessed, however, and therefore the estimate of size remains imprecise. Hysteroscopy alone cannot differentiate between a septate uterus and a bicornuate uterus; laparoscopy or SHG is required to complete the evaluation. Hysteroscopic surgery is currently considered the method of choice for correcting the various types of intrauterine pathology.

DIAGNOSTIC LAPAROSCOPY

Laparoscopy allows the surgeon to assess the outer surface of the uterus and other pelvic structures. It is used to establish the precise diagnosis of the various congenital and acquired anomalies. Laparoscopy is also used for the removal of subserosal and intramural fibroids.[48,49] Currently, laparoscopy is rarely used just to clarify uterine anatomy, and is generally reserved for women in whom interventional therapy is likely to be undertaken.

CHOICE OF METHOD FOR IMAGING UTERINE MORPHOLOGY

Ultrasonography is currently the most readily available and least invasive mode of imaging in cases of suspected uterine abnormalities (Table 11.2). 2D sonography allows excellent assessment of myometrial morphology, and is especially useful for determining the number, size and location of myomas. Filling the uterine cavity with fluid facilitates the use of SHG for accurate delineation of

Table 11.2 Imaging modalities for assessing uterine anomalies in women with recurrent pregnancy loss

Imaging modalities	Advantages	Disadvantages	Cost
Ultrasonography	• Readily available • Least invasive • Excellent assessment of the myometrial morphology	• Poor demonstration of uterine contour • Uterine cavity not clearly demonstrated	Low
Hysterosalpingography	• Shows the contour of the uterine cavity, cervical canal, and tubal lamina	• Exposure to radiation • Iodine sensitivity risk • Painful • Pelvic inflammatory disease risk • High false-positive rates	Moderate
3D sonography	• Allows visualization of both the uterine cavity and the myometrium • Enables easy differentiation between subseptate and bicornuate uteri	• Equipment not readily available • Requires experienced operator	Moderate
Sonohysterography	• Good evaluation of uterine cavity • Tubal patency assessed	• Time-consuming • High false-positive diagnosis rate for intrauterine adhesions	Low
Diagnostic hysteroscopy	• Most accurate assessment of the uterine cavity • Simple outpatient procedure	• Limited efficiency to differentiate between a uterine septum and a bicornuate uterus • No information on tubal patency • Invasive: risk of infection, perforation	Moderate
Magnetic resonance imaging (MRI)	• Useful in clarifying details of soft tissue anatomy	• No information on tubal patency • Not easy to interpret results	High
Diagnostic laparoscopy	• Accurate for differentiating between a uterine septum and a bicornuate uterus	• Invasive • Requires general anesthesia • Low postoperative morbidity	High

intrauterine polyps, and improves the accuracy of identifying submucous myomas encroaching on the cavity and to assess the size of uterine septa. 3D sonography greatly enhances our ability to differentiate between a uterine septum and a bicornuate uterus (Figures 11.2–11.5). HSG can help delineate the integrity of the uterine cavity, but, due to its invasive nature and the associated exposure to radiation, it is limited to infertility investigation where evaluation of tubal patency is required.

Hysteroscopy can be performed nowadays with 2–3 mm scopes without the need for speculum, tenaculum, or anesthesia.[50] This simple outpatient procedure provides an accurate assessment of the uterine cavity. It remains the method of choice for assessment of the presence and extent of intrauterine adhesions. It is also the optimal method to evaluate the size and extension of polyps and submucous myomas.

However, hysteroscopy cannot fully differentiate between a uterine septum and a bicornuate uterus.

The role of MRI is limited due to its cost. However, in selected and complicated cases, MRI may help to clarify the details of soft tissue anatomy and may be especially useful when planning surgical correction. Laparoscopy used to be the gold standard for differentiating between a uterine septum and a bicornuate uterus, but with modern imaging modalities, it is rarely needed for determination of uterine anatomy and is usually only used when a decision has been made to attempt surgical correction.

TREATMENT

As stated above, little evidence can be found in the current literature demonstrating that uterine factors, including intrauterine adhesions, septa, myomas, and endometrial polyps, are causally linked with reproductive loss. However, there are reports suggesting that treatment of these abnormalities may improve fertility outcome.[51] The published evidence includes several observational series that demonstrate successful fertility, with term pregnancy rates ranging from 32% to 87% following hysteroscopic division of intrauterine adhesions.[51] The evidence supporting a direct link between a septate uterus and reproductive loss is derived from the results of metroplasty. Several case series have demonstrated a reduction in the spontaneous abortion rate (from 91% to 17%), after hysteroscopic metroplasty. Furthermore, following metroplasty, the mean pregnancy rate in previously infertile patients is 47%. However, there are no prospective controlled trials that have provided conclusive evidence that the correction of uterine anatomical abnormalities benefits the next pregnancy.[52] Furthermore, the above data are mostly based on observational, retrospective studies with small sample sizes and heterogeneous patient populations, and are therefore a far cry from the type of evidence required for current treatment guidelines. A recent review of all published large randomized controlled trials and meta-analyses undertaken by the ESHRE Special Interest Group for Early Pregnancy (SIGEP) protocol for the investigation and medical management of recurrent miscarriage concluded that the only interventions that do not require more randomized controlled trials are tender loving care and health advice.[1]

Surgery is the main treatment offered to patients with uterine anomalies (Table 11.3). However, not all anatomical defects can be surgically corrected, and not all anomalies require surgical intervention. The most crucial step before making any treatment decision is accurate imaging in order to determine the exact anomaly. Currently, endoscopic procedures are the main approach used to correct most uterine defects. Operative hysteroscopy currently allows a technically straightforward method of correcting intrauterine pathology such as septum, fibroids, or polyps. Laparotomy currently has a very limited role in the management of congenital uterine anomalies in women with recurrent abortion.

There are many questions regarding the optimal management of patients with recurrent abortions and uterine anomalies, such as the indications for resection of a uterine septum and whether small intrauterine polyps significantly influence reproductive performance. It is debatable whether surgical reconstruction such as Strassman's metroplasty

Table 11.3 The role of surgical intervention in women with uterine anomalies and recurrent pregnancy loss

Study	Postoperative morbidity	Technical difficulty	Likelihood of benefit	Cost
Hysteroscopic polypecomy	+	+	++	+
Hysteroscopic adhesiolysis	+	+ to ++	+++	+
Hysteroscopic myomectomy	+ to ++	++ to +++	++	+ to ++
Hysteroscopic metroplasty for septate uterus	+	+	++	+ to ++
Hysteroscopic metroplasty for hypoplastic/DES-exposed uterus	+	++	+	++
Abdominal metroplasty	+++	+++	++	+++
Cervical cerclage	++	++	+	++
Interruption of a fallopian tube with hydrosalpinx	++	++	++?	++

+ low; +++ high.

should be performed for bicornuate uterus. When should myomectomy be performed? What is the role of non-surgical management of myomas? When should cervical cerclage be offered? We will try to discuss these questions in the light of the currently available data.

SHOULD INTRAUTERINE POLYPS BE EXCISED?

Although the association between endometrial polyps and pregnancy loss has not been proven, polyps are more common in patients with recurrent spontaneous abortion.[53] Surgical excision is usually recommended,[2] since there are data suggesting that hysteroscopic polypectomy can increase fertility.[31,32] A prospective randomized study in 215 infertile women scheduled to undergo intrauterine insemination (IUI) showed that hysteroscopic polypectomy improved the likelihood of conception, with a relative risk of 2.1 (95% confidence interval (CI) 1.5–2.9).[32] Pregnancies in the patients who underwent polypectomy were obtained before the first IUI in 65% of cases.

There is a consensus that hysteroscopy is the optimal method to perform polypectomy. Hysteroscopic polypectomy can be performed by several techniques, including excision with forceps or gentle curettage. A recent study[54] has assessed 240 cases of hysteroscopic polypectomy using microscissors, grasping forceps, or electrosurgery either with a monopolar probe or a resectoscope. Resectoscopic polypectomy required more operating time, had more glycine absorption and complications, but had a lower recurrence rate than other hysteroscopic techniques. The resectoscope had a 0% recurrence rate and the grasping forceps had a 15% recurrence rate.[54] The introduction of bipolar electrodes may increase the safety of hysteroscopic endometrial polypectomy in an outpatient setting.[55]

DOES THE RESECTION OF A UTERINE SEPTUM IMPROVE PREGNANCY OUTCOME?

Septate uterus is more prevalent in women with repeated pregnancy loss.[56] However, it may be difficult to differentiate between a 'normal' arcuate

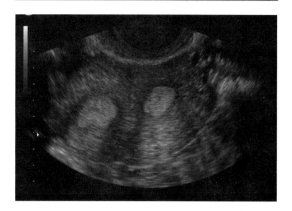

Figure 11.6 Two-dimensional transvaginal ultrasound of a septated uterus. (Courtesy of Professor Yaron Zalael MD, Sheba Medical Center, Tel-Hashomer, Israel.)

uterus and a septate uterus (Figures 11.6 and 11.7). In order to justify metroplasty, reliable diagnosis is required.

Although no randomized controlled studies are available, observational studies have reported impressive results following incision of a septum in patients with recurrent abortion. Fedele et al[57] studied the reproductive outcome in 102 patients with a complete ($n = 23$) or partial ($n = 79$) septate uterus and infertility or repeated abortion. Following hysteroscopic metroplasty, the cumulative pregnancy and birth rates at 36 months were 89% and 75%, respectively, in the septate uterus group and 80% and 67% in the subseptate uterus group. Fedele et al[57] concluded that after hysteroscopic metroplasty, the reproductive prognosis was favorable and not influenced by the malformation subclass.[57]

A meta-analysis of published retrospective data comparing pregnancy outcome before and after hysteroscopic septoplasty indicated a marked improvement after surgery.[56] However, the significance of this meta-analysis remains limited by the nonrandomized observational methodology used by the studies that were assessed. Grimbizis et al[58] summarized the results of a a highly selected group of symptomatic patients drawn from a large number of reports. They had previously had term

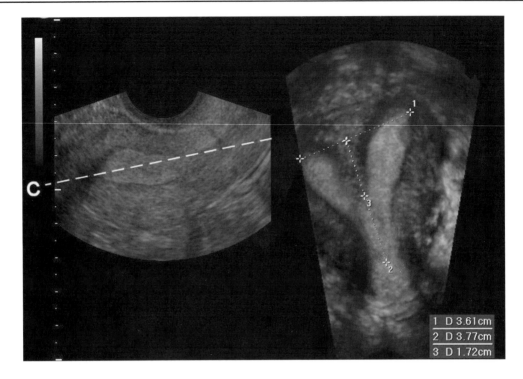

Figure 11.7 Two- and three-dimensional transvaginal ultrasound of a septated uterus of the same patient as in Figure 11.6 using volume contrast imaging in plane C. (Courtesy of Professor Yaron Zalael MD, Sheba Medical Center, Tel-Hashomer, Israel.)

delivery and live birth rates of only 5%. After hysteroscopic septum resection, the outcome was remarkable, in that the subsequent term delivery rate was approximately 75% and the live birth rate about 85%.[58] However, this was not a randomized trial.

Transabdominal surgical techniques, such as the modified Tompkins metroplasty, are still occasionally used to repair uterine septa.[59] However, in light of the low morbidity associated with hysteroscopic resection and the possibility of performing the procedure on an ambulatory basis, abdominal surgery seems to be rarely, if ever, indicated.[52] However, hysteroscopic metroplasty is associated with a substantial, and as yet non-quantified, increased risk of uterine rupture during subsequent pregnancies.[60] This is especially significant when the risk of uterine rupture after hysteroscopic metroplasty is compared with that of women who underwent

uncomplicated hysteroscopic resection of submucous myomas or endometrial polyps.[60] Uterine perforation and/or the use of electrosurgery increase this risk, but are not considered independent risk factors.[60]

Homer et al[56] have suggested that a septate uterus per se is not an indication for surgical intervention, because it is not always associated with a poor obstetric outcome. This approach is supported by a recent retrospective study of 67 patients who had a complete septate uterus including the cervix and a longitudinal vaginal septum.[61] There was no association with primary infertility, and pregnancy was reported to progress successfully without surgical treatment. The results did not support elective hysteroscopic incision of the septum in asymptomatic patients before the first pregnancy.[61] In women with one miscarriage, the situation remains controversial, and a conservative approach has been suggested, since it is expected that after a single miscarriage 80–90% will have a live birth in the next pregnancy.[56] However, a more liberalized approach to treatment is currently advocated by most authorities in light of the simplicity, minimal postoperative sequelae, and improved reproductive outcome associated with hysteroscopic metroplasty.[56,58]

SHOULD THE CERVICAL PORTION OF THE SEPTUM BE SPARED IN PATIENTS WITH A COMPLETE SEPTATE UTERUS?

It was previously believed that the in patients with a complete septate uterus, the cervical portion of the septum should be spared and the dissection started at the level of the internal os to avoid secondary cervical incompetence.[36] However, a recent multicenter randomized controlled clinical trial by Parsanezhad et al[62] examined whether division of the cervical portion of a uterine septum is associated with intraoperative bleeding, cervical incompetence, or secondary infertility. Twenty-eight women with complete uterine septum and a history of pregnancy wastage or infertility were randomized to undergo metroplasty including division of the cervical portion of the septum or the same procedure with preservation of the cervical portion. Resection of the cervical portion was reported to make the procedure safer, easier, and less complicated than preservation of the cervical septum.[62]

MANAGEMENT OF MYOMAS IN RECURRENT PREGNANCY LOSS

Myomas are frequently found in women of reproductive age, and are more prevalent in women over 35 years of age Although myomas are more prevalent in women with recurrent spontaneous abortion,[34,53] the causal association remains poorly established. It is therefore still undetermined which women will benefit most from surgical excision of uterine myomas. Evidence – mostly from the in vitro fertilization (IVF) literature – suggests that only those myomas that distort the endometrial cavity impair fertility.[63] Patients with distorted uterine cavities due to submucous fibroids larger than 2 cm have

higher pregnancy rates following hysteroscopic resection. Since submucous myomas are easily treatable in recurrent pregnancy loss, it has been suggested that these patients should be identified early after other potential causes of recurrent pregnancy loss have been eliminated.[34]

The location and size of the myomas are the two parameters that influence the success of a future pregnancy.[63] At present, it seems that subserosal myomas have little, if any, effect on reproductive outcome, especially if they are up to 5–7 cm in diameter. The impact of intramural myomas on the outcome of pregnancy is still disputed.[28,64] However, intramural myomas that do not encroach upon the endometrium also can be considered to be relatively harmless to reproduction, if they are less than 4–5 cm in diameter. Myomectomy is therefore currently recommended for intramural myomas that compress the uterine cavity and submucous myomas significantly reduce pregnancy rates.[63]

Hysteroscopic myomectomy is the gold standard for the treatment of submucous myomas. Size and intramural extension can limit its success, although this greatly depends on the operator's experience. The removal of larger fibroids may require two procedures to avoid intraoperative complications. Fibroids with significant intramural extension present a challenge during the procedure.

Laparoscopic myomectomy is gradually being accepted as the gold standard for the removal of most intramural and subserosal uterine myomas in women who desire to preserve their uterus.[48] Traditionally, laparotomy used to be indicated for the surgical management of fibroids in such locations, but laparoscopy can be used to manage most of these cases. Pregnancy rates following myomectomy, both via laparoscopy and laparotomy, are in the 50–60% range, with most having good outcomes.[49] It is should be noted that spontaneous uterine rupture during pregnancy has been reported following laparoscopic myomectomy.[65]

Laparoscopic-assisted myomectomy (LAM) is another new approach that is often a very convenient and less invasive form of surgery.[66] By decreasing the technical demands, and thereby the operative time, LAM may be offered more widely to patients. In carefully selected cases, LAM is a safe and efficient alternative to both laparoscopic myomectomy and myomectomy by laparotomy. These cases include patients with numerous large or deep intramural myomas. LAM allows easier repair of the uterus and rapid morcellation of the myomas. In women who desire a future pregnancy, LAM may be a better approach, because it allows meticulous suturing of the uterine defect in layers and thereby eliminates excessive electrocoagulation.[66]

Laparoscopy is also being expanded to include such techniques as laparoscopic uterine artery ligation and directed laparoscopic cryomyolysis. However, many of these treatment options are still associated with significant concerns regarding future reproductive performance. Additional non-surgical techniques recently introduced to treat myomas include uterine artery embolization and transabdominal interventional MRI-guided cryoablation.[48] Furthermore, the first MRI-guided focused ultrasound surgery system used to treat myomas was recently approved by the US Food and Drug Administration. It is apparent the physician's skills and experience, as well as local availability of these new techniques, will largely determine patient assignment to therapy.[48]

Uterine fibroid embolization is an increasingly popular, minimally invasive technique that has been successfully used in the management of symptomatic myomas.[49,67] This procedure is not without risk for women desiring to enhance their reproductive outcome. Following uterine fibroid embolization, transient ovarian failure has been reported, as has permanent amenorrhea associated with endometrial atrophy. Amenorrhea seems to occur after the procedure in approximately 1% of patients and is highly age-dependent, with a reported incidence of 3% (range 1–7%) in women under 40 years of age and 41% (range 26–58%) in women over 50.

The pregnancy rate has not been established following uterine artery embolization. However, higher rates of pregnancy complications have been reported following uterine artery embolization compared with myomectomy.[49] These complications include preterm delivery (odds ratio (OR) 6.2;

95% CI 1.4–27.7), malpresentations (OR 4.3; 95% CI 1.0–20.5), spontaneous abortion, abnormal placentation, and postpartum hemorrhage. At present, it seems that although most pregnancies following uterine artery embolization are expected to have good outcomes, myomectomy should still be recommended as the treatment of choice over uterine artery embolization in most patients desiring future fertility.[49,67]

IS CERVICAL CERCLAGE INDICATED IN WOMEN WITH UTERINE ANOMALIES?

Cervical incompetence has been associated with uterine anomalies, as well as following in utero exposure to DES.[2] Furthermore, cervical incompetence is of special concern in women with RPL, as weakening of the cervix may occasionally be due to repeated trauma to the cervix, following overdilatation during repeated curettage.

Seidman et al[68] have studied the effect of cervical cerclage on the survival rate of the fetus in 86 pregnancies in women with congenital uterine anomalies and a random group of 106 pregnancies in women with normally shaped uteri.[68] The uterine morphological factors were determined in all by HSG, and, when necessary, hysteroscopy and laparoscopy were combined. The incidence of HSG-proven cervical incompetence (23%) was similar in the two groups. In the respective groups, 67 and 29 pregnancies were managed with cervical cerclage. The fetal outcome was stratified by cervical incompetence and obstetric history. The percentage of viable newborns was significantly higher in women with malformed uteri who underwent cerclage (88%) compared with those without cerclage (47%). No statistically significant beneficial effect of cerclage was found for normal uteri, even when only those patients with a history of recurrent fetal loss were considered.[68]

The precise indications for cervical cerclage remain controversial. The Cervical Incompetence Prevention Randomized Cerclage Trial (CIPRACT) found that therapeutic cerclage with bed rest reduces preterm delivery before 34 weeks of gestation and compound neonatal morbidity in women with risk factors and/or symptoms of cervical incompetence and a cervical length of less than 25 mm before 27 weeks of gestation.[69] Risk factors for cervical incompetence included in this major study included, among others, DES exposure and uterine anomaly.

Levine and Berkowitz[70] studied the effect of conservative management on pregnancy outcome in 120 DES-exposed women with and without gross structural lesions of the genital tract. Cerclage was limited to two women with a history of cervical incompetence or acute cervical change in the second trimester. Women with cervical change occurring after 25 weeks of gestation were managed with bed rest. It was found that the majority of pregnancy losses in DES-exposed patients occurred in the first trimester. Patients exposed in utero to DES who had conservative management had good pregnancy outcomes.[70]

Cervical incompetence is a challenging clinical diagnosis, and is an infrequent cause of pregnancy loss even in patients with gross structural abnormalities of the genital tract. Prophylactic cerclage for patients with uterine anomalies and DES exposure should be recommended only when other risk factors, such as three or more midtrimester pregnancy losses or preterm deliveries, are present.[68,70]

DOES STRASSMAN METROPLASTY STILL HAVE A ROLE IN PATIENTS WITH A BICORNUATE UTERUS?

The Strassman procedure involves the unification of the two uterine horns of a bicornuate uterus, and is carried out via laparotomy. This procedure often leaves a small cavity with scarring, which makes implantation difficult, and may also cause pelvic adhesions resulting in secondary infertility. However, the postmetroplasty reproductive capacity of women with a bicornuate uterus has been reported to be good.[71,72] Furthermore, the role of abdominal metroplasty has been suggested as a valid approach[72] (using the Jones or Strassman techniques) in patients with bicornuate, T-shaped, or septate uteri, when associated with other pelvic lesions not amenable to the transcervical hysteroscopic approach. However, surgical correction of a

bicornuate uterus for pregnancy maintenance is poorly supported by data and rarely seems warranted. As a bicornuate uterus is usually associated with problems during the third trimester of pregnancy, the procedure should thus be limited to very few well-selected cases with recurrent second- and third-trimester problems. The development of a laparoscopic approach to metroplasty for bicornuate uterus needs further study, since this new technique may be associated with less postoperative morbidity.

DOES HYDROSALPINX AFFECT PREGNANCY OUTCOME AFTER EARLY RECURRENT MISCARRIAGE?

It is well established that tubal disease, particularly hydrosalpinx, has a detrimental effect on the outcome of IVF. Although no randomized trial has shown a significant benefit from surgical intervention for tubal disease prior to IVF,[73] a recent meta-analysis concluded that laparoscopic salpingectomy should be considered for all women with hydrosalpinges prior to IVF. It was also stated that further randomized trials are required to assess other treatment modalities for hydrosalpinx, such as salpingostomy, tubal occlusion, or aspiration at oocyte retrieval.[73]

A recent prospective randomized controlled trial[74] enrolled 13 patients with a history of unexplained recurrent early spontaneous abortion and a unilateral hydrosalpinx diagnosed by sonography or HSG and in whom other causes of abortion had been excluded. The patients were randomized to undergo laparoscopic unilateral tubal fulguration or no surgical intervention. Six of the seven patients in the treatment group and five of the six in the control group conceived. Five patients in the treatment group and none in the control group had a pregnancy progress beyond the first trimester. The progressing pregnancies in the treatment group reached 36–40 weeks of gestation – a statistically significant difference. The authors concluded that laparoscopic tubal fulguration improves pregnancy outcome in selected patients with previous recurrent early abortion and a unilateral hydrosalpinx. This study urgently needs confirmation in a larger patient sample.[74]

IS HYSTEROSCOPIC METROPLASTY INDICATED IN DES-EXPOSED WOMEN?

Hysteroscopic metroplasty has been reported as a safe and feasible method to improve reproductive performance in patients with DES-exposed and hypoplastic malformed uteri suffering from severe infertility, recurrent pregnancy loss, or implantation failures in an IVF programme.[75–77] In one series,[75] eight patients referred for infertility, recurrent pregnancy loss, or both with an abnormal uterine contour as seen by HSG underwent hysteroscopic metroplasty. Each patient served as their own control. Three of five patients with secondary infertility and RPL had live births, as did a patient with secondary infertility.[75]

In a larger study[76] with a similar design, 24 patients with hypoplastic uterus and/or uterine deformity as seen by HSG underwent hysteroscopic metroplasty. Postoperative HSG showed an improved uterine cavity in 23 cases. The final result was considered to be excellent in terms of anatomical correction in 15 patients. Eleven pregnancies occurred, the abortion rate decreased from 88% in previous pregnancies to 12.5%, and the rate of term deliveries increased from 3% to 87.5%.[76] Ten patients delivered healthy infants after 30 weeks of gestation; one patient delivered more prematurely. Six deliveries were normal and four required cesarean section.[76]

At present, it seems that hysteroscopic metroplasty, with its simplicity and minimal postoperative sequelae, seems to be an operation of choice in women with a hypoplastic malformed uterus and a history of severe infertility and/or RPL.[77] However, the previously quoted series used historical controls. Larger series with a better study design are necessary before hysteroscopic metroplasty can be recommended for all women with DES-exposed or hypoplastic malformed uterus and recurrent miscarriage.

CONCLUSIONS

A contemporary review of the current literature shows that the prevalence and impact of uterine malformations on reproduction are still not clearly established.[49] Consequently, the investigation of women with recurrent abortion should be limited in most cases to screening with ultrasonography, preferably utilizing 3D techniques and in selected cases benefiting from the application of hydrosonography (Table 11.2). More invasive and expensive imaging modalities, including hysteroscopy, laparoscopy, and MRI, should be reserved for inconclusive cases with a suspected uterine deformity.

Surgical intervention for uterine malformations remains poorly supported by randomized controlled trials (Table 11.3). It is generally agreed that adhesions, polyps, and protruding submucous myomas should be hysteroscopically resected. However, the need for hysteroscopic division of a uterine septum remains debatable, but may be indicated in a patient with two or more pregnancy losses, as its associated morbidity is low. Abdominal metroplasty for bicornuate uterus is even more difficult to support in the light of its significant associated morbidity and the lack of controlled data. Abdominal metroplasty is currently recommended only in selected cases with recurrent severe problems in the second and third trimesters. Cervical cerclage is only indicated in women with uterine anomalies in the presence of a clinical diagnosis of cervical incompetence or additional risk factors. In women with hydrosalpinges and early recurrent abortion, laparoscopic salpingectomy or proximal tubal occlusion should be considered.

Miscarriages – clinically detectable pregnancies that fail to progress – seem to be the inevitable byproduct of the limited efficiency of human reproduction, and do not always point to the presence of a correctable defect. Thus, surgical intervention should be carefully considered based on the patient's clinical history and not merely as an attempt to correct all anatomical uterine defects now more commonly diagnosed by modern imaging modalities.

REFERENCES

1. Jauniaux E, Farquharson RG, Christiansen OB, Exalto N, On behalf of ESHRE Special Interest Group for Early Pregnancy (SIGEP). Evidence-based guidelines for the investigation and medical treatment of recurrent miscarriage. Hum Reprod 2006; 21:2216–22.

2. Devi Wold AS, Pham N, Arici A. Anatomic factors in recurrent pregnancy loss. Semin Reprod Med 2006; 24:25–32.

3. The American Fertility Society classifications of adnexal adhesions, distal tubal occlusion, tubal occlusion secondary to tubal ligation, tubal pregnancies, müllerian anomalies and intrauterine adhesions. Fertil Steril 1988; 49:944–55.

4. Homer HA, Li TC, Cooke ID. The septate uterus: a review of management and reproductive outcome. Fertil Steril 2000; 73:1–4.

5. Proctor JA, Haney AF. Recurrent first trimester pregnancy loss is associated with uterine septum but not with bicornuate uterus. Fertil Steril 2003; 80:1212–15.

6. Salim R, Regan L, Woelfer B, et al. A comparative study of the morphology of congenital uterine anomalies in women with and without a history of recurrent first trimester miscarriage. Hum Reprod 2003; 18:162–6.

7. Simon C, Martinez L, Pardo F, et al. Müllerian defects in women with normal reproductive outcome. Fertil Steril 1991; 56:1192–3.

8. Jurkovic D, Geipel A, Gruboeck K, et al. Three-dimensional ultrasound for the assessment of uterine anatomy and detection of congenital anomalies: a comparison with hysterosalpingography and two-dimensional sonography. Ultrasound Obstet Gynecol 1995; 5:233–7.

9. Raga F, Bauset C, Remohi J, et al. Reproductive impact of congenital müllerian anomalies. Hum Reprod 1997; 12:2277–81.

10. Dabirashrafi H, Bahadori M, Mohammad K, et al. Septate uterus: new idea on the histologic features of the septum in this abnormal uterus. Am J Obstet Gynecol 1995; 172:105–7.

11. Nakada K, Makino T, Tabuchi S, et al. Analysis of congenital uterine anomalies in habitual abortions, evaluation of metroplasty. Jpn J Fertil Steril 1989; 34:842–7.

12. Golan A, Ron-El R, Herman A, et al. Diagnostic hysteroscopy: its value in an in-vitro fertilization/embryo transfer unit. Hum Reprod 1992; 7:1433–4.

13. Acien P. Reproductive performance of women with uterine malformations. Hum Reprod 1993; 8:122–6.

14. Woelfer B, Salim R, Banerjee S, et al. Reproductive outcomes in women with congenital uterine anomalies detected by three-dimensional ultrasound screening. Obstet Gynecol 2001; 98:1099–103.

15. Fedele L, Bianchi S, Agnoli B, et al. Urinary tract anomalies associated with unicornuate uterus. J Urol 1996; 155:847–8.

16. Heinonen PK, Saarikoski S, Pystynen P. Reproductive performance of women with uterine anomalies. An evaluation of 182 cases. Acta Obstet Gynecol Scand 1982; 61:157–62.

17. Fedele L, Bianchi S, Tozzi L, et al. Fertility in women with unicornuate uterus. Br J Obstet Gynaecol 1995; 102:1007–9.

18. Heinonen PK. Unicornuate uterus and rudimentary horn. Fertil Steril 1997; 68:224–30.

19. Surico N, Ribaldone R, Arnulfo A, et al. Uterine malformations and pregnancy losses: Is cervical cerclage effective? Clin Exp Obstet Gynecol 2000; 27:147–9.

20. Fedele L, Bianchi S, Zanconato G, et al. Laparoscopic removal of the cavitated noncommunicating rudimentary uterine horn: surgical aspects in 10 cases. Fertil Steril 2005; 83:432–6.

21. Heinonen P. Clinical implications of the didelphic uterus: long-term follow-up of 49 cases. Eur J Obstet Gynecol Reprod Biol 2000; 91:183–90.

22. Lin PC. Reproductive outcomes in women with uterine anomalies. J Womens Health (Larchmt) 2004; 13:33–9.

23. Kaufman RH, Adam E, Hatch EE, et al. Continued follow-up of pregnancy outcomes in diethylstilbestrol-exposed offspring. Obstet Gynecol 2000; 96:483–9.

24. Veurink M, Koster M, Berg LT. The history of DES, lessons to be learned. Pharm World Sci 2005; 27:139–43.

25. Goldberg JM, Falcone T. Effect of diethylstilbestrol on reproductive function. Fertil Steril 1999; 72:1–7.

26. Eldar-Geva T, Meagher S, Healy DL, et al. Effect of intramural, subserosal, and submucosal uterine fibroids on the outcome of assisted reproductive technology treatment. Fertil Steril 1998; 70:687–91.

27. Casini ML, Rossi F, Agostini R, et al. Effects of the position of fibroids on fertility. Gynecol Endocrinol 2006; 22:106–9.

28. Oliveira FG, Abdelmassih VG, Diamond MP, et al. Impact of subserosal and intramural uterine fibroids that do not distort the endometrial cavity on the outcome of in vitro fertilization–intracytoplasmic sperm injection. Fertil Steril 2004; 81:582–7.

29. Ribeiro SC, Reich H, Rosenberg J, et al. Laparoscopic myomectomy and pregnancy outcome in infertile patients. Fertil Steril 1999; 71:571–4.

30. Rossetti A, Sizzi O, Soranna L, et al. Long-term results of laparoscopic myomectomy: recurrence rate in comparison with abdominal myomectomy. Hum Reprod 2001; 16:770–4.

31. Neuwirth RS, Levin B, Keltz MD. Pregnancy rates after hysteroscopic polypectomy and myomectomy in infertile women. Obstet Gynecol 1999; 94:168–71.

32. Perez-Medina T, Bajo-Arenas J, Salazar F, et al. Endometrial polyps and their implication in the pregnancy rates of patients undergoing intrauterine insemination: a prospective, randomized study. Hum Reprod 2005; 20:1632–5.

33. lton VK, Saunders NA, Harris LH, et al. Intrauterine adhesions after manual vacuum aspiration for early pregnancy failure. Fertil Steril 2006; 85:1823.

34. Ventolini G, Zhang M, Gruber J. Hysteroscopy in the evaluation of patients with recurrent pregnancy loss: a cohort study in a primary care population. Surg Endosc 2004; 18:1782–4.

35. Royal College of Obstetricians and Gynaecologists. The Investigation and Treatment of Recurrent Miscarriage. Guideline No. 17. London: RCOG Press, 2003.

36. Kupesic S. Clinical implications of sonographic detection of uterine anomalies for reproductive outcome. Ultrasound Obstet Gynecol 2001; 18:387–400.

37. Baramki TA. Hysterosalpingography. Fertil Steril 2005; 83:1595–606.

38. Salim R, Woelfer B, Backos M, et al. Reproducibility of three-dimensional ultrasound diagnosis of congenital uterine anomalies. Ultrasound Obstet Gynecol 2003; 21:578–82.

39. Valenzano MM, Mistrangelo E, Lijoi D, et al. Transvaginal sonohysterographic evaluation of uterine malformations. Eur J Obstet Gynecol Reprod Biol 2006; 124:246–9.

40. Sylvestre C, Child TJ, Tulandi T, et al. A prospective study to evaluate the efficacy of two- and three-dimensional sonohysterography in women with intrauterine lesions. Fertil Steril 2003; 79:1222–5.

41. Alborzi S, Dehbashi S, Parsanezhad ME. Differential diagnosis of septate and bicornuate uterus by sonohysterography eliminates the need for laparoscopy. Fertil Steril 2002; 78:176–8.

42. Soares SR, Barbosa dos Reis MM, Camargos AF. Diagnostic accuracy of sonohysterography, transvaginal sonography, and hysterosalpingography in patients with uterine cavity diseases. Fertil Steril 2000; 73:406–11.

43. Marten K, Vosshenrich R, Funke M, et al. MRI in the evaluation of müllerian duct anomalies. Clin Imaging 2003; 27:346–50.

44. Troiano RN, McCarthy SM. Müllerian duct anomalies: imaging and clinical issues. Radiology 2004; 233:19–34.

45. Pui MH. Imaging diagnosis of congenital uterine malformation. Comput Med Imaging Graph 2004; 28:425–33.

46. Zupi E, Marconi D, Vaquero E, et al. Hysteroscopic findings in 344 women with recurrent spontaneous abortion. J Am Assoc Gynecol Laparosc 2001; 8:398–401.

47. Weiss A, Shalev E, Romano S. Hysteroscopy may be justified after two miscarriages. Hum Reprod 2005; 20:2628–31.

48. Seidman DS, Nezhat CH, Nezhat F, et al. Minimally invasive surgery for fibroids. Infert Reprod Med Clin North Am 2002; 13:375–91.

49. Goldberg J, Pereira L. Pregnancy outcomes following treatment for fibroids: uterine fibroid embolization versus laparoscopic myomectomy. Curr Opin Obstet Gynecol 2006; 18:402–6.

50. Sagiv R, Sadan O, Boaz M, et al. A new approach to office hysteroscopy compared with traditional hysteroscopy: a randomized controlled trial. Obstet Gynecol 2006; 108:387–92.

51. Sanders B. Uterine factors and infertility. J Reprod Med 2006; 51:169–76.

52. Management of recurrent early pregnancy loss. ACOG Practice Bulletin, No. 24, February 2001. Int J Gynecol Obstet 2002; 78:179–90.

53. Valli E, Zupi E, Marconi D, et al. Hysteroscopic findings in 344 women with recurrent spontaneous abortion. J Am Assoc Gynecol Laparosc 2001; 8:398–401.

54. Preutthipan S, Herabutya Y. Hysteroscopic polypectomy in 240 premenopausal and postmenopausal women. Fertil Steril 2005; 83:705–9.

55. Marsh F, Rogerson L, Duffy S. A randomised controlled trial comparing outpatient versus daycase endometrial polypectomy. BJOG 2006; 113:896–901.

56. Homer HA, Li TC, Cooke ID. The septate uterus: a review of management and reproductive outcome. Fertil Steril 2000; 73:1–14.

57. Fedele L, Arcaini L, Parazzini F, et al. Reproductive prognosis after hysteroscopic metroplasty in 102 women: life-table analysis. Fertil Steril 1993; 59:768–72.

58. Grimbizis GF, Camus M, Tarlatzis BC, et al. Clinical implications of uterine malformations and hysteroscopic treatment results. Hum Reprod Update 2001; 7:161–74.

59. Patton PE, Novy MJ, Lee DM, et al. The diagnosis and reproductive outcome after surgical treatment of the complete septate uterus, duplicated cervix and vaginal septum. Am J Obstet Gynecol 2004; 190:1669–75.

60. Sentilhes L, Sergent F, Roman H, et al. Late complications of operative hysteroscopy: predicting patients at risk of uterine rupture during subsequent pregnancy. Eur J Obstet Gynecol Reprod Biol 2005; 120:134–8.

61. Heinonen PK. Complete septate uterus with longitudinal vaginal septum. Fertil Steril 2006; 85:700–5.

62. Parsanezhad ME, Alborzi S, Zarei A, et al. Hysteroscopic metroplasty of the complete uterine septum, duplicate cervix, and vaginal septum. Fertil Steril 2006; 85:1473–7.

63. Kolankaya A, Arici A. Myomas and assisted reproductive technologies: when and how to act? Obstet Gynecol Clin North Am 2006; 33:145–52.

64. Benecke C, Kruger TF, Siebert TI, et al. Effect of fibroids on fertility in patients undergoing assisted reproduction. A structured literature review. Gynecol Obstet Invest 2005; 59:225–30.

65. Seidman DS, Nezhat CH, Nezhat FR, Nezhat C. Spontaneous uterine rupture in pregnancy 8 years after laparoscopic myomectomy. J Am Assoc Gynecol Laparoscop 2001; 8:333–5.

66. Seidman DS, Nezhat FR, Nezhat CH, Nezhat CR. The role of laparoscopic-assisted myomectomy (LAM). JSLS 2001; 5:299–303.

67. Mara M, Fucikova Z, Maskova J, et al. Uterine fibroid embolization versus myomectomy in women wishing to preserve fertility: preliminary results of a randomized controlled trial. Eur J Obstet Gynecol Reprod Biol 2006; 126:226–33.

68. Seidman DS, Ben-Rafael Z, Bider D, et al. The role of cervical cerclage in the management of uterine anomalies. Surg Gynecol Obstet 1991; 173:384–6.

69. Althuisius SM, Dekker GA, Hummel P, et al. Final results of the Cervical Incompetence Prevention Randomized Cerclage Trial (CIPRACT): therapeutic cerclage with bed rest versus bed rest alone. Am J Obstet Gynecol 2001; 185:1106–12.

70. Levine RU, Berkowitz KM. Conservative management and pregnancy outcome in diethylstilbestrol-exposed women with and without gross genital tract abnormalities. Am J Obstet Gynecol 1993; 169:1125–9.

71. Lolis DE, Paschopoulos M, Makrydimas G, et al. Reproductive outcome after Strassman metroplasty in women with a bicornuate uterus. J Reprod Med 2005; 50:297–301.

72. Khalifa E, Toner JP, Jones HW Jr. The role of abdominal metroplasty in the era of operative hysteroscopy. Surg Gynecol Obstet 1993; 176:208–12.

73. Johnson NP, Mak W, Sowter MC. Surgical treatment for tubal disease in women due to undergo in vitro fertilisation. Cochrane Database Syst Rev 2004; (3):CD002125.

74. Zolghadri J, Momtahan M, Alborzi S, et al. Pregnancy outcome in patients with early recurrent abortion following laparoscopic tubal corneal interruption of a fallopian tube with hydrosalpinx. Fertil Steril 2006; 86:149–51.

75. Nagel TC, Malo JW. Hysteroscopic metroplasty in the diethylstilbestrol-exposed uterus and similar nonfusion anomalies: effects on subsequent reproductive performance; a preliminary report. Fertil Steril 1993; 59:502–6.

76. Garbin O, Ohl J, Bettahar-Lebugle K, et al. Hysteroscopic metroplasty in diethylstilboestrol-exposed and hypoplastic uterus: a report on 24 cases. Hum Reprod 1998; 13:2751–5.

77. Barranger E, Gervaise A, Doumerc S, et al. Reproductive performance after hysteroscopic metroplasty in the hypoplastic uterus: a study of 29 cases. BJOG 2002; 109:1331–4.

12. Immunobiology of recurrent miscarriage

Marighoula Varla-Leftherioti

INTRODUCTION

Initially, recurrent spontaneous abortions (RSA) were considered to be due either to chromosomal aberrations of the fetus that are incompatible with its development or to maternal causes such as uterine anatomical abnormalities, hormonal or metabolic disturbances, hereditary thrombophilias, and infectious agents. When all the above causes of miscarriage were excluded, the miscarriages were characterized as 'unexplained miscarriages'. During the last 20 years, it has become clear that a large proportion of unexplained RSA (possibly more than 80%) may be due to immunological causes.[1]

In the 1980s, immune-mediated abortions were considered as a syndrome characterized by (a) more than two miscarriages with the same partner, (b) a higher frequency of ectopic pregnancies, (c) a tendency to infertility (because of miscarriages), and (d) a higher frequency of fetal growth retardation (in the case of live birth followed by recurrent losses).[2] Today, immune-mediated abortions are known to be characterized by either autoimmune or alloimmune disturbances.[3] In autoimmune abortions, the development of the placenta and the embryo is affected by maternal autoantibodies and autoreactive cells, which target decidual and trophoblastic molecules. In alloimmune abortions, the maternal immune system reacts against the embryo and damages trophoblast through allogeneic, rejection-type reactions.

AUTOIMMUNE ABORTIONS

Maternal autoimmune disturbances may be the cause of a high percentage of hitherto-unexplained miscarriages. Approximately 30% of women with 'unexplained' RSA have increased serum levels of autoantibodies, with antiphospholipid antibodies (aPL) predominating.[4] The observation that most of these women with abnormal autoimmune function have no other symptoms except reproduction-related symptoms led to the definition of a separated diagnostic entity: reproductive autoimmune failure syndrome (RAFS).[5] In 1999, the American Society of Reproductive Immunology, considering autoimmune abortions as one of the manifestations not only of RAFS but also of antiphospholipid syndrome (APS), suggested that these two syndromes should be included in a broader clinical entity: reproductive autoimmune syndrome (RAS).[6,7] Clinical and laboratory findings of APS and RAFS are presented in Table 12.1.

Given the clinical findings of RAS, an autoimmune cause of miscarriages should be suspected in women with a history of (1) three or more consecutive preembryonic or embryonic pregnancy losses, and (2) one or more unexplained fetal deaths above 10 weeks of gestation. Testing for autoimmune disturbances should be also considered in women with fewer miscarriages if they have experienced thrombosis or autoimmune thrombocytopenia (criteria for APS), or they have a history of endometriosis or unexplained difficulty in conceiving, or even a history of fetal growth retardation, severe preeclampsia or other obstetric complications (i.e., abruptio placentae, chorea gravidarum, herpes gestationis, HELLP syndrome (hemolysis, elevated liver enzymes, and low platelet count)) in previous successful pregnancies (criteria for RAFS). The workup in autoimmune abortions must include testing for aPL gammopathies (mainly immunoglobulin M (IgM)), antinuclear antibodies (ANA), and organ-specific autoantibodies. The most important among the above disturbances is the increase in aPL, which are recognized to have the strongest association with pregnancy loss. There is evidence that 2–20% of

Table 12.1 Clinical and laboratory findings in reproductive autoimmune syndrome (RAS)

	Antiphospholipid syndrome (APS)	Reproductive autoimmune failure syndrome (RAFS)

CLINICAL FEATURES	• Thrombosis (≥1 unexplained venous or arterial thrombosis, including stroke)
	• Autoimmune thrombocytopenia
	• Recurrent pregnancy loss:
	  ≥1 consecutive and otherwise unexplained fetal deaths (≥ 10 weeks)
	  ≥ 3 consecutive and otherwise unexplained preembryonic or embryonic pregnancy losses
		• Fetal growth retardation (<34 weeks)
		• Severe preeclampsia
		• Obstetric complications (abruptio placentae, chorea gravidarum, herpes gestationis, HELLP syndrome[a])
		• Unexplained infertility
		• Endometriosis
		• Recurrent pregnancy loss:
		  ≥1 consecutive and otherwise unexplained fetal deaths (≥ 10 weeks)
		  ≥ 3 consecutive and otherwise unexplained preembryonic or embryonic pregnancy losses

LABORATORY FINDINGS	• Anticardiolipin antibodies (aCL) (>20 GPL or MPL units) • Lupus anticoagulant (LA)	• Antiphospholipid antibodies (aPL) • Lupus anticoagulant (LA) • Gammopathy (usually polyclonal, mostly immunoglobulin M (IgM)) • Antinuclear antibodies (ANA) (including antibodies against histones) • Organ-specific autoantibodies (antithyroid antibodies (ATA), anti-smooth muscle antibodies (ASMA))

[a]Hemolysis, elevated liver enzymes, and low platelet count.

women with recurrent preembryonic or embryonic pregnancy losses have increased titers of aPL and that these women have an 80–90% pregnancy loss rate, with half of their pregnancies being lost in the first trimester.[8,9]

AUTOIMMUNE ABORTIONS ASSOCIATED WITH ANTIPHOSPHOLIPID ANTIBODIES

FORMATION AND CHARACTERIZATION OF ANTIPHOSPHOLIPID ANTIBODIES

Phospholipids (PL) are the basic components of all cell membranes, where they are present in two layers. Each PL consists of a glycerol moiety attached to two esterified fatty acid chains (one saturated and one unsaturated) as well as a phosphodiester-linked alcohol side-chain. In normal situations, the inner leaflet of the phospholipid bilayers is composed of negatively charged or anionic alcohol groups facing the cytoplasm, whereas the outer layer is composed of neutral or zwitterionic alcohol groups facing the

extracellular fluid or bloodstream.[10] In situations of ischemia, cell injury or abnormal immunregulation (autoimmunity), negatively charged PL can be exteriorized to the outer leaflet, while in the presence of excess calcium or low pH, cone-shaped, hexagonal-phase phospholipid configurations can be formed. These changes may either provide an antigenic stimulus for the production of aPL or permit a number of serum proteins with procoagulant activity (β_2-glycoprotein I (β_2GPI), prothrombin, protein C, protein S, and annexin V) to bind PL epitopes and to be presented to the immune system in unique 'neoantigenic' conformations, which are recognized and give rise to aPL.[11] In the latter case, aPL may recognize either only the PL region of the complex or an epitope consisting of the portion of the PL and neighboring amino acids on the protein carrier or they clearly act with the protein alone. The most important among the proteins that bind to PLs is β_2GPI, the antibodies against which are usually enlisted in the group of aPL.[3,4] Recently, Kuwana et al[12] were able to detect β_2GPI-specific CD4[+] and human leukocyte antigen

(HLA) class II restricted autoreactive T cells, which preferentially recognize the antigenic peptide containing the major pPL-binding site and have the capacity to stimulate B cells to produce pathogenic anti-β_2GPI antibodies.[12]

Because of the different methods whereby induction can occur, aPL are a heterogeneous group of autoantibodies.[11] aPL that bind to PL, present in unique hexagonal phases either alone or complexed with prothrombin or β_2GPI, prolong pPL-dependent clotting assays and are known as lupus anticoagulants (LA). The subgroup of aPL that bind to PL/protein complexes and may or may not prolong PL-dependent clotting assays include antibodies against cardiolipin (aCL), phosphatidylethanolamine (aPE), phosphatidylserine (aPS), phosphatidylcholine (aPC), phosphatidylglycerol (aPG), phosphatidylinositol (aPI), and phosphatidic acid (aPA). These antibodies are detected by immunoassays using PL-coated surfaces, and there is no agreement if there is a correlation between them and LA or discordance between their prevalence.

FORMATION OF aPL DURING PREGNANCY

Pregnancy itself appears to be a triggering event that allows protein cofactors to bind PL and become antigenic for aPL production. Placental tissues continuously change, and this major tissue remodeling results in externalization of inner surface PL, which, when appearing on the outer membrane, may either be a direct stimulus for aPL production or permit plasma proteins to bind them so that neoantigens give rise to aPL. This has been documented for phosphatidylserine (PS). Despite the presence of an active membrane-associated adenosine triphosphate (ATP)-dependent aminophospholipid translocase that normally relocates PS from the outer to the inner monolayer, PS is exteriorized during trophoblast differentiation.[13] When exposed to the blood, PS allows β_2GPI to be immobilized and become antigenic for pathogenic aPL production. Infusion of aPS into pregnant mice results in an increased fetal resorption rate and lower mean weights of the placentas and fetuses.[14]

The main cause of fetal loss in the presence of aPL is hypoxia to the placenta because of uteroplacental blood supply insufficiency resulting from multiple intervillous thromboses, intravillous infractions, and decidual vasculopathy. Additionally to thrombosis, aPL directly target trophoblastic cells and may affect pregnancy by inhibiting normal PL functions related to trophoblastic cell division (aPE), intertrophoblastic fusion, hormone secretion and trophoblast invasion (aPS).[15]

AUTOIMMUNE ABORTIONS NOT ASSOCIATED WITH aPL

The following autoantibodies other than aPL are included in the diagnostic criteria for RAFS and are associated with pregnancy loss.

ANTINUCLEAR ANTIBODIES AND ANTIBODIES TO NUCLEAR ANTIGENS

ANA and antibodies against single- and double-stranded DNA (ssDNA and dsDNA) appear to be increased in about 35% of women with RSA, while their percentage is less than 10% in fertile women with no abortion history. Antibodies against histones or non-DNA nuclear components (Sm, RNP, SSA, SSB, and Scl70) are also found in some of these women.[16] The presence of ANA is associated with inflammation around the placenta, so that the environment does not enhance the 'acceptance' of the embryo. In these cases, anti-inflammatory prevention therapy with corticosteroids has been reported, but remains controversial.[17]

ANTI-THYROID ANTIBODIES

Anti-thyroid autoantibodies (ATA) have been suggested to be independent markers of 'at-risk' pregnancy. Euthyroid women with RSA have increased levels of autoantibodies either against thyroglobulin (TG) or thyroid peroxidase (TPO) (22–37%, vs 7–19% in controls), while the probability of abortion in women with ATA has been shown to be 10–32% versus 3–16% in controls.[18–21] The mechanism whereby ATA affect pregnancy is not known.

It is possible that the high rate of miscarriage is related to a very mild thyroid 'underfunction', with the thyroid gland being less able to adapt to the increased requirements of pregnancy; thus, these women would benefit from thyroid replacement therapy.[20] Furthermore, it has been suggested that ATA may coexist with activated T cells in the uterus that secret abortogenic cytokines, or that their presence may reflect an underlying immunological dysfunction (possibly a T-lymphocyte defect).[19] This suggestion is supported by the coexistence of ATA with non-organ-specific autoantibodies as well as with increased natural killer (NK) cells in habitual aborters.[21] In terms of this last explanation, treatment with intravenous immunoglobulin (IVIG) is expected not only to neutralize the antibodies, but also to provide the required modulation of immune functioning.

OTHER AUTOANTIBODIES AND IMMUNE DISTURBANCES ASSOCIATED WITH RAS

Several 'non-classical' aPL (directed against prothrombin or thromboplastin, or mitochondrial antibodies of M5 type) have been observed in women with recurrent miscarriages, but their clinical significance remains unclear.[22]

Another interesting finding in aborters with ANA or ATA is the increased presence of peripheral CD19⁺CD5⁺ cells,[23] which are believed to produce polyvalent antibodies (mainly IgM) that are also directed against hormones (estradiol, progesterone, and human chorionic gonadotropin (hCG)) and neurotransmitters (endorphins and serotonin), and may be responsible for insufficient decidualization and decreased blood supply to the endometrium, respectively.

Finally, a genetic background may predispose to fetal loss in women with autoimmune-mediated abortions. Beer et al[24] have reported an increase in the HLA-DQA1*0501 allele (currently assigned as 0505) in women with recurrent pregnancy losses who are aPL-positive. They have suggested that fetuses compatible with their mothers for this allele are autoimmune-unacceptable to the mother and trigger her to develop aPL when the pregnancy fails

and to be most prone to miscarriage in subsequent pregnancies. According to our experience, the preliminary results from the 13th International Histocompatibility Workshop,[25] and data from the 14th International Histocompatibility Workshop, an HLA-DQA1*0505 sharing is found in couples with autoimmune RSA rather than those with alloimmune abortions, and could possibly be used as a marker for the autoimmune etiology of miscarriages.

ALLOIMMUNE ABORTIONS

The observations that, in some cases of abortion, the embryo is infiltrated by lymphocytes and the lesions found to the placenta resemble the allogeneic reactions found in transplanted grafts indicate that in these cases the embryo is 'rejected' by the mother.[26] To assess the mechanisms causing such type of abortion (*alloimmune abortion*), it is necessary to know the nature of the immune response in normal pregnancy, since it is the disturbances in normal pregnancy immunological mechanisms that result in allogeneic antifetal reactions.

THE IMMUNE RESPONSE IN NORMAL PREGNANCY

The conseptus is a *semiallogeneic graft*, because it is produced by the contribution of both the mother and the father. Although fetal alloantigens encoded by genes inherited from the father should provoke maternal responses and lead to fetal loss, normally this does not happen. This natural miracle, known as the *immunological paradox of pregnancy*, is considered to be the result of a particular immune response of the pregnant woman, and for more than 50 years it has been a challenge for reproductive immunologists to attempt to elucidate the underlying immunological mechanisms.

FACILITATION REACTION

The first reliable explanation for fetal tolerance was the suggestion that in allogeneic reactions such as transplantation and pregnancy, the immune response is a bipolar one that can be either harmful or favorable to the target cells expressing alloantigens. The harmful effect (rejection reaction observed in transplantation) is characterized by cytotoxic antibodies and cytotoxic cells that damage the antigenic target. The enhancing effect (facilitation reaction) is characterized by a predominance of humoral responses, which may counteract the rejection reaction and have a beneficial effect on the antigenic target.[27] Predominance of this facilitation reaction over the rejection reaction appears in pregnancy, where enhancing non-complement-fixing antibodies and suppressor cells favor the acceptance of the embryo because they prevent complement-mediated cell lysis, while they block allogeneic reactions, either by covering the alloantigens or through the function of an idiotype–anti-idiotype antibody network.[28] If the coexisting but suppressed rejection reaction is upregulated, the embryo is rejected. The suggestion that the facilitation reaction prevails over the rejection reaction and succeeds in fetal tolerance has been followed by a plethora of studies that have focused on the mechanisms mediating this specific response.

Th2-TYPE IMMUNE RESPONSE

In 1987, Wegmann[29] presented the 'immunotrophic' theory, according to which the normal development of the placenta is the result of the influence of cytokines (placenta immunotrophic cytokines, such as granulocyte–macrophage colony-stimulating factor (GM-CSF), transforming growth factor β (TGF-β), and interleukin-3 (IL-3)). In 1993, Wegman et al[30] suggested that during pregnancy there is a change of the T-helper 1(Th1)/Th2 equilibrium so that Th2-type cytokines (IL-4, IL-5, and IL-10) predominate over Th1-type cytokines (IL-2 and interferon γ (IFN-γ)) and benefit the developing embryo by enhancing placental growth and function as well as by preventing inappropriate anti-trophoblast cytotoxic reactions.

The important role of cytokines in a fruitful maternal–fetal symbiosis has been well documented through the years. However, the trophoblastic antigenic stimulus, the maternal cells that are stimulated for the initiation of the enhancing response,

and the exact factors modulating Th2 shift remain unclarified. Several studies have examined the significance of molecules of several antigenic systems, that are expressed on the trophoblast (molecules of the major histocompatibility complex (MHC), erythrocyte antigens, complement regulatory proteins, Fc receptors, various isoenzymes, adhesion molecule, R80K protein, etc.), but no specific antigenicity has been proven.[31] Nevertheless, specific trophoblastic molecules as well as various proteins produced by the trophoblast appear to modulate the cytokine pattern towards preferential expression of Th2 cytokines. Heat-shock proteins (Hsp), pregnancy-specific β_1-glycoprotein, and increased expression of the non-classical MHC class I HLA-G molecule have been suggested to stimulate endometrial macrophages for IL-10 production, which enhances a Th2 shift.[32,33] Decidual cells may also produce high levels of Th2-type cytokines after interacting with trophoblastic CD1d molecules, which present glycolipid antigens to specific cell populations bearing T- and NK-cell receptors.[34] Moreover, binding of leukemia inhibitory factor (LIF), which is produced by decidual cells, to its receptor (LIF-R) on the syncytiotrophoblast may enhance placental growth and differentiation and a Th2 shift.[35] Finally, hCG produced by the trophoblast induces the production of progesterone by the corpus luteum. Through an immunoregulatory protein known as progesterone-induced blocking factor (PIBF), progesterone may induce the production of IL-4 by γδ T lymphocytes and thus enhance a Th2 response.[36]

CYTOKINE AND HORMONE NETWORK

The acceptance of a Th2 shift alone for the maintenance of pregnancy must be considered as a simplification of the cytokine-mediated mechanisms enhancing pregnancy at the fetomaternal interface. It must not be ignored that in the first stages of pregnancy, IFN-γ, a Th1 cytokine, contributes to the vascular development and remodeling of uterine spiral arteries required for implantation and successful gestation.[37] In addition, it must be remembered that the cytokine network at the fetomaternal interface is extremely complicated and the embryo has been successfully described as 'bathing in a sea of cytokines'.[38] Different cell populations are potentially involved in the production not only of Th2 cytokines but also of Th1 cytokines, as well as other cytokines (i.e., IL-12, IL-15, and IL-18), chemokines, and growth factors that control the differentiation and the activation of immune cells locally. A cytokine that controls the shift to a Th1 response (i.e., IL-12) coexists with one enhancing the Th2 response(i.e., IL-10), and these are possibly controlled by primary regulatory factors on a competitive basis. This regulatory and competitive role is attributed to homones (i.e., hCG, progesterone, and relaxin), the secretion of which is induced by cytokines at the same time that the hormones themselves control the production of cytokines. For example, Th2-type cytokines induce the secretion of hCG by the trophoblast, which stimulates the corpus luteum to produce progesterone. Progesterone enhances the production of Th2 cytokines by competing with relaxin, which is also produced by the corpus luteum and which enhances the production of Th1 cytokines.[39]

OTHER MECHANISMS ENHANCING FETAL TOLERANCE

Although Th2 cytokines characterize the immune response in normal pregnancy, the Th2 shift is just part of this particular immune response. Many different mechanisms acting locally or at a distance ensure tolerance to the semiallogeneic graft by the maternal natural and adaptive immune defences. Thus, tolerance is modulated by the cumulative effect of preimplantation factors, molecules expressed on the trophoblast as well as decidual immune cells. Changes in metabolic factors, hormones, and cytokines during ovulation, coitus, and fertilization result in local immunosuppression within the maternal genital tract and prepare the uterus for the implantation of the blastocyst.[40] Trophoblastic molecules may be specifically recognized by maternal immune cells as alloantigens or may act as antigen-presenting molecules or have an immunosuppressive/immunomodulatory function. Decidual immune cells may regulate the immune

response not only by producing cytokines and growth factors, but also by specific recognition of trophoblastic molecules, suppression of cytotoxic reactions, and control of trophoblast invention and NK-cell toxicity.

Several specific immunosuppressive and cytotoxicity-blocking mechanisms have been suggested to contribute to fetal tolerance.[41] Sperm may promote local immunosuppression via prostaglandins, while TGF-β contained in seminal plasma may play a critical role in providing the necessary antigenic and environmental signals for the production of growth factors (GM-CSF) by the uterine epithelium and the initiation of an appropriate maternal immune response to the conceptus if pregnancy is achieved.[42] The maternal innate immune system, which is the first to confront the embryo, actively reacts to the 'invader' by developing an inflammatory response, which may enhance conditions for tolerance.[43] Decidual macrophages, apart from a tendency to express their activation by the production of anti-inflammatory rather than proinflammatory cytokines, appear to have an immunosuppressive action and a limited antigen-presenting capacity.[44] Another protective mechanism involves (at least in animals) indoleamine 2,3-deoxygenase (IDO), an enzyme for tryptophan catabolism. IDO expressed by trophoblastic cells may catabolize tryptophan in placental immune cells (maternal T cells) and prevent them from activating lethal antifetal immune responses.[41] Apoptotic mechanisms may also contribute to the protection of the embryo. For example, the presence of the CD95L (FasL) molecule (CD95 (Fas) ligand) on trophoblastic cells seems to protect them by inducing apoptosis of activated CD95[+] T lymphocytes.[45] Finally, modulation of local placental immunity during pregnancy has been ascribed to HLA-G, whose distribution is mainly restricted to the placenta. It has been suggested that HLA-G is an immunosuppressive molecule inducing apoptosis of activated cytotoxic T lymphocytes (CTL) and downregulating the proliferation of helper T cells. In addition, soluble HLA-G molecules may block receptors on CTL and prevent their action on target cells expressing paternally derived alloantigens.[46]

THE ROLE OF NK CELLS IN THE MAINTENANCE OF PREGNANCY

In 1996, an important role was attributed to decidual NK (dNK) cells in the allorecognition mechanisms acting in pregnancy, and it was suggested that the concept of 'the fetus as an allograft' required redefinition to encompass these cells.[47] NK-like cells (CD3⁻CD16⁻CD56⁺ᵇʳⁱᵍʰᵗ) are the dominant decidual cell population from the first stages of pregnancy through the first trimester. Due to their increased presence and direct contact with invading trophoblast, they have been considered as important for the establishment of normal pregnancy. There is evidence that, coincident with blastocyst implantation and decidualization, uterine NK cells become activated and produce IFN-γ, perforin, and other molecules, including angiogenetic factors. In this way, they can control trophoblast invasion through their cytotoxic activity; and they also initiate vessel instability and remodeling of decidual arteries to increase the blood supply to the fetoplacental unit.[37] Furthermore, dNK cells may be involved in cytokine-mediated immunoregulation of the maternal immune response, producing Th2-type cytokines and growth factors, which result in placental augmentation and local immunosuppression and immunomodulation.[48,49]

As in any other population of NK cells, the mode of action of dNK cells involves a repertoire of activating and inhibitory receptors belonging to three main families: the KIR family (killer immunoglobulin-like receptors), the C-type lectin family (CD94/NKG) and the immunoglobulin-like transcripts (ILT or LIR). Through their receptors, dNK cells may recognize selected epitopes on HLA class I molecules expressed on the invading trophoblast. It is interesting that the specific ligands for most of the receptors are the non-classical HLA class I molecules G and E as well the classical HLA class I antigen C, which are the only HLA molecules expressed on the extravillous trophoblast. Moreover, some of the receptors recognizing HLA-G and HLA-C epitopes are selectively expressed on dNK cells. The specific interaction of NK-cell receptors with trophoblastic antigens led to the concept of an embryo recognition model through an 'NK-cell allorecognition system'. High-affinity interactions of NK-cell receptors with their ligands may provide self-signals to either a cytotoxic NK-cell activation (Th1 response) or inhibition of activation and protection of the trophoblast (Th2 response). Which one of the two responses will predominate depends on the action of the inhibitory receptors, which prevails over the action of the activating ones. So, if the inhibitory dNK receptors recognize their specific ligands on the trophoblast, they are expected to inhibit dNK cell activation for trophoblast damage, otherwise dNK cells are allowed to develop anti-trophoblast activity (reviewed by Varla-Leftherioti[43]).

Most studies that have investigated the effect of dNK-cell receptors in the maintenance of pregnancy have specifically focused on the interactions involving HLA-G molecules, because of their restricted distribution to placental tissues. HLA-G has been shown to be the ligand for at least three inhibitory receptors, and the expression of some HLA-G isoforms has been shown to protect trophoblastic cells from lysis by activated cytotoxic cell clones.[50] Nevertheless, the control of the anti-trophoblast activity of dNK cells is probably the result of the cumulative interaction of several receptors on maternal dNK cells, with different self and non-self class I molecules appearing on the HLA haplotypes expressed on the trophoblast. Among the different NK-cell receptor interactions with their specific counterparts on the trophoblast, the interactions between inhibitory receptors of the KIR family (inhKIR) and their ligands (HLA-C molecules) appear to be those mainly involved in the function of an NK-cell-mediated allorecognition system in pregnancy.[51] Given the differences in both the inhKIR repertoire and the HLA-C allotypes among unrelated individuals, each pregnancy presents a different combination of maternal inhKIR receptors on dNK cells and self and non-self HLA-C allotypes on the trophoblast. This combination is expected to ensure the appropriate receptor–ligand interactions to inhibit dNK-cell anti-trophoblast activity, thus favoring pregnancy.

IMMUNOPATHOLOGY OF ALLOIMMUNE ABORTION

In contrast to normal pregnancy, a predominant Th1-type response or defective production of Th2-type cytokines appears in spontaneous abortion.[52] In response to the conceptus or other antigens, decidual lymphocytes secrete proinflammatory Th1-type cytokines such as IL-2, IFN-γ, and tumor necrosis factor α (TNF-α), which adversely affect the development of the embryo. Fetal rejection occurs through immune-induced inflammation (delayed-type hypersensitivity reactions resulting in lymphocyte infiltration of the trophoblast), tissue degradation (cytotoxic reactions resulting in damage of the trophoblast by NK cells and cytotoxic antibodies produced by specific subpopulations of B lymphocytes), and coagulation (upregulation of a novel prothrombinase fgl2, which results in vasculitis affecting the maternal blood supply to the implanted embryo).[33,48,53] In addition to the Th1-type response, other mechanisms thought to be involved in the response to normal pregnancy have also been found in abortions (namely, disturbances in tryptophan catabolism and reduced apoptosis).[53]

Unfortunately, the specific mechanism causing fetal rejection is as yet undefined, since no relevant single specific mechanism has been recognized as essential for a successful pregnancy. We speculate that the disruption of one or more of the mechanisms leading to tolerance in normal pregnancy may occur in stress situations and can lead to rejection. These disturbances may include (a) absence of immunosuppressive proimplantation factors in the woman's genital tract, (b) absence of immunodependent specific suppression at the fetomaternal interface, and (c) inappropriate expression or defective recognition of trophoblastic and immunoregulatory molecules by decidual cells, including disturbances in the NK allorecognition system. Alone or in combination, the above disturbances seem to deregulate the sensitive balance of maternal tolerance to the embryo and lead to its 'rejection'.

Figure 12.1 is a diagram of the response in a normal pregnancy:

- Preimplantation factors cause local immunosuppression in the genital tract and prepare the endometrium to accept the semiallogeneic embryo.
- In an environment of hormone-dependent maternally and fetally derived immunosuppression, specific decidual cells recognize specific molecules on the trophoblast.
- Activated decidual cells secrete growth factors (GM-CSF, TGF-β, and IL-3) that enhance placental growth (immunotrophism).
- Specific lymphocytes of the pregnant woman are also activated and secrete anti-inflammatory cytokines (IL-4, IL-10, and IL-13), so that a Th2-type immune response is developed.
- Produced antibodies block cytotoxic reactions that would harm the embryo.

In abortion (Figure 12.2), tolerance enhancing preimplantation factors may be absent, trophoblastic antigens may be inappropriately expressed, and the recognition of trophoblastic antigens and/or immunoregulatory molecules may be defective. Th1 cells produce proinflammatory cytokines (IL-2, IFN-γ, and TNF-a), which generate a Th1-type response. In the absence of blocking factors, cytotoxic antibodies and cytotoxic cells (mainly NK cells) damage the trophoblast.

FACTORS INDUCING A Th1 RESPONSE IN ABORTION

Although the immunopathology underlying Th1 preponderance in abortion is unknown, it is widely accepted that situations such as stress, infection, and autoimmunity may cause Th1 cytokine-triggered abortions. Stress has been suggested to alter the endocrine system (corticotrophin-releasing hormone, adrenocorticotropin, and progesterone), which triggers an immune bias towards an abortogenic Th1 cytokine profile.[54] Infections may also cause Th1 cytokine-triggered abortions. Clark et al[55] have suggested that this kind of abortion depends on the availability/presence of bacterial endotoxins such as lipopolysacharide (LPS). Infectious agents may trigger a Th1 response when they are recognized by specific decidual T cells bearing $V_{\delta 2}$ receptors, which when activated secrete abortogenic cytokines. Barakonyi et al[56] have shown

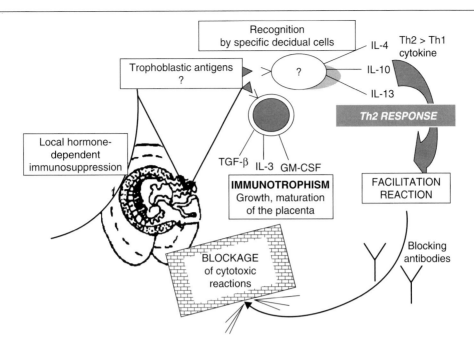

Figure 12.1 Immunologic mechanisms in normal pregnancy. IL, interleukin; Th, T-helper; TGF-β, transforming growth factor β; GM-CSF, granulocyte–macrophage colony-stimulating factor.

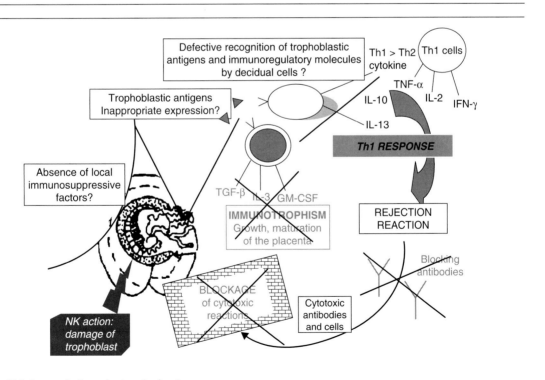

Figure 12.2 Immunologic mechanisms in abortion.

that peripheral blood $\gamma\delta^+$ T cells from women with RSA preferentially express the $V_{\gamma9}V_{\delta2}$ T-cell receptor combination. $V_{\gamma9}V_{\delta2}$ T cells are known to recognize non-peptide organophosphate and alkylamine antigens and eliminate bacteria and parasites. We have investigated the bias towards these cells in women with unexplained pregnancy losses and have found that the majority had undiagnosed genital tract or even systematic bacterial infections (unpublished data).

Genetic factors may also predispose to Th1-triggered abortion. It has been suggested that the cytokine balance is determined by maternal genes, which regulate the response to stress, LPS, and paternally inherited trophoblastic antigens.[33,37] Furthermore, cytokine gene polymorphisms (i.e., TNF and IFN-γ) have been associated with recurrent abortion in women with Th1 immunity to the trophoblast.[57]

ROLE OF NK CELLS IN ABORTION

Decidual NK cells appear to be the main cell population involved in alloimmune abortion. Under the influence of Th1-type cytokines, they are stimulated to become classical NK cells expressing CD16 ($CD3^-CD16^+CD56^+$), which can damage the trophoblast either directly by releasing cytolytic substances or indirectly by producing inflammatory cytokines.[58] Clinical studies have demonstrated that women who tend to abort have increased numbers of NK cells of the conventional $CD3^-CD56^+CD16^+$ type in the uterus,[59,60] as well as increased blood NK-cell subsets and NK-cell activity, all of which have been associated with abortion of chromosomally normal embryos.[61,62]

Considering the function of dNK-cell receptors, the rejection of the embryo may be the result of a defect in the NK allorecognition system. Studies in RSA couples as well as in cases of sporadic abortion have suggested that aborting women have a limited repertoire of inhKIR receptors and many of them lack the appropriate inhKIR to interact with trophoblastic HLA-Cw molecules (lack of maternal inhKIR–fetal HLA-C epitope matching). Hence, the triggering signals that the dNK cells may receive to attack the trophoblast (including activation signals provided through interactions of activating NKR–trophoblastic HLA-Cw pairs), are not inhibited and the embryo is not protected.[63,64] Although these suggestions have not been confirmed, recent data from the 14th International Histocompatibility Workshop provide evidence on the role of KIR haplotypes (activating KIR) in abortion. A high percentage of women with RSA of alloimmune etiology were found to have a divergence of the common AA KIR repertoire to a rather uncommon repertoire where A KIR haplotypes contain 'extra' activating KIR, while the ratio of inhibitory to activating KIR was slightly lower than that in fertile women or women with autoimmune abortions. It is possible that this imbalance in favor of activating KIR gives to these women a high potential for dNK-cell activation, which may damage trophoblast and avert pregnancy.[65]

WORKUP IN ALLOIMMUNE ABORTIONS

The diagnosis of alloimmune abortions is complex, as the pathophysiology is far from certain. To approach it, one has to keep in mind the various different immunological mechanisms involved in normal pregnancy, and to look for relevant disturbances that could damage the trophoblast. Immunological tests that have been used include the following:

- partner's HLA typing, since increased HLA sharing between both spouses has been considered as a marker of insufficient alloantigenic stimulus for the initiation of the appropriate immune response
- detection of lymphocytotoxic antibodies against paternal cells (antipaternal antibodies), the absence of which may indirectly indicate a maternal under-responsiveness and lack of pregnancy enhancing humoral factors in women's serum
- mixed lymphocyte cultures to evaluate whether the maternal antipaternal response is inhibited in the presence of maternal serum – an indication that the woman's serum does not contain satisfactory levels of antibodies that would block antitrophoblast cytotoxic responses.

However, none of the above tests has been shown to be diagnostic.

In the light of current knowledge, the workup in women suspected to have alloimmune abortion should include tests to detect the Th1 response (increased serum levels or intracellular predominance of IL-2, IFN-γ, and TNF-α), but the diagnostic value of these measurements is also doubtful. In practice, alloimmune abortions are most often diagnosed by the study of peripheral blood NK cells, which, when occurring in increased numbers or activity, have been associated with the abortion of chromosomally normal embryos. NK-cell levels have also been used as markers for the selection of women for immunotherapy.[61,62] Finally, diagnosis can be supported by allogeneic-type reactions (villitis and increase in CD3⁻CD16⁺CD56⁺ dNK cells) detected by histology and/or immunohistochemistry of previously aborted placental tissue.[60]

PREVENTIVE IMMUNOTHERAPY IN ALLOIMMUNE ABORTION

For the prevention of recurrent alloimmune abortions, two main types of immunotherapy have been used:

1. *Active immunization of women using paternal or third-party lymphocytes.* The application of this type of immunotherapy started in the early 1980s, when it was considered that some unexplained abortions are due to increased HLA sharing between partners. In these cases, it was expected that the administration of lymphocytes expressing paternal antigens that are inherited by the embryo would reinforce the alloantigenic stimulus for the initiation of the enhancing pregnancy response. According to a series of studies, including multicenter ones, this therapy has given varying results, ranging from very good to doubtful.[66] Today, its application is rather limited. Suggested mechanisms of action include the induction of effective presentation of paternally derived fetal antigens (amplification of the alloeantigenic stimulus) and the regulation of the maternal response mainly through the suppression of NK-cell activity[67] and the enhancement of a Th2-type immune response.[68]

2. *Passive immunization in the form of intravenous administration of immunoglobulin G (IVIG)* (immunomodulation for the blockage of allogeneic cytotoxic reactions). IVIG appears to suppress NK-cell activity and subsets,[69] and it has been suggested as the only therapeutic solution for women having increased percentage and activity of peripheral NK cells. Recently, it was shown that, in women with alloimmune abortion, IVIG enhances a shift to a Th2-type response.[70]

In addition to immunotherapy, hormonal support (progesterone or hCG supplements) has been used to improve the live birth rate in recurrently aborting women by modulating the balance between Th1 and Th2 cytokines and possibly by preventing inappropriate apoptosis.[39]

EPILOGUE

It is conceivable that the two categories of autoimmune- and alloimmune-mediated abortions may not really represent distinct immunological pathologies. Abortogenic cytokines known to mediate alloimmune abortions may also mediate those with autoimmune pathology. The paradigm of miscarriages associated with ATA is a good example of combined autoimmune and Th1 disturbances. As suggested by Gleicher,[71] the disturbances in the two types of abortion as well as of other immune-mediated reproductive diseases may reflect a misdirection of a more broadly based immune response (reproductive Immune Failure Syndrome, RIFS). Nevertheless, at present, the classification of the immunological disturbances as autoimmune or alloimmune helps to explain a high percentage of abortions that were previously considered as 'unexplained', to identify candidates for immune testing, and to offer immunological treatments. In autoimmune abortions – especially those associated with aPL – the immunopathology is better defined, the diagnosis is relatively simple, and the therapy has been widely described and shown to be beneficial.

In alloimmune abortions, there are still many questions to be answered concerning the exact underlying mechanisms, since, even in normal pregnancy, many stages of the maternal immune response remain unclarified. Available diagnostic methods can only provide indirect markers of the underlying pathology – hence, the results must be interpreted with caution, in order that the 'diagnosis' be established and the appropriate immunointervention administered.

REFERENCES

1. Mc Intyre JA, Coulam CB, Faulk WP. recurrent spontaneous abortion. Am J Reprod Immunol 1989; 21:100–4.
2. Clark DA, Daya S. Trials and tribulation in the treatment of recurrent spontaneous abortion. Am J Reprod Immunol 1991; 25:18–24.
3. Stern JJ, Coulam CB. Current status of immunologic recurrent pregnancy loss. Curr Opin Obstet Gynecol 1993; 5:252–9.
4. Matzner W, Chong P, Xu G, et al. Characterization of antiphospholipid antibodies in women with recurrent spontaneous abortions. J Reprod Immunol 1994; 33:31–9.
5. Gleicher N, el-Roeiy A. The reproductive autoimmune failure syndrome. Am J Obstet Gynecol 1988; 159:223–7.
6. Coulam CB, Branch DW, Clark DA, et al. American Society for Reproductive Immunology: report of the committee for establishing criteria for diagnosis of reproductive autoimmune syndrome. Am J Reprod Immunol 1999; 41:121–32.
7. Coulam CB. The role of antiphospholipid antibodies in reproduction: questions answered and raised at the 18th Annual Meeting of the American Society of Reproductive Immunology. Am J Reprod Immunol 1999; 41:1–4.
8. Kutteh WH. Antiphospholipid antibodies and reproduction. J Reprod Immunol 1997; 35:151–71.
9. Branch W. Antiphospholipid antibodies and reproductive outcome: the current status of affairs. J Reprod Immunol 1998; 38:75–87.
10. Cullis PR, Hope MJ, Tilcockn CP. Lipid polymorphism and the roles of lipids in membranes. Chem Phys Lipids 1986; 40:127–44.
11. Lockwood CJ, Rand JH. The immunobiology and obstetrical consequences of antiphospholipid antibodies. Obstet Gynecol Surv 1994; 49:432–41.
12. Kuwana M, Matsuura E, Kobayashi K, et al. Binding of β_2-glycoprotein I to anionic phospholipids facilitates processing and presentation of a cryptic epitope that activates pathogenic autoreactive T cells. Blood 2005;105:1552–7.
13. Lyden TW, Vogt E, Ng AK, et al. Monoclonal antiphospholipid antibody reactivity against human placental trophoblast. J Reprod Immunol 1992; 22:1–14.
14. Blank M, Tincani A, Shoenfeld Y. Induction of experimental antiphospholipid syndrome in naive mice with purified IgG antiphosphatidylserine antibodies. J Rheumatol 1994; 21:100–4.
15. Emoto K, Kobayashi T, Yamaji A, et al. Redistribution of phosphatidylethanolamine at the cleavage furrow of dividing cells during cytokinesis. Proc Natl Acad Sci USA 1996; 93:12867–72.
16. Kaider AS, Kaider BD, Janowicz PB, et al. Immunodiagnostic evaluation in women with reproductive failure. Am J Reprod Immunol 1999; 42:335–46.
17. Kwak JY, Gilman-Sachs A, Beaman KD, et al. Reproductive outcome in women with recurrent spontaneous abortions of alloimmune and autoimmune causes: preconception versus postconception treatment. Am J Obstet Gynecol 1992; 166:1787–95.
18. Stagnaro-Green A, Roman SH, Cobin RH, et al. Detection of at-risk pregnancy by means of highly sensitive assays for thyroid autoantibodies. JAMA 1990; 264:1422–5.
19. Pratt DE, Kaberlein G, Dudkiewicz A, et al. The association of antithyroid antibodies in euthyroid nonpregnant women with recurrent first trimester abortions in the next pregnancy. Fertil Steril 1993; 60:1001–5.
20. Vaquero E, Lazzarin N, De Carolis C, et al. Mild thyroid abnormalities and recurrent spontaneous abortion: diagnostic and therapeutical approach. Am J Reprod Immunol 2000; 43:204–8.
21. Marai I, Carp H, Shai S, et al. Autoantibody panel screening in recurrent miscarriages. Am J Reprod Immunol 2004; 51:235–40.
22. Sherer Y, Tartakover-Matalon S, Blank M, et al. Multiple autoantibodies associated with autoimmune reproductive failure. J Assist Reprod Genet 2003; 20:53–7.
23. Beer AE, Kwak JY, Ruiz JE. Immunophenotypic profiles of peripheral blood lymphocytes in women with recurrent pregnancy losses and in infertile women with multiple failed in vitro fertilization cycles. Am J Reprod Immunol 1996; 35:376–82.
24. Beer AE, Kwak JYH, Gilman-Sacks A, et al. New horizons in the evaluation and treatment of recurrent pregnancy loss. In: Hunt JS, ed. Immunobiology of Reproduction. New York: Serono Symposia USA, 1994: 316–34.
25. Varla-Leftherioti M. Reproductive immunology component. In: Hansen J, Dupont B, eds. HLA 2004: Immunobiology of the Human MHC: Proceedings of the 13th IHWC. Seattle: IHWC, 2006.
26. Labarrere CA. Allogeneic recognition and rejection reactions in the placenta. Am J Reprod Immunol 1989; 21:94–9.
27. Voisin GA. Immunological facilitation, a broadening of the concept of the enhancement phenomenon. Prog Allergy 1971; 15:328–485.
28. Chaouat G, Voisin GA, Escalier D, et al. Facilitation reaction (enhancing antibodies and suppressor cells) and rejection reaction (sensitized cells) from the mother to the paternal antigens of the conceptus. Clin Exp Immunol 1979; 35:13–24.
29. Wegmann TG. Placental immunotrophism: maternal T cells enhance placental growth and function. Am J Reprod Immunol 1987; 15: 67–9.
30. Wegmann TG, Lin H, Guilbert L, et al. Bidirectional cytokine interactions in the maternal–fetal relationship: Is successful pregnancy a TH2 phenomenon? Immunol Today 1993; 14:353–6.
31. Clark DA. Immunobiological characterization of the trophoblast–decidual interface in human pregnancy. In: Kurpisz M, Fernandez N, eds. Immunology of Human Reproduction. Oxford: BIOS, 1995: 301–11.
32. Clark D. Editorial. Signaling at the fetomaternal interface. Am J Reprod Immunol 1999; 41:169–73.
33. Clark DA, Arck PC, Chaouat G. Why did your mother reject you? Immunogenetic determinants of the response to environmental selective pressure expressed at the uterine level. Am J Reprod Immunol 1999; 41:5–22.
34. Boyson JE, Rybalov B, Koopman LA, et al. CD1d and invariant NKT cells at the human maternal–fetal interface. Proc Natl Acad Sci 2002; 99:13741–6.
35. Kojima K, Kanzaki H, Iwai M, et al. Expression of leukaemia inhibitory factor (LIF) receptor in human placenta: a possible role for LIF in the growth and differentiation of trophoblasts. Hum Reprod 1995; 10:1907–11.

36. Szekeres-Bartho J, Barakonyi A, Polgar B, et al. The role of γ/δ T cells in progesterone-mediated immunomodulation during pregnancy. A review. Am J Reprod Immunol 1999; 42:44–8.

37. Ashkar AA, Di Santo JP, Croy BA. Interferon gamma contributes to initiation of uterine vascular modification, decidual integrity, and uterine natural killer cell maturation during normal murine pregnancy. J Exp Med 2000; 92:259–70.

38. Chaouat G, Ledee-Bataille N, Dubanchet S, et al. TH1/TH2 paradigm in pregnancy: paradigm lost? Cytokines in pregnancy/early abortion: reexamining the TH1/TH2 paradigm. Int Arch Allergy Immunol 2004; 134:93–119.

39. Carp H, Torchinsky A, Fein A, et al. Hormones, cytokines and fetal anomalies in habitual abortion. Gynecol Endocrinol 2001; 15:472–83.

40. Mellor AL, Munn DH. Immunology at the maternal–fetal interface: Lessons for T cell tolerance and suppression. Annu Rev Immunol 2000; 18:367–91.

41. Thellin O, Coumans B, Zorzi W, et al. Tolerance to the foeto–placental 'graft': ten ways to support a child for nine months. Curr Opin Immunol 2000; 12:731–7.

42. Robertson SA. Seminal plasma and male factor signalling in the female reproductive tract. Cell Tissue Res 2005; 322:43–52.

43. Varla-Leftherioti M. The significance of women's NK cell receptors' repertoire in the maintenance of pregnancy. Chem Immunol Allergy 2005; 89:84–95.

44. Mizuno M, Aoki K, Kimbara T. Functions of macrophages in human decidual tissue in early pregnancy. Am J Reprod Immunol 1994; 3:180–8.

45. Zorzi W, Thellin O, Coumans B, et al. Demonstration of the expression of CD95 ligand transcript and protein in human placenta. Placenta 1998; 19:269–77.

46. Le Bouteiller P. HLA-G and local placental immunity. Gynecol Obstet Fertil 2003; 31:782–5.

47. King A, Loke YW, Chaouat G. NK cells and reproduction. Immunol Today 1997; 18:64–6.

48. Clark D, Arck PC, Jallili R, et al. Psycho–neuro–cytokine/endocrine pathways in immunoregulation during pregnancy. Am J Reprod Immunol 1996; 35:330–7.

49. Chaouat G, Tranchot Diallo J, Volumenie JL, et al. Immune suppression and Th1/Th2 balance in pregnancy revisited: a (very) personal tribute to Tom Wegmann. Am J Reprod Immunol 1997; 37:427–34.

50. Menier C, Riteau B, Dausset J, et al. HLA-G truncated isoforms can substitute for HLA-G1 in fetal survival. Hum Immunol 2000; 61:1118–25.

51. Varla-Leftherioti M. Role of a KIR/HLA-C allorecognition system in pregnancy. J Reprod Immunol 2004; 62:19–27.

52. Raghupathy R. TH1-type immunity is incompatible with successful pregnancy. Immunol Today 1997; 18:478–82.

53. Thellin O, Heinen E. Pregnancy and the immune system: between tolerance and rejection. Toxicology 2003; 185:179–84.

54. Arck PC. Stress and pregnancy loss: role of immune mediators, hormones and neurotransmitters. Am J Reprod Immunol 2001; 46:117–23.

55. Clark DA, Chaouat G, Gorczynski RM. Thinking outside the box: mechanisms of environmental selective pressures on the outcome of the materno–fetal relationship. Am J Reprod Immunol 2002; 47:275–82.

56. Barakonyi A, Polgar B, Szekeres-Bartho J. The role of γ/δ T-cell receptor-positive cells in pregnancy: Part II. Am J Reprod Immunol 1999; 42:83–7.

57. Daher S, Shulzhenko N, Morgun A, et al. Associations between cytokine gene polymorohisms and recurrent pregnancy loss. J Reprod Immunol 2003; 58:69–77.

58. King A, Wheeler R, Carter NP, et al. The response of human decidual leukocytes to IL-2. Cell Immunol 1992; 141:409–42.

59. Vassiliadou N, Bulmer JN. Immunohistochemical evidence for increased numbers of 'classic' CD57+ natural killer cells in the endometrium of women suffering spontaneous early pregnancy loss. Hum Reprod 1996; 11:1569–74.

60. Kwak JY, Beer AE, Kim SH, et al. Immunopathology of the implantation site utilizing monoclonal antibodies to natural killer cells in women with recurrent pregnancy losses. Am J Reprod Immunol 1999; 41:91–8.

61. Coulam CB, Goodman C, Roussev RG, et al. Systemic CD56+ cells can predict pregnancy outcome. Am J Reprod Immunol 1995; 33:40–6.

62. Aoki K, Kajiura S, Matsumoto Y, et al. Preconceptual natural killer cell activity as a predictor of miscarriage. Lancet 1995; 345:1340–2.

63. Varla-Leftherioti M, Spyropoulou-Vlachou M, Niokou D, et al. Natural killer (NK) cell receptors' repertoire in couples with recurrent spontaneous abortions. Am J Reprod Immunol 2003; 49:183–91.

64. Varla-Leftherioti M, Spyropoulou-Vlachou M, Keramitsoglou T, et al. Lack of the appropriate natural killer cell inhibitory receptors in women with spontaneous abortion. Hum Immunol 2005; 66:65–71.

65. Varla-Leftherioti M, Keramitsoglou T, Spyropoulou-Vlachou M, et al. Report from the Reproductive Immunology Component at the 14th International HLA and Immunogenetics Workshop. Tissue Antigens 2007; 69 suppl 1:1–7.

66. Coulam CB, Clark DA, Collins J, et al. The Recurrent Miscarriage Immunotherapy Trialists. Worldwide collaborative observational study and meta-analysis on allogenic leukocyte immunotherapy for recurrent spontaneous abortion. Am J Reprod Immunol 1994; 32:55–72.

67. Gafter U, Sredni B, Segal J, et al. Suppressed cell-mediated immunity and monocyte and natural killer cell activity following allogeneic immunization of women with spontaneous recurrent abortion. J Clin Immunol 1997; 17:408–19.

68. Hayakawa S, Karasaki, Suzuki M, et al. Effects of paternal lymphocyte immunization on peripheral TH1/TH2 balance and Tcr Vβ and Vγ repertoire usage of patients with recurrent spontaneous abortions. Am J Reprod Immunol 2000; 43:107–15.

69. Ruiz JE, Kwak JY, Baum L, et al. Intravenous immunoglobulin inhibits natural killer cell activity in vivo in women with recurrent spontaneous abortion. Am J Reprod Immunol 1996; 35:370–5.

70. Graphou O, Chioti A, Pantazi A, et al. Effect of intravenous immunoglobulin treatment on the Th1/Th2 balance in women with recurrent spontaneous abortions. Am J Reprod Immunol 2003; 49:21–9.

71. Gleicher N. Some thoughts on the reproductive autoimmune failure syndrome (RAFS) and Th-1 versus Th-2 immune responses. Am J Reprod Immunol 2002; 48:252–4.

DEBATE

12a. Should paternal leukocyte immunization be used in RPL?
–For

David A Clark

There are two types of arguments put forward to support offering paternal leukocyte immunization to women with recurrent early pregnancy loss.[1] The first relies on evidence-based medicine: if there is adequate evidence from controlled clinical trials for efficacy, it is reasonable to offer treatment. The second relies on rationale: if there is a credible mechanism, then treatment should work, and hence should be offered. Side effects and cost–benefit are usually also considered in making a positive recommendation and in the patient's decision. In 1994, the results of the Recurrent Miscarriage Immunotherapy Trialists Group (RMITG) meta-analysis were published.[2] The meta-analysis was conducted by two independent teams under the aegis of the ASRI Ethics Committee. John Collins and Robin Roberts headed the first team; Jim Scott headed the second. Using an intention-to-treat analysis, the first team found that paternal leukocyte immunization increased the live birth rate by a statistically significant 10%.[2,3] The second team arrived at the same conclusion, in an intention-to-treat analysis, that allogeneic leukocyte immunotherapy significantly improved the live birth rate.[2,4] The effect of maternal age and number of previous abortions that impact on probability of a successful next pregnancy were taken into account.[2]

As for the rationale behind paternal leukocyte immunization, a 2001 article[5] in Human Reproduction Update[5] explained the current knowledge of mechanisms of spontaneous abortion, and mechanisms whereby administration of mononuclear leukocytes bearing paternal antigens can counter loss. We know more now about how allogeneic leukocytes work. However, our understanding of the mechanism(s) by which a treatment may work has no bearing on whether or not it does work.[1] It follows that the empirical data from clinical trials is crucial. Commonly, these form the basis for a systematic review, as exemplified by the Cochrane Database. A recent updated review by Porter et al[6] concluded that none of the proposed immunological interventions for recurrent pregnancy loss were effective. If one is unfamiliar with the flaws and pitfalls of a systematic review (as described by Christiansen et al[7]) and is influenced by publication in a respected venue, one might be persuaded to accept the negative point of view. However, the tenets of evidence-based medicine treat authority with justifiable suspicion, and there is an established tradition from Galileo and Luther to the effect that we can find the truth ourselves if we have access to the data and have a knack for the critical thinking required.[8] Therefore, the paper in Human Reproduction Update[5] carefully evaluated the biological factors in the design and outcome of individual clinical trials.

Table 12a.1 compares the meta-analysis of paternal leukocyte immunotherapy from the recent Cochrane Database review with my own updated analysis, also using the Peto method. The data utilizing only published information (without having the raw data describing the individual patients) are shown in italics. For non-italicized authors, I have

Table 12a.1 Two meta-analyses of paternal leukocyte immunotherapy (LIT) for recurrent unexplained recurrent miscarriages (Peto method)

Study	Scott analysis (2006)			Clark analysis (2006)		
	LIT	Placebo	OR	LIT	Placebo	OR
Mowbray (London)	23/37	14/30	2.33	25/37	14/30	2.33
Cauchi (Melbourne)	13/20	16/22	0.70	13/20	16/22	0.70
Ho (Taiwan)	33/42	32/49	1.90	33/42	32/49	1.90
Gatenby (Newtown)	13/19	12/20	1.43	13/19	12/20	1.43
Christiansen (Aarlborg)	4/8	16/28	0.75	4/8	15/29	0.94
Daya (Hamilton)				5/10	1/6	3.75
Kilpatrick (Edinburgh)	8/12	6/10	1.32	8/12	6/10	1.32
Reznikoff (Paris)	17/26	14/26	1.60	17/26	14/26	1.60
Illeni (Milan)	10/16[c]	11/14[c]	**0.48**[c]	10/22	11/22	0.84
Stray Pedersen (Oslo)	*24/33*	*22/31*	*1.09*	*24/33*	*22/31*	*1.09*
Scott (Utah)	*6/10*	*5/12*	*2.01*	*6/10*	*5/12*	*2.01*
Ober (Chicago)	*31/68*	*41/63*	*0.46*	*31/68*	*41/63*	*0.46*
Pandey (Minnesota)	*21/25*[c]	*6/20*[c]	**9.03**[c]	*21/32*	*6/47*	*10.17*
Total patients	210/326	196/331		210/339	195/367	
OR and 95% CI		1.27 (0.92–1.74)[a]			1.41 (1.04–1.92)[b]	
Heterogeneity		$\chi^2 = 24.58, p < 0.01$			$\chi^2 = 32.24, p < 0.01$	

OR, odds ratio; CI, confidence interval.

[a]As the 95% CI includes 1.0, an OR of 1.27 *is not* statistically different from 1.0 at $2p \leq 0.05$.

[b]OR *is* significantly different from 1.0 at $2p \leq 0.028$. As the null hypothesis was that LIT does not increase the live birth rate in those to whom it is given, $p \leq 0.014$.

[c]Figures in bold differ from intentions to treat figures in Clark's meta-analysis.

used the numbers from the intention-to-treat analysis by John Collins and Robin Roberts in the RMITG meta-analysis. In the dataset in Table 12a.1 the figures from Illeni et al have been updated, based on their subsequently published paper.[9] Two of the trials are included even though they are problematic. The trial by Illeni et al[9] included many women with a long interval between treatment and pregnancy.[4] Mowbray and Underwood[10,11] had shown that women lost protection after 3 months unless they made antipaternal antibodies, and that boosting was required in most women (who do not make antibodies) when pregnancy did occur. In the trial by Cauchi et al, a purportedly ineffective treatment dose was given and the controls had had fewer prior abortions than the treated patients.[2,12] Hence, the two groups were unmatched for the most significant prognostic factor, the number of previous miscarriages. For italicized entries, one is relying solely on published data. It was not possible to obtain the raw data from Stray Pederson or Scott et al, or from the trial by Ober et al.[13] The trial by

Pandey and Agrawal[14] has been published fairly recently, and data have not yet been requested. It can be seen that the result of my analysis differs from that in the Cochrane database, and achieves statistical significance. I used intention-to-treat data from Pandey and Agrawal as had been used for other data, whereas only the patients who achieved pregnancy in the study by Pandey and Agrawal were included in the Cochrane meta-analysis[6] as shown in Table 12a.1. Such post hoc selection can lead to misleading conclusions.

A major problem with both analyses shown in Table 12a.1 is a χ^2 value for heterogeneity that is less than 0.05. Purists say one cannot combine the data in a meta-analysis when that happens. One either has to omit the results of Ober et al[13] or those of Pandey and Agrawal.[14] There are many problems concerning the trial of Ober et al[13] that strongly suggest that it should be excluded from the meta-analysis. Scott was involved in the trial by Ober et al.[13] His own data should not have been included in the Cochrane database meta-analysis, in order to avoid a perception of bias.[6] Additionally, the original Ober et al[13] database has been closed to outside inspection. Hence, it has been impossible to determine if the patients were matched for the results of autoantibody tests, or if all of the patients had the testing done. This is important, because a post hoc non-intention-to-treat analysis by Ober et al[13] suggested that the abortion rate in patients who achieved pregnancy was significantly greater than those who received control treatment, although by intention-to-treat analysis, these was no significant effect on live birth rate.[13] It was known from a logistic regression analysis performed as part of the RMITG[2] study that patients with secondary recurrent abortion did not benefit from allogeneic leukocyte treatment, and those with antinuclear antibody or anticardiolipin antibody had a reduced chance of success.[2,3] Indeed, analysis of primary recurrent

miscarriage patients in randomized trials *excluding* autoantibody-positive patients showed a clear benefit of treatment, and it has been argued that patients aborting after treatment are losing karyotype abnormal embryos that die from non-immunological mechanisms[15,16] (Figure 12a.1). Other problems with the trial by Ober et al[13] have been detailed elsewhere.[1,5,17] Ober et al[13] stored the purified husband mononuclear leukocytes at 4°C overnight before use, and storage can cause loss of effectiveness due to shedding of surface CD200 molecules into the supernatant.[5,18] Whole blood was used by Unander,[19] in an uncontrolled study of recurrent spontaneous abortion patients. This study also used 2 or more units of blood (which contains more cells than used by Ober et al[13]), and 2 or more units of whole blood is sufficient to cause transfusion-related immunomodulation in humans, and CD200 molecules

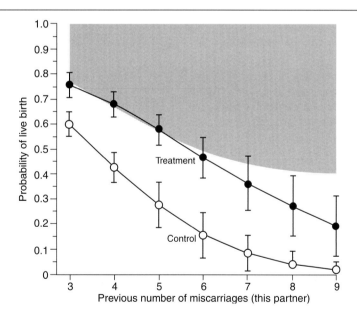

Figure 12a.1 Expected chance of a live birth with leukocyte immunotherapy. Expected chance of a livebirth with (filled circles) or without (open circles) leukocyte immunotherapy in relationship to previous number of spontaneous abortions with partner in women with no autoimmunity (antinuclear antibodies or anticardiolipin antibodies) who achieved a pregnancy. Based on seven randomized (and usually blinded) controlled trials. Total sample of 230 women: of 123 immunized, 111 became pregnant, of 135 controls, 119 became pregnant. The shaded area shows the proportion of losses in the untreated controls that were expected to fail due to karyotype abnormalities in the embryo. This is an intention-to-treat analysis that included patients who were immunized but did not achieve pregnancy. (Reproduced from Clark DA et al. Am J Reprod Immunol 1996; 35:495–8,[15] with permission from Blackwell Munksgaard.)

released into the plasma may exert suppression.[18] Pandey and Agrawal,[14] however, stored purified blood mononuclear leukocytes at 37°C and obtained a strong anti-abortive effect. Small numbers of cells were given repeatedly until the women developed antibodies, detected in a blocking assay. Such antibodies, via immunological enhancement, can prolong survival of donor cells that would otherwise be rejected.[5] We have recently shown[20] that human mononuclear leukocytes stored at 4°C lose CD200, but that storage at 37°C greatly increases CD200 expression. Thus, there are important biological explanations for the different outcomes shown in Table 12a.1 Focus on the rigor of randomization, blinding, concealment of allocation, analysis by intention to treat, etc. (i.e., high quality) misses key biological factors that impact on the result. Indeed, including biologically flawed data in a meta-analysis can swamp out significant effects. Giving penicillin to 100 patients with fever and a sore throat will show little difference from placebo, whereas if 25 patients with such symptoms and a positive culture for a penicillin-sensitive pathogen are treated, a positive result can be obtained. Of course, if the penicillin has been stored so as to render it inactive, one should not be surprised if one's null belief is confirmed. It should be noted that when the result of the double-blinded trials in the RMITG register were compared with unblinded and cohort-controlled trials (not included in Table 12a.1), there was actually a greater benefit of leukocyte immunotherapy in the double-blinded trials.[21] It has also been reported[22] for a variety of different types of treatments of non-fertility problems that the results of cohort-controlled trials and blinded randomized trails are not significantly different. Tender loving care (TLC) has been touted as effective for recurrent miscarriage, and the mechanisms of stress-triggered loss (which can be prevented by leukocyte immunization) are well worked out in mice; none of the human studies of TLC has had appropriate controls or has tested for non-inferiority to immunotherapy in a randomized controlled trial.

In the USA the Food and Drug Administration (FDA) has decided to regulate leukocyte immunotherapy, and requires further clinical trials to show efficacy and safety. The issue of safety was addressed in the RMITG[2] meta-analysis, and more recently in a long-term follow-up study on 2687 patients immunized in Germany.[23] In both series, the incidence of side effects was minimal. However, the FDA does not accept trial data not performed on US soil. There have been some attempts to start a new US multicenter trial, but there have been a number of political roadblocks. The cost of the study by Ober et al[13] (estimated as $US2.2. million) has reduced National Institutes of Health (NIH) funding for basic science research grants, and, given current low NIH funding rates, the prospect of mounting another large multicenter trial is vanishingly small. In my opinion, there are sufficient data to argue that paternal leukocyte immunotherapy should be offered to selected subgroups of patients: primary recurrent spontaneous abortion, no evidence of autoimmunity, and with karyotyping of any miscarriages to be sure that only karyotypically normal embryos are being lost. By 'spontaneous recurrent miscarriage', I refer to patients whose loss process (as detected by serial β human chorionic gonadotropin (β-hCG) values) does not begin before 6 weeks of gestation.[10] Losses at earlier time points raise the specter of autoimmune problems, where different treatments, (e.g., intravenous immunoglobulin, IVIG) merit consideration.[5]

The Cochrane review[6] also concludes that IVIG is ineffective, but again patient selection (i.e., heterogeneity), timing of treatment, and choice of IVIG product impact on the outcome – all important factors that render the Cochrane analysis suspect.[24] IVIG, like leukocyte immunotherapy, appears to include a CD200-dependent activity that results in suppression of natural killer (NK) cells.[18] Elevated blood NK-cell activity (even when in the upper end of the so-called 'normal' range) is known to be a predictor of subsequent miscarriage[25,26] and elevated levels may reflect an abnormal response to stress in primary recurrent miscarriage patients.[26] Furthermore, peripheral blood NK cells include a heterogeneous group of distinct types of cells. Elevation of the NKT subset of NK cells has been reported to bias the local cytokine environment towards a pro-abortive T-helper (Th1) pattern.[27]

Some authors have focused on the problem of validity of the 'blocking antibody' theory as a basis for disbelieving that paternal leukocyte immunotherapy can work.[1] It has been established that antibodies can enhance the survival of grafts of allogeneic cells by 'immunological enhancement', but Mowbray[10] showed that an antibody response was *not required* for an anti-abortion effect – only for prolonged protection after paternal leukocyte immunotherapy. As previously mentioned, immunological enhancement of survival of paternal cells bearing CD200 could explain Mowbray's observation.[1,5] CD200 can have a variety of effects, including stimulation of development of regulatory T cells of the type being recently proposed to play a role in pregnancy success in mice and humans.[28] Immunization with allogeneic leukocytes can stimulate the development of regulatory T cells.[29] Antibodies are not required for these processes. A full understanding of the mechanism of action of paternal leukocytes and the underlying abortive processes that may be antagonized[5] may improve patient selection and methods of treatment – but this is not a prerequisite for the demonstration of efficacy based on the existing *evidence*.

Tissue therapies such as paternal leukocytes and IVIG may be replaced in the future by treatment with cytokines such as granulocyte–macrophage colony-stimulating factor (GM-CSF) and transforming growth factor β (TGF-β).[24,30,31] However, these must be tested in randomized controlled trials that pay proper attention to the biological as well as the methodological factors. Until then, it remains reasonable for cognoscenti to offer paternal leukocyte therapy to *appropriately selected patients*.

REFERENCES

1. Clark DA. Shall we properly re-examine the status of allogeneic therapy for recurrent early pregnancy failure? Am J Reprod Immunol 2004; 51:7–15.
2. Recurrent Miscarriage Immunotherapy Trialists Group. Worldwide collaborative observational study and meta-analysis on allogeneic leukocyte immunotherapy for recurrent spontaneous abortion. Am J Reprod Immunol 1994; 32:55–72.
3. Collins JA, Roberts RM. Reports of independent analyses of data from the worldwide prospective collaborative study on immunotherapy for recurrent unexplained abortion: Immunotherapy for recurrent spontaneous abortion: Analysis 1. Am J Reprod Immunol 1994; 32:275–80.
4. Scott JR. Immunotherapy for recurrent spontaneous abortion: Analysis 2. Am J Reprod Immunol 1994; 32:279–80.
5. Clark DA, Coulam CB, Daya S, et al. Unexplained sporadic and recurrent miscarriage in the new millennium: A critical analysis of immune mechanisms and treatment. Hum Reprod Update 2001; 7:501–11.
6. Porter TF, LaCoursiere Y, Scott JR. Immunotherapy for recurrent miscarriage. Cochrane Database Syst Rev 2006; (2):CD000112.
7. Christiansen OB, Nybo Andersen AM, Bosch E, et al. Evidence-based investigations and treatments of recurrent pregnancy loss. Fertil Steril 2005; 83:821–39.
8. Vamvakas EC, Blajchman MA, eds. Immunomodulatory Effects of Blood Transfusion. Bethesda, MD: AAAB Press, 1999.
9. Illeni MT, Marelli G, Parazzini F, et al. Immunotherapy and recurrent abortion: a randomized clinical trial. Hum Reprod 1994; 9:1247–9.
10. Mowbray JF. Immunology of early pregnancy. Hum Reprod 1988; 3:79–82.
11. Mowbray JF, Underwood JL. Effect of paternal lymphocyte immunization on birthweight and pregnancy outcome. In: Chaouat G, Mowbray JF, eds. Cellular and Molecular Biology of the Materno–Fetal Relationship. Paris: INSERM/John Libby Eurotext, Colloque 212, 1991:295–302.
12. Clark DA, Daya S. Trials and tribulations in the treatment of recurrent spontaneous abortion. Am J Reprod Immunol 1991; 25:18–24.
13. Ober C, Karrison T, Odem RR, et al. Mononuclear-cell immunization in prevention of recurrent miscarriages: a randomized trial. Lancet 1999; 354:365–9.
14. Pandey MJ, Agrawal S. Induction of MLR-Bf and protection of fetal loss: a current double blind randomized trial of paternal lymphocyte immunization for women with recurrent spontaneous abortion. Int Immunopharmacol 2004; 4:289–98.
15. Daya S, Gunby J, and the Recurrent Miscarriage Immunotherapy Trialists Group. The effectiveness of allogeneic leukocyte immunization in unexplained primary recurrent spontaneous abortion. Am J Reprod Immunol 1994; 32:294–303.
16. Clark DA, Daya S, Coulam CB, et al. Implications of abnormal human trophoblast karyotype of the evidence-based approach to the understanding, investigation, and treatment of recurrent spontaneous abortion. Am J Reprod Immunol 1996; 35:495–8.
17. Carp HJA. Immunization with refrigerated paternal cells did not prevent recurrent miscarriage. Evidence Based Obstet Gynecol 2000; 2:49.
18. Clark DA, Chaouat G. Loss of surface CD200 on stored allogeneic leukocytes may impair anti-abortive effect in vivo. Am J Reprod Immunol 2004; 53:13–20.
19. Unander M. In: Beard RW, Sharp, F eds. Early Pregnancy Loss: Mechanisms and Treatment. London: RCOG/Ashton-under-Lyne, UK: Peacock Press, 1988: 400–3.
20. Clark DA, Banwatt D. Altered expression of cell surface CD200 tolerance-signaling molecule on human PBL stored at 4°C or 37°C correlates with reduced or increased efficacy in controlled trials of treatment of recurrent spontaneous abortion. Am J Reprod Immunol 2006; 55:392–3.
21. Clark DA, Gunby J, Daya S. The use of allogeneic leukocytes or IVIg G for the treatment of patients with recurrent spontaneous abortion. Transfus Med Rev 1997; 11:65–94.
22. Benson K, Hartz AJ. A comparison of observational studies and randomized controlled trials. N Engl J Med 2000; 342:1878–86.
23. Kling C, Steinmann J, Westphal E, et al. Adverse effects of intradermal allogeneic lymphocyte immunotherapy: acute reactions and role of autoimmunity. Hum Reprod 2006; 21:429–35.
24. Clark DA, Coulam CB, Stricker RB. Is intravenous immunoglobulins (IVIG) efficacious in early pregnancy failure? A critical review and

meta-analysis for patients who fail in vitro fertilization and embryo transfer (IVF). J Assist Reprod Genet 2006; 23:1–13.

25. Aoki K, Kajijura S, Matsumoto Y, et al. Preconceptional natural-killer-cell activity as a predictor of miscarriage. Lancet 1995;345:1340–2.

26. Shakhar K, Rosenne E, Lowenthan R, et al. High NK cell activity in recurrent miscarriage: what are we really measuring? Hum Reprod 2006; 21:2421–5.

27. Tsuda H, Sakai M, Michimata T, et al. Characterization of NKT cells in human peripheral blood and decidual lymphocytes. Am J Reprod Immunol 2001; 45:295–302.

28. Sasaki Y, Sasaki M, Miyazaki S. Decidual and peripheral blood CD4+CD25+ regulatory T cells in early pregnancy subjects and spontaneous abortion cases. Mol Hum Reprod 2004; 10:347–53.

29. Kitade H, Kawai M, Rutgeerts O, et al. Early presence of regulatory cells in transplanted rats rendered tolerant by donor-specific blood transfusion. J Immunol 2005; 175:4963–70.

30. Scarpellini F, Grasso JA, Sbracia M, et al. GM-CSF treatment of women with habitual abortion showing low expression of IL-10 in secretory endometria. Am J Reprod Immunol 2005; 53:307–8.

31. Clark DA, Fernandes J, Banwatt D. Prevention of abortion in the CBA ×DBA/2 model by intravaginal TGF-β is associated with local recruitment of predominantly CD8+ Foxp3+ T cells to the genital tract. Am J Reprod Immunol 2006; 55:392.

DEBATE

12b. Should IVIG treatment be used in RPL? – For

Carolyn B Coulam

INTRODUCTION

Recurrent pregnancy loss (RPL) is a significant clinical problem for which there is no known treatment. It includes recurrent spontaneous abortion and recurrent occult preclinical pregnancy or losses. The reason for this lack of effective treatment involves the multiple causes of RPL, in that one treatment will not treat all causes. Thus, the key to successful treatment is to determine the cause of the RPL. If the cause can be modulated by intravenous immunoglobulin (IVIG), then treatment with IVIG will be effective. This chapter will discuss the causes of recurrent pregnancy loss, how to identify those individuals most likely to respond to treatment with IVIG, and published success rates of IVIG therapy.

CAUSES OF RECURRENT SPONTANEOUS ABORTIONS

There are two major reasons for RPL. One is that there is something wrong with the pregnancy itself, such as a chromosomal abnormality that prohibits the pregnancy from implanting or growing properly. The other reason is a problem in the maternal environment in which the pregnancy grows that does not allow an otherwise-normal embryo to implant or grow properly. However, if fetal chromosomal aberrations explained all of recurrent miscarriage, the probability of three or more miscarriages in a row resulting from (accidents) would account for 5% or less of the observed incidence of losses.[1]

Maternal causes of pregnancy loss have been classified as anatomical, hormonal, immunological, and thrombophilic.

Immunological mechanisms have recently been proposed as a major cause of RPL associated with the loss of chromosomally normal pregnancies. Forty-five percent of miscarriages and 95% of late pregnancy losses from women experiencing RPL are chromosomally normal. Literature is developing that suggests a role of the immune system in the majority of these losses.[1–3] The end-result of the immunological processes that leads to loss of the pregnancy involves interference with the blood supply to the pregnancy. Thrombophilias also lead to vasculopathy of the vessels in and around the placenta and to secondary thrombosis, leading to inadequate perfusion of the intervillous space.[4] About 30% of obstetric complications, including RPL, are associated with inherited thrombophilia.[5,6] An immune trigger may combine with an underlying thrombophilic tendency that has been otherwise non-pathogenic to cause pregnancy loss.

HOW TO IDENTIFY THOSE INDIVIDUALS MOST LIKELY TO RESPOND TO TREATMENT WITH IVIG

Of all of the causes of RPL discussed above, the ones that would be expected to respond to IVIG treatment would be the etiologies that involve a mechanism that can be modulated by IVIG. The mechanisms by which IVIG is believed to enhance live birth rates include:[7]

- IVIG decreases killing activity of natural killer (NK) cells.
- IVIG increases the activity of suppressor T cells.
- IVIG suppresses B-cell production of autoantibody.
- IVIG contains antibodies to antibodies or anti-idiotypic antibodies.
- IVIG act on Fc receptors, including binding of complement by the Fc component of immunoglobulin G (IgG).

Based upon these mechanisms, IVIG would be expected to enhance live birth rates in individuals who had elevated circulating NK cells or elevated NK cytotoxicity, activated T-cell activity, excess of proinflammatory T-helper 1 (Th1)-type cytokines, elevated production of autoantibodies that can cause endothelial damage and clotting, and increased activation of complement. Indeed, all of these findings have been reported among women experiencing RPL.[8–14] Proinflammatory cytokines at the maternal–fetal surface can cause clotting of the placental vessels and subsequent pregnancy loss. One source of these cytokines is the NK cell. Biopsies of the lining of the uterus from women experiencing RPL reveal an increase in activated NK cells.[15] Peripheral blood NK cells are also elevated in women with RPL compared with women without a history of pregnancy loss.[16] Measurement of NK cells in peripheral blood of women with a history of RPL and a repeated failing pregnancy has shown a significant elevation associated with loss of a normal karyotypic pregnancy and a normal level associated with loss of embryos that are karyotypically abnormal.[17,18] Furthermore, increased NK-cell activity in the blood of non-pregnant women is predictive of recurrence of pregnancy loss.[9] T cells with a CD8+ marker are required for protection against NK cytokine-dependent miscarriage.[19] IVIG has been shown to decrease NK killing activity and enhance CD8+ cell activity. Both of these events are necessary for pregnancy to be successful.

IVIG would not be expected to be effective in enhancing live birth rates in women who had chromosomally abnormal pregnancies or anatomical, hormonal, or thrombotic risk factors contributing to their losses. Therefore, to select the person most likely to respond to IVIG treatment would require documentation of an immunological risk factor and the absence of non-immunological risk factors. An example of testing included in evaluation for RPL would include:

- chromosome analysis of previous pregnancy losses or both partners
- hysterosonogram, hysterosalpingogram, or hysteroscopy
- blood drawn for antiphospholipid antibodies (aPL), antinuclear antibodies (ANA), antithyroid antibodies (ATA), lupus-like anticoagulant (LA), reproductive immunophenotype, NK activation assay, and tests for embryotoxins (embryotoxicity assay), including Th1 cytokines.
- thrombophilia panel.

SUCCESS RATES OF IVIG THERAPY

Originally, IVIG therapy was used to treat women with postimplantation pregnancy losses who had not been successful in pregnancies previously treated with aspirin and prednisone or heparin. The rationale for the use of IVIG in the original studies was the suppression of LA in a woman being treated for severe thrombocytopenia. IVIG was often given with prednisone or heparin plus aspirin. More recently, IVIG therapy alone has been used to successfully treat women with aPL as well as women who become refractory to conventional autoimmune treatment with heparin or prednisone and aspirin.[20] IVIG has been reported to successfully treat women with elevated circulating levels of NK cells, NK-cell killing activity, and embryotoxins, with live birth rates between 70% and 80%.[21]

IVIG has also been used to treat women with unexplained RPL. Ten controlled trials of IVIG for treatment of RPL have been published.[21–30] Four of these reported significant enhancement in the live birth rate with IVIG treatment and six were unable to show benefit of treatment. The number of patients participating in each trial, the time of first IVIG administration (pre- or postconception), whether the patients were selected for treatment with IVIG based on obstetric history alone or obstetric history and immunological test results, and whether the trial showed benefit or no benefit from treatment are summarized in Table 12b.1. Five trials gave IVIG before conception, and four of these five showed significant benefit in enhancing live birth rates, whereas five trials delayed treatment until pregnancy was established, and of these none demonstrated benefit of treatment ($p = 0.04$, Fisher's exact test). Among the trials showing benefit of treatment with IVIG, three out of four used immune test results to select patients for IVIG treatment, and among trials showing no benefit from treatment, none of six selected patients for treatment using immune testing ($p = 0.03$). By waiting until 5–8 weeks of pregnancy to begin treatment, women with pathology occurring earlier would have been excluded and those pregnancies destined to succeed would be included, leading to selection bias. Indeed, a negative correlation with delay in treatment is significant. Only one study took into account the pregnancies lost as a result of chromosomal abnormalities.[23] Approximately 60% of the pregnancies lost in the clinical trial would be expected to have chromosomal abnormalities that would not be corrected by IVIG. It has also recently

been shown that some brands of IVIG can be as much as eight times more potent in suppressing NK cells than others (that were used in 'negative' trials).[31] Indeed, IVIG can increase the success rate in in vitro fertilization failure patients based on meta-analysis of controlled clinical trials, provided treatment is given prior to conception/embryo transfer, and a value for immunological testing is suggested by higher rates of efficacy in patients selected for treatment using these tests.[31] One would not expect IVIG to benefit patients lacking a condition that IVIG could correct, especially if given after the process causing the pregnancy loss had occurred or if the IVIG lacked the necessary activity. Pooling flawed randomized clinical trials with adequate randomized clinical trial in a meta-analysis (such as the Cochrane data[32]) would be expected to block detection of a beneficial effect for patients.

CONCLUSION

IVIG is effective treatment for women experiencing recurrent pregnancy loss if the patients treated actually have a condition that IVIG is expected to correct and if the IVIG is given in a manner that would reasonably be expected to correct the underlying pathophysiology.

Table 12b.1 Classification of outcome of controlled trials of IVIG in RPL

Trial	N	IVIG started	Selection	Outcome benefit ($p<0.05$)
Coulam and Goodman et al [21]	63	Preconception	Immunological testing	Yes
Coulam et al[23]	95	Preconception	Obstetric history	Yes
Kiprov et al[26]	35	Preconception	Immunological testing	Yes
Stricker et al[27]	47	Preconception	Immunological testing	Yes
Stevenson et al[25]	39	Preconception	Obstetric history	No
Mueller-Eckhart et al[22]	64	Postconception	Obstetric history	No
Christiansen et al[24]	34	Postconception	Obstetric history	No
Christiansen et al[28]	58	Postconception	Obstetric history	No
Perino et al[29]	46	Postconception	Obstetric history	No
Jablonowska et al[30]	41	Postconception	Obstetric history	No

REFERENCES

1. Clark DA. Is there any evidence for immunologically mediated or immunologic modifiable early pregnancy failure? J Assist Reprod Genet 2003; 20:62–71.

2. Clark DA, Lea RG, Podor T, et al. Cytokines determining the success or failure of pregnancy. Ann NY Acad Sci 1991; 626:524–36.

3. Raghupathy R. Th1 type immunity is incompatible with successful pregnancy. Immunol Today 1997; 18:478–82.

4. Many A, Schrieber L Rosner S, et al. Pathologic features of the placenta in women with severe pregnancy complications and thrombophilia. Obstet Gynecol 2001; 98:1041–4.

5. Hiller E, Pihusch R. Thrombophilia caused by congenital disorders of blood coagulation. Semin Thromb Hemost 1998; 116:26–32.

6. Coulam CB, Jeyendran RS, Fishel LA, et al. Multiple thrombophilic gene mutations rather than specific gene mutations are risk factors for recurrent miscarriage. Am J Reprod Immunol 2006; 55:360–8.

7. Sewell WAC, Jolles S. Immunomodulatory action of intravenous immunoglobulins. Immunology 2002; 107:387–93.

8. Coulam CB, Roussev RG. Correlation of NK cell activation and inhibition markers with NK cytotoxicity among women experiencing immunological implantation failure after in vitro fertilization and embryo transfer. J Assist Reprod Genet 2003; 20:58–62.

9. Aoki K, Kajijura S, Matsumoto Y, et al. Preconceptional natural killer cell activity as a predictor of miscarriage. Lancet 1995; 135:1340–2.

10. Yamada H, Morikawa M, Kato EH, et al. Preconceptional natural killer cell activity and percentage as predictors of biochemical pregnancy and spontaneous abortion with a normal karyotype. Am J Reprod Immunol 2003; 50:351–4.

11. Ruiz JE, Kwak JY, Baum L, et al. Intravenous immunoglobulins inhibits natural killer activity in vivo in women with recurrent spontaneous abortion. Am J Reprod Immunol 1996; 35:370–5.

12. Kwak JY, Kwak FM, Ainbinder SW, et al. Elevated peripheral blood natural killer cells are effectively downregulated by immunoglobulin G infusion in women with recurrent spontaneous abortions. Am J Reprod Immunol 1996; 35:363–9.

13. Ruiz JE, Kwak JY, Baum L, et al. Effects of intravenous immunoglobulin G on natural killer cell cytotoxicity in vitro in women with recurrent spontaneous abortion. J Reprod Immunol 1996; 31:125–41.

14. Graphou O, Chioti A, Pantazi A, et al. Effect of intravenous immunoglobulins treatment on the Th1/Th2 balance in women with recurrent spontaneous abortions. Am J Reprod Immunol 2003; 49:21–9.

15. Lachapelle MH, Miron P, Hemmings R, et al. Endometrial T, B, and NK cells in patients with recurrent spontaneous abortion. J Immunol 1996; 158:4886–91.

16. Yamada H, Morikawa M, Kato EH, et al. Preconceptional natural killer cell activity and percentage as predictors of biochemical pregnancy and spontaneous abortion with a normal karyotype. Am J Reprod Immunol 2003; 50:351–4.

17. Coulam CB, Stephenson M, Stern JJ, Clark DA. Immunotherapy for recurrent pregnancy loss: analysis of results from clinical trials. Am J Reprod Immunol 1996; 35:352–9.

18. Clark DA, Daya S, Coulam CB, et al. Implications of abnormal human trophoblast karyotype for the evidence-based approach to the understanding, investigation, and treatment of recurrent spontaneous abortion. Am J Reprod Immunol 1996; 35:495–8.

19. Coulam CB, Roussev RG. Increasing circulating T-cell activation markers are linked to subsequent implantation failure after transfer of in vitro fertilized embryos. Am J Reprod Immunol 2003; 50:340–5.

20. Mac Lachlan NA, Letsky E, De Sweit M. The use of intravenous immunoglobulin therapy in the management of antiphospholipid antibody associated pregnancies. Clin Exp Rheumatol 1990; 8:221–4.

21. Coulam CB, Goodman C. Increased pregnancy rates after IVF/ET with intravenous immunoglobulin treatment in women with elevated circulating CD56+ cells. Early Pregnancy Biol Med 2000; 4:90–8.

22. Mueller-Eckhart G, Mallmann P, Neppert J, et al. Immunogenetic and serological investigations of nonpregnancy and pregnant women with a history of recurrent spontaneous abortion. German RSA/IVIG Trialist Group. J Reprod Immunol 1994; 27:95–109.

23. Coulam CB, Krysa LW, Stern JJ, et al. Intravenous immunoglobulin for treatment of recurrent pregnancy loss. Am J Reprod Immunol 1995; 34:333–7.

24. Christiansen OB, Pedersen B, Rosgaard A, et al. A randomized, double-blind, placebo controlled trial of intravenous immunoglobulin in the prevention of recurrent miscarriage: evidence for a therapeutic effect in women with secondary recurrent miscarriage. Hum Reprod 2002; 17:809–16.

25. Stephenson MD, Dreher K, Houlihan E, et al. Prevention of unexplained recurrent spontaneous abortion using intravenous immunoglobulin: a prospective, randomized, double-blinded, placebo-controlled trial. Am J Reprod Immunol 1998; 39:82–8.

26. Kiprov DD, Nachtigall RD, Weaver RC, et al. The use of intravenous immunoglobulin in recurrent pregnancy loss associated with combined alloimmune and autoimmune abnormalities. Am J Reprod Immunol 1996; 36:228–34.

27. Stricker RB, Steinleitner A, Bookoff CN, et al. Successful treatment of immunological abortion with low-dose intravenous immunoglobulin. Fertil Steril 2000; 73:536–40.

28. Christiansen OB, Mathiesen O, Husth M, et al. Placebo-controlled trial of treatment of unexplained secondary recurrent spontaneous abortions and recurrent late spontaneous abortions with i.v. immunoglobulin. Hum Reprod 1995; 10:2690–5.

29. Perino A, Vassiliadis A, Vucetich A, et al. Short-term therapy for recurrent abortion using intravenous immunoglobulins: results of a double-blind placebo-controlled Italian study. Hum Reprod 1997; 12:2388–92.

30. Jablonowska B, Selbing A, Palfi M, et al. Prevention of recurrent spontaneous abortion by intravenous immunoglobulin: a double-blind placebo-controlled study. Hum Reprod 1999; 14:838–41.

31. Clark DA, Coulam CB, Stricker RB. Is intravenous immunoglobulins (IVIG) efficacious in early pregnancy failure? A critical review and meta-analysis for patients who fail in vitro fertilization and embryo transfer (IVF). J Assist Reprod Genet 2006; 23:1–13.

32. Porter TF, LaCoursiere Y, Scott JR. Immunotherapy for recurrent miscarriage. Cochrane Database Syst Rev. 2006; (2):CD000112.

DEBATE

12c. Should immunotherapy be used in RPL? – Against

Raj Rai

INTRODUCTION

The investigation and treatment of women with recurrent pregnancy loss (RPL) has historically been based on anecdotal evidence, personal bias of physicians, and the results of small uncontrolled studies.[1] This has led to the situation where women have been subjected to treatments of no proven benefit, some of which have subsequently been demonstrated to be harmful.[2] This is unacceptable. Indeed, in the current climate in which patient demands and expectations for a 'treatment/cure' of their reproductive failure are ever-increasing, it is incumbent upon clinicians to reject previous practice and embrace an evidence-based approach to the management of RPL.

The concept of immune dysfunction as a basis for miscarriage is an attractive one. However, while pregnancy has traditionally been viewed as a battle between the semiallogenic fetus and the mother, from an evolutionary viewpoint this is not advantageous.[3] Regardless, immunotherapy has been introduced into clinical practice as a treatment for RPL based on the hypotheses that either alloimunity or autoimmunity is responsible for pregnancy failure. In order to critically evaluate the use of paternal leukocyte immunization (active immunization) and intravenous immunoglobulin (IVIG, passive immunization) as treatments for RPL, it is necessary to examine the rationale for their use.

RATIONALE (OR NOT) FOR IMMUNOTHERAPY

PATERNAL WHITE CELL IMMUNIZATION

One concept of an alloimmune basis for RPL is based on an increased sharing of human leukocyte antigens (HLA) between both partners that prevents the maternal production of a 'blocking' antibody that protects the fetus against immunological attack.[4] Women with successful pregnancies produce this 'blocking' antibody and those whose pregnancy ends in miscarriage do not. Leukocyte immunization has been reported to induce production of the 'blocking' antibody.[5] However, the 'blocking antibody' hypothesis has never been validated, and an increased sharing of HLA class I alleles between partners has been refuted in a recent meta-analysis.[6] Further, (a) production of a 'blocking' antibody is usually not evident until after 28 weeks' gestation and may disappear between pregnancies;[7] (b) miscarriage occurs despite the presence of 'blocking' antibody;[8,9] and (c) women who exhibit no production of 'blocking' antibodies do experience successful pregnancies.

IVIG

Current concepts on the etiology of RPL focus on autoimmune-mediated pregnancy loss (e.g., antiphospholipid syndrome, APS), natural killer (NK) cells, and a disordered cytokine balance at the fetomaternal interface. IVIG has a number of immunomodulatory effects on cytokine production, antigen neutralization, Fc receptor blockade, alteration in the distribution and function of T-cell subsets, antibodies, and autoantigens that may potentially ameliorate a dysregulated immune response causal of pregnancy loss. However, the role of autoantibodies, apart from antiphospholipid antibodies (aPL), in the pathogenesis of RPL is unproven.[2] The relationship between peripheral blood NK (PBNK) cells and reproductive failure is one of the most controversial fields in reproductive immunology. This relationship has been examined in several small observational studies.[10–16] Although the underlying etiology of reproductive failure among women in individual studies may well be different, the reports are consistent in associating enhanced NK-cell activity with subsequent failure to conceive or miscarriage. Hence, amid much publicity, peripheral blood NK-cell testing is being promoted as a useful diagnostic test to guide the initiation of a variety of immunosuppressive therapies among patients with either RPL or infertility.

There are fundamental flaws in the methodologies used in the published studies. The level and activation of NK cells are dependent on other variables, such as whether whole blood or fractionated mononuclear cells are used in the assay, the time of day a sample is taken, whether any physical exercise has been performed, the parity of the patient, and whether the samples have been previously frozen.[17–21] Different NK-cell assays have also been employed, and results may vary depending on whether the chromium-51 (^{51}Cr)-release cytotoxicity assay is used or CD69 expression is assayed. Importantly, it is not known which in vitro assay most accurately reflects in vivo function, and indeed what biological relevance such activity has. Furthermore, it is unclear what an abnormal NK-cell number is. While traditionally a peripheral NK-cell level greater than 12% of all lymphocytes has been regarded as the cut-off between a raised and a normal level,[22] this figure is well within the normal range (up to 29%) published by others.[23] Hence individuals with entirely normal results are being labelled as having raised NK-cell numbers.

A recent fascinating study has cast further doubt on the validity of PBNK cell testing in women with RPL.[24] The authors reported that immediately after insertion of an intravenous cannula for blood withdrawal, women with RPL show an increased proportion of NK cells within lymphocytes, elevated blood NK-cell concentrations, and augmented NK activity per milliliter of blood compared with control women who have no known fertility problems. However, these differences disappear after 20 minutes, when blood is drawn again from the same cannula. The authors concluded that the elevated NK indices previously observed in women with RPL are due to a transient increase in NK-cell numbers, rather than a chronic state.

EFFICACY OF IMMUNOTHERAPY

It is important when evaluating the effect of any intervention proposed as a treatment for RPL to be cognisant of the fact that the two most important determinants of the outcome of a particular pregnancy are the mother's age and the number of miscarriages she has previously experienced. The rate of sporadic fetal aneuploidy is in the region of 50% among women between 40 and 44 years of age, rising to 75% among those older than 45 years. On the basis of a 15% clinical miscarriage rate, 35% of women with three consecutive miscarriages will have done so purely by chance alone. Such women have an excellent chance of a future successful pregnancy. Among those less than 39 years, a live birth rate of 65–70% with supportive care alone can be expected.[25] It is against this high spontaneous resolution rate that the efficacy of any putative treatment for RPL has to be judged.

PATERNAL WHITE CELL IMMUNIZATION

A number of studies have examined the efficacy of paternal leukocyte immunization as a treatment for RPL. These studies, which have used differing methodologies, entry criteria, and analyses, have reported conflicting results. The largest study (183 women), which was a double-blinded, multicenter, randomized clinical trial, reported that, on an intention-to-treat basis, the success rate was 36% in the treatment group versus 48% in the control group (odds ratio (OR) 0.60; 95% confidence interval (CI) 0.33–1.12).[26] If analysis was restricted to only those who conceived, the corresponding success rates were 46% with immunization but 65% with placebo saline injections (OR 0.45; 95% CI 0.22–0.91), suggesting that immunization may *increase* the rate of clinically recognized pregnancy loss. Partly on the basis of this large study and the lack of scientific validity underlying paternal white cell immunization, the US Food and Drug Administration (FDA) issued guidance in 2002 highlighting the lack of efficacy of this treatment and reminding clinicians that it should only be offered in the context of therapeutic studies and will require Investigational New Drug Approval (http://www.fda.gov/CBER/ltr/lit013002.htm).

The conclusions of several published meta-analyses have also been conflicting. The largest and most recent – a Cochrane review published in 2006, based on 12 trials (641 women) – reported an OR of 1.23 (95% CI 0.89–1.70) among those administered paternal leukocytes compared with controls.[27] Intention-to-treat analysis did not result in a significant difference between treatment and controls (4 trials; 350 women; OR 1.35; 95% CI 0.89–2.05).

IVIG

Studies using IVIG have used different preparations, doses, starting times, frequency, and duration of administration. In addition, differing entry criteria have been used. Some studies have included those with an autoimmune disturbance only, while others have included those with 'unexplained' RPL. Hence, at present, the only reasonable basis for the assessment of the efficacy of IVIG as a treatment for RPL would be to examine the results of meta-analyses. The Cochrane review[27] reports that, irrespective of whether analysis is performed on an intention-to-treat basis (OR 1.18; 95% CI 0.72–1.93) or not (OR 0.98; 95% CI 0.61–1.58), IVIG does not improve pregnancy outcome among women with RPL.

CONCLUSION

The lack of scientific rationale for immunotherapy has not stopped its introduction into clinical practice. However, despite the limitations of meta-analyses, the use of either paternal leukocyte immunization or IVIG as a treatment for RPL has not been shown to be of benefit. The use of these immunomodulatory agents should be resisted.

REFERENCES

1. Rai R, Clifford K, Regan L. The modern preventative treatment of recurrent miscarriage. Br J Obstet Gynaecol 1996; 103:106–10.
2. Rai R, Regan L. Recurrent miscarriage. Lancet 2006; 368:601–11.
3. Parham P. NK cells and trophoblasts: partners in pregnancy. J Exp Med 2004; 200:951–5.
4. Rocklin RE, Kitzmiller JL, Carpenter CB, et al. Maternal-fetal relation. Absence of an immunologic blocking factor from the serum of women with chronic abortions. N Engl J Med 1976; 295:1209–13.
5. Takakuwa K, Kanazawa K, Takeuchi S. Production of blocking antibodies by vaccination with husband's lymphocytes in unexplained recurrent aborters: the role in successful pregnancy. Am J Reprod Immunol Microbiol 1986; 10:1–9.
6. Beydoun H, Saftlas AF. Association of human leucocyte antigen sharing with recurrent spontaneous abortions. Tissue Antigens 2005; 65:123–35.
7. Regan L, Braude PR, Hill DP. A prospective study of the incidence, time of appearance and significance of anti-paternal lymphocytotoxic antibodies in human pregnancy. Hum Reprod 1991; 6:294–8.
8. Pena RB, Cadavid AP, Botero JH, et al. The production of MLR-blocking factors after lymphocyte immunotherapy for RSA does not predict the outcome of pregnancy. Am J Reprod Immunol 1998; 39:120–4.
9. Jablonowska B, Palfi M, Ernerudh J, et al. Blocking antibodies in blood from patients with recurrent spontaneous abortion in relation to pregnancy outcome and intravenous immunoglobulin treatment. Am J Reprod Immunol 2001; 45:226–31.
10. Aoki K, Kajiura S, Matsumoto Y, et al. Preconceptional natural-killer-cell activity as a predictor of miscarriage. Lancet 1995; 345:1340–2.
11. Beer AE, Kwak JY, Ruiz JE. Immunophenotypic profiles of peripheral blood lymphocytes in women with recurrent pregnancy losses and in infertile women with multiple failed in vitro fertilization cycles. Am J Reprod Immunol 1996; 35:376–82.
12. Emmer PM, Nelen WL, Steegers EA, et al. Peripheral natural killer cytotoxicity and CD56+CD16+ cells increase during early pregnancy in women with a history of recurrent spontaneous abortion. Hum Reprod 2000; 15:1163–9.
13. Fukui A, Fujii S, Yamaguchi E, et al. Natural killer cell subpopulations and cytotoxicity for infertile patients undergoing in vitro fertilization. Am J Reprod Immunol 1999; 41:413–22.
14. Ntrivalas EI, Kwak-Kim JY, Gilman-Sachs A, et al. Status of peripheral blood natural killer cells in women with recurrent spontaneous abortions and infertility of unknown aetiology. Hum Reprod 2001; 16:855–61.

15. Putowski L, Darmochwal-Kolarz D, Rolinski J, et al. The immunological profile of infertile women after repeated IVF failure (preliminary study). Eur J Obstet Gynecol Reprod Biol 2004; 112:192–6.

16. Yamada H, Morikawa M, Kato EH, et al. Pre-conceptional natural killer cell activity and percentage as predictors of biochemical pregnancy and spontaneous abortion with normal chromosome karyotype. Am J Reprod Immunol 2003; 50:351–4.

17. Pross HF, Maroun JA. The standardization of NK cell assays for use in studies of biological response modifiers. J Immunol Meth 1984; 68:235–49.

18. Plackett TP, Boehmer ED, Faunce DE, et al. Aging and innate immune cells. J Leukoc Biol 2004; 76:291–9.

19. Reichert T, DeBruyere M, Deneys V, et al. Lymphocyte subset reference ranges in adult Caucasians. Clin Immunol Immunopathol 1991; 60:190–208.

20. Porzsolt F, Gaus W, Heimpel H. The evaluation of serial measurements of the NK cell activity in man. Immunobiology 1983; 165:475–84.

21. Strong DM, Ortaldo JR, Pandolfi F, et al. Cryopreservation of human mononuclear cells for quality control in clinical immunology. I. Correlations in recovery of K- and NK-cell functions, surface markers, and morphology. J Clin Immunol 1982; 2:214–21.

22. Beer AE, Kwak JY, Ruiz JE. Immunophenotypic profiles of peripheral blood lymphocytes in women with recurrent pregnancy losses and in infertile women with multiple failed in vitro fertilization cycles. Am J Reprod Immunol 1996; 35:376–82.

23. Eidukaite A, Siaurys A, Tamosiunas V. Differential expression of KIR/NKAT2 and CD94 molecules on decidual and peripheral blood CD56^{bright} and CD56^{dim} natural killer cell subsets. Fertil Steril 2004; 81 (Suppl 1):863–8.

24. Shakhar K, Rosenne E, Loewenthal R, et al. High NK cell activity in recurrent miscarriage: What are we really measuring? Hum Reprod 2006; 21:2421–5.

25. Clifford K, Rai R, Regan L. Future pregnancy outcome in unexplained recurrent first trimester miscarriage. Hum Reprod 1997; 12:387–9.

26. Ober C, Karrison T, Odem RR, et al. Mononuclear-cell immunisation in prevention of recurrent miscarriages: a randomised trial. Lancet 1999; 354:365–9.

27. Porter TF, LaCoursiere Y, Scott JR. Immunotherapy for recurrent miscarriage. Cochrane Database Syst Rev 2006; (2):CD000112.

13. Infections and recurrent pregnancy loss

David Alan Viniker

INTRODUCTION

Any acute severe infection can be associated with occasional pregnancy loss. The role of infection in recurrent pregnancy loss (RPL) has been unclear.[1] In recent years, there has been increasing interest in microorganisms as possible causes of pathology in previously unexplained medical conditions.[2] In this chapter, the evidence for and against infection as a cause of RPL is presented. Specific infections are discussed, and the recent developments in molecular biology are discussed as they relate to future investigation.

TUBERCULOSIS

Chronic infection, notably tuberculosis, is more commonly related to infertility, with only sporadic reports of pregnancy loss.[3,4] Saracoglu et al[3] diagnosed 72 patients with pelvic tuberculosis from 1979 to 1989. The most common presentations were infertility (47.2%), pelvic or abdominal pain (32%), and abnormal bleeding (11%). There was one case of RPL. Physical examination was normal in 32% of the patients and chest X-ray was normal in 81%. The most common site of infection was the fallopian tubes, with occlusion in 32 of the 34 patients having hysterosalpingography.

In a series of 25 cases of genital tuberculosis, 21 presented with infertility, 3 had postmenopausal bleeding, and 1 was admitted with an acute abdomen.[4] Two women subsequently conceived, but both aborted.

LISTERIOSIS

Romana et al[5] have put forward the case that latent listeriosis may cause recurrent miscarriage, as anti-listeric antibodies have been detected by direct immunofluorescence studies. Romana et al[5] investigated 309 women: 207 had a total of 334 miscarriages, 67 delivered prematurely, 75 had stillbirths, and 43 had malformed living or stillborn infants. Treatment resulted in the birth of 152 normal babies, all negative on immunofluorescence for anti-listeric antibodies. Manganiello and Yearke[6] attempted to isolate *Listeria monocytogenes* from the cervix and endometrium of patients presenting with a history of two or more fetal losses. Endometrial tissue and endocervical swabs were cultured. During a 10-year study period, none of the patients with recurrent fetal loss were found to harbor the organism in their genital tract. Hence, *L. monocytogenes* could account for occasional fetal loss, but not on a recurring basis. Manganiello and Yearke[6] concluded that routinely culturing for *L. monocytogenes* in patients with recurrent miscarriage is not warranted.

TORCH INFECTIONS

There have been conflicting opinions on the role of cytomegalovirus (CMV) in recurrent miscarriage. Szkaradkiewicz et al[7] found significantly elevated immunoglobulin G (IgG) in most of 11 women on the first day after a second consecutive trimester miscarriage. The control group were 15 women in the second trimester of a normal pregnancy. They concluded that in the majority of the studied women, reactivation of chronic CMV infection occurred. Cook et al[8] used the polymerase chain reaction (PCR) to detect CMV in gestational tissue of women with recurrent miscarriage. DNA was extracted from 25 samples of gestational tissue from 21 women with at least three unexplained spontaneous miscarriages. None of these specimens contained evidence of CMV DNA, demonstrating that CMV is not a common direct cause of recurrent miscarriage.

Screening for TORCH infections (toxoplasmosis, rubella, CMV, and herpes simplex virus (HSV)) is unhelpful in the investigation of recurrent miscarriage. While these infections can be associated with an individual pregnancy loss, they are illnesses generally contracted once and therefore should not result in RPL. The current recommendation is that TORCH screening in the investigation of RPL should be abandoned.[1]

CHLAMYDIAE

Mezinova et al[9] have reported that chlamydiae have been found in 41.7% of 163 women with habitual miscarriage in their series. The miscarriage rate was 59.1% in the presence of chlamydiae. However, all women treated for chlamydial infection went on to deliver at term. It was concluded that women with habitual miscarriage and chlamydiae should receive appropriate therapy. Endometrial, endocervical, and urethral specimens have been obtained from 16 non-pregnant women with a history of RPL.[10] Chlamydiae were isolated from the endometria of five women. No chlamydiae were isolated from the cervix or urethra of two patients with proven endometrial involvement. This study demonstrated that eradicating intrauterine chlamydial infection before pregnancy improved pregnancy outcome in women with RPL. It was suggested that asymptomatic chlamydial infection might have an adverse effect on placentation.

An association between positive chlamydia serology and RPL has been reported by Kishore et al.[11] Rhesus incompatibility and anatomical, endocrine,

and chromosome abnormalities were excluded from the study by Kishore et al.[11] Serum anti-*Chlamydia trachomatis* IgM positivity was found in 46.5% of 47 patients with RPL miscarriages, compared with 13.8% of 29 age-matched controls of normal pregnant women ($p < 0.001$). The relationship between high-titer IgG antibodies to *C. trachomatis* and recurrent miscarriage has been investigated.[12] It was found that 7 (41%) of 17 women with three miscarriages and 6 (60%) of 10 women with four miscarriages had anti-chlamydial antibodies, compared with 20 (14%) of 148 women with no miscarriages, 6 (13%) of 47 women with one miscarriage, and 4 (12%) of 33 women with two miscarriages. The incidence of three or more miscarriages was 31.8% for women with high-titer IgG, compared with 7.5% among women who were seronegative ($p < 0.001$). It was concluded that high-titer IgG to *C. trachomatis* was associated with recurrent miscarriage and it was suggested that the mechanism might involve reactivation of latent chlamydial infection, endometrial damage from previous infection, or an immune response to an epitope shared by chlamydial and fetal antigens.

In contrast, a study of 101 women with RPL did not find an association with chlamydiae.[13] Screening involved direct examination, culture, and serological testing. The culture-positive and serology-positive rates of 15% and 35% did not differ from those of other unselected populations. The time from last miscarriage or type of miscarriage was unrelated to *C. trachomatis* infection. The unselected population rates for chlamydiae in this study were noticeably higher than generally expected. Others have also failed to find an association between IgG anti-chlamydial antibodies and RPL.[14–16] Rae et al[14] looked at IgG to chlamydiae in 106 women with unexplained RPL and compared their findings with sera from a general antenatal population of 3890. Twenty-six (24.5%) women with RPL had positive serology compared with 788 (20.3%) of controls. Anti-chlamydial antibody seropositivity did not correlate with subsequent pregnancy outcome. It was concluded that there is no association between IgG antibodies to *C. trachomatis* and recurrent spontaneous abortion.

In a prospective study,[15] 70 patients with RPL attending a specialist recurrent miscarriage clinic were selected. The controls were 40 normal pregnant women and 94 asymptomatic sexually active women. There was no statistical difference in the frequencies of anti-chlamydial IgG or IgA antibodies between women with recurrent miscarriage and controls. In another study[16] of 504 patients with a history of two or more consecutive first-trimester miscarriages, the presence of IgA and IgG antibodies to *C. trachomatis* did not influence subsequent pregnancy outcome.

There does not appear to be robust evidence to support serological investigations for chlamydiae as part of the routine investigation of RPL, but direct swab tests from the cervix may be taken and positive results treated appropriately.

SYPHILIS

In some parts of Africa, the incidence of syphilis seroreactivity in pregnant women is at least 10%, and this is associated with spontaneous abortion, perinatal mortality, or a viable infant with congenital syphilis.[17] Screening for syphilis should be considered in at-risk populations.

BACTERIAL VAGINOSIS

In women of reproductive age, lactobacilli are normally the predominant bacteria in the vagina. Lactobacilli are responsible for reducing the vaginal pH by metabolizing glycogen from squamous cells to lactic acid. The resulting acidic milieu provides protection against infection. Bacterial vaginosis (BV) has become the adopted nomenclature to describe a clinical condition characterized by an overgrowth of predominantly anaerobic bacteria within the vagina and a concomitant reduction or absence of lactobacilli. BV is recognized as the most common cause of vaginal discharge. The discharge tends to be malodorous, particularly after sexual intercourse. A remarkable feature of BV is the absence of a host reaction – hence the suffix 'osis' rather than 'itis', as signs of inflammation are absent.

In gram-stained smears of vaginal fluid, BV is diagnosed when three out of four of Amsel's criteria[18] are present: namely the presence of clue cells (vaginal epithelial cells heavily coated with bacilli on wet preparation microscopy), vaginal pH>4.5; a homogenous discharge; and a strong fishy odor, which may be amplified on adding alkali to the vaginal fluid. The organisms most often associated with BV are *Gardnerella vaginalis*, *Mycoplasma hominis*, *Ureaplasma urealyticum*, *Mobiluncus* spp., *Prevotella*, *Porphyromonas*, *Bacteroides,* and *Peptostreptococcus* spp. It has been suggested that the clinical manifestations of BV depend on a synergistic interaction of a variety of microorganisms. The gram-negative organisms, including *Bacteroides,* are sensitive to metronidazole, whereas *Mycoplasma, Ureaplasma,* and *Mobiluncus* are sensitive to macrolides such as erythromycin and to the tetracyclines.

In a study by Wilson et al,[19] 749 consecutive women undergoing in vitro fertilization had a vaginal smear taken at the time of egg collection in a study comparing the prevalence of BV according to causation of infertility.[1] The smears were gram-stained and graded as normal, intermediate, or BV. The smears were normal in 63.6%, intermediate in 12.1%, and BV in 24.3%. The rates of BV were 36.4% in tubal factor, 15.6% in male factor, 33.3% in anovulation, 12.5% in endometriosis, and 18.9% in unexplained infertility. Women with tubal infertility were three times more likely to have BV than women with male factor infertility, endometriosis, or unexplained infertility. Women with anovulation were also three times more likely to have BV compared with women with endometriosis or male factor infertility, which the authors suggested supports the theory that there is a hormonal influence on vaginal flora.

The detrimental effects on pregnancy associated with BV may be due to the bacteria ascending into the uterus.[20,21] One hypothesis suggests that microorganisms, possibly those associated with BV, may surreptitiously inhabit the uterine cavity (bacteria endometrialis), where they are the culprits behind some common gynecological and obstetric enigmas.[21] Relatively little has been written about

Table 13.1 A comparison of the bacteriology of the vagina and the uterine cavity

Vagina	Uterine cavity
• Rich in microorganisms	• Relatively sterile
• High vaginal swabs: routine clinical investigation	• Samples mainly confined to research centers
• BV: diagnosis by microscopy of wet preparation or gram stain	• Wet preparations and gram stain not studied
• Culture unhelpful for BV diagnosis	• Cultures only. Specialist centers required for *Mycoplasma hominis* and *Ureaplasma urealyticum*
• Possible marker for bacteria endometrialis	• Microorganisms can be present even with negative cervical cultures
• BV: no clinical inflammation	• Microorganisms can occur with negative clinical examination

BV, bacterial vaginosis.

bacterial colonization of the endometrial cavity. Bacteriological investigations of the vagina and endometrial cavity are compared in Table 13.1. The healthy vagina is rich in microorganisms, whereas the endometrial cavity is considered to be relatively sterile. Many microorganisms colonize the vagina without necessarily being pathogenic. High vaginal swabs are frequently obtained in routine clinical practice, whereas the bacteriology of the endometrium has been studied almost entirely in research projects. The bacteriological diagnosis of BV is dependent on microscopic assessment of a wet preparation of the discharge or a gram stain rather than culture, whereas investigation of the uterine cavity has depended on culture alone. The clinical significance of the varied patterns of bacteria found in the vagina remains controversial. Our knowledge about intrauterine microorganisms is comparatively spartan and more difficult to interpret. Pathogenic microorganisms can be found in the endometrial cavity without evidence of pelvic infection being visible at laparoscopy and with negative cervical cultures.[22] The bacteriology of the endometrial cavity has been investigated[23] immediately after hysterectomy in 99 women. Nearly a quarter of all the patients in this study by Moller et al[23] harbored one or more microorganisms in the uterus, mostly *G. vaginalis*, *Enterobacter*, or *Streptococcus agalactiae*. The samples were not tested for mycoplasmas or *Mobiluncus*.

The prevalence of BV in pregnancy varies from 9% to 23%.[24] Coitus during pregnancy is not related to BV or premature delivery. Pregnant women do not commonly develop BV after 16 weeks' gestation. If present at 16 weeks, BV spontaneously remits in approximately 30–50% of those reaching term.[25,26]

PREMATURE DELIVERY

There is a substantial body of evidence indicating that BV is associated with premature delivery.[24,27–32] The association with premature delivery may have implications for miscarriage, and raise the possibility that antibiotics may reduce this complication. BV diagnosed in early pregnancy is particularly significant,[27] as the presence of BV in early pregnancy is associated with a two- to threefold increased risk of preterm labor. Women who have abnormal vaginal flora that spontaneously return to normal and who are not treated have as many abnormal outcomes as those treated with placebo, suggesting that the damage occurs in early pregnancy[28] or that the responsible microorganisms have ascended into the uterine cavity. In order to determine whether abnormal vaginal microflora are associated with premature labor, a study was conducted by McDonald et al[29] in Australia. The assessment included cultures for aerobic and anerobic bacteria, yeasts, genital mycoplasmas, and *G. vaginalis*. The results of 428 women in preterm labor were compared with those of 568 women in labour at term. Two distinct bacteriological groupings were associated with preterm labor: the BV group of organisms and a group of enteropharyngeal organisms. *G. vaginalis* was found in 12% of women in preterm labour, compared with 6% at term. The prevalence of *G. vaginalis* was even higher (17%) in women in preterm labour at less than 34 weeks' gestation. In an analysis of 12 937 women screened for BV, the odds ratio (OR) for preterm birth (<37 weeks' gestation) for asymptomatic BV-positive versus BV-negative women ranged from 1.1 to 1.6 and did not vary significantly with the gestational age at the time of screening.[30]

Vaginal fluid was collected for gram staining from 354 women admitted in preterm labour with intact membranes between 24 and 34 weeks' gestation in a prospective blinded study in Paris.[33] Normal flora were found in 254 women of the 354 women tested (72.3%). Intermediate changes were found in 76 (21.7%) and BV in 24 (6.8%). Women with normal, intermediate, and abnormal flora had 27 (10.6%), 14 (18.4%), and 6 (25.0%) births before 33 weeks, respectively. A history of spontaneous miscarriage after 14 weeks was the only risk factor associated with BV. Preterm delivery before 33 weeks was significantly associated with the flora grade ($p = 0.02$). It was concluded that the frequency of BV and its association with preterm delivery are variable and should be interpreted differently for different populations. Although an association was found between BV and delivery before 33 weeks, the authors considered the predictive value of BV to be disappointing, and the usefulness of testing for BV in women with premature labor was not demonstrated.

TREATMENT AND PREMATURE DELIVERY

EFFECT OF ANTIBIOTICS ON THE PREVALENCE OF BV

Antibiotics have been shown to affect the presence of BV. Clindamycin has been shown to be effective in eradicating the bacteria, whether used intravaginally[34] or orally.[26] Abnormal flora were found after oral clindamycin in 10% of treated patients compared with 93% of placebo patients ($p < 0.001$) in the trail conducted by Ugwumadu et al[26] involving 462 women (231 in the clindamycin group and 231 in a placebo group). Normal flora were maintained in two-thirds of women throughout pregnancy. The results of four weekly smears were compared in 135 women: 69 clindamycin-treated and 66 placebo-treated. For the clindamycin group, the prevalence of abnormal flora was 15% at 20 weeks' and 17% at 36 weeks' gestation, compared with 69% at 20 weeks' and 43% at 36 weeks' in

the placebo group. Borisov et al[34] compared the effect of intravaginal clindamycin with the effect of metronidazole in 128 pregnant women with BV. BV was eradicated in 93% of the women using intravaginal clindamycin and in 87% of the group receiving the metronidazole. Both treatments were more effective than oral ampicillin for 7 days, which had a cure rate of 62%.

Ugwumadu et al[26] concluded that as previous research had shown that spontaneous resolution of BV does not modify the risk of preterm birth, early screening and treatment should be advocated.

EFFECT OF ANTIBIOTICS IN WOMEN WITH PREVIOUS PREMATURE LABOR

The effect of antibiotics has been assessed in women at high risk of premature labor with BV. The results of two studies indicate that antibiotics may reduce the incidence of premature labor. Both metronidazole and metronidazole together with erythromycin have been assessed in double-blinded placebo-controlled trials.

In the study by Morales et al[35] women with premature labor or premature rupture of the membranes in the preceding pregnancy were screened for BV between 13 and 20 weeks' gestation. Patients with a positive screen were randomized to receive metronidazole orally or placebo. Forty-four patients received metronidazole and 36 received placebo. The metronidazole group had fewer hospital admissions for preterm labor (27% vs 78%), preterm births (18% vs 39%), low-birth-weight infants (<2500 g: 14% vs 33%), and premature rupture of the membranes (5% vs 33%).

Hauth et al[36] performed BV testing at 23 weeks in 624 pregnant women at risk of delivering prematurely. Patients were randomized on a 2:1 basis to receive treatment with erythromycin and metronidazole ($n = 426$) or placebo ($n = 190$). A second course of treatment was instituted for those women who still had BV at 28 weeks. In the antibiotic group, 110 women delivered prematurely (26%), compared with 68 women in the placebo group (36%; $p = 0.01$). The association between treatment and lower rates of prematurity was observed only among the 258 women who had BV (31% with treatment vs 49% with placebo; $p = 0.006$).

The effects of both metronidazole and clindamycin have been assessed on premature labour in randomized placebo studies and meta-analyses in low-risk patients in whom BV was an incidental finding.

McDonald et al[37] reported a trial of metronidazole in women with a heavy growth of G. vaginalis or a gram stain indicative of BV at 19 weeks in 879 women. Metronidazole was administered at 24 weeks and at 29 weeks if G. vaginalis persisted. There was no difference in overall preterm births between metronidazole and placebo groups. In a subset of 46 women with a previous preterm birth, metronidazole showed a significant reduction in spontaneous preterm birth: 2/22 (9.1%), versus 10/24 (41.7%) in placebo-treated patients. In this study, antibiotics were most effective when there was a history of previous premature labor.

In the study by Camargo et al[38] of 785 low-risk Brazilian pregnant women, 134 women with BV were treated with metronidazole, tinidazole, or secnidazole; 71 women with BV received no treatment. Premature delivery occurred in 5.5% of women without BV, in 22.5% of women with untreated BV, and in 3.7% of treated women. Perinatal complications were significantly higher in those women with untreated BV. The risk ratios were 7.5 for premature rupture of the membranes 3.4 for preterm labor 3, 6.0 for preterm birth, and 4.2 for low birthweight.

Mothers with singleton pregnancies and no history of preterm delivery in whom BV was diagnosed by gram stain at 12 weeks' gestation were randomized to receive vaginal clindamycin or placebo in the study by Kurkinen-Raty et al[39] of 101 women with BV. Of 51 women, 17 (33%) were cured after clindamycin treatment, compared with 17 out of 50 (34%) of the placebo-treated group. The failure rate of clindamycin to cure BV was particularly high in this study. The preterm birth rate was 13.7% (7/51) in the clindamycin-treated patients and 6.0%

(3/50) in the placebo group. Premature delivery occurred in 20.7% (6/29) in those in whom BV persisted, compared with 0% (0/26) where BV was successfully treated. Hence, it is not sufficient to treat BV – the bacteria must be eradicated.

Intravaginal clindamycin was also assessed by Rosenstein et al[28] Thirty-four women had normal vaginal flora at their first antenatal clinic visit, compared with 268 women who had abnormal vaginal flora. Follow-up assessed for pregnancy outcome, vaginal flora, and detection of M. hominis and U. urealyticum after treatment. There were no significantly different outcomes in pregnancy between the treated and placebo groups. Women with grade III flora responded better to clindamycin than women with grade II flora by number of abnormal outcomes ($p = 0.03$) and return to normal vaginal flora. Women whose abnormal vaginal flora had spontaneously returned to normal and who were therefore not treated had as many abnormal outcomes as those receiving placebo, suggesting that damage by abnormal bacterial species occurred early in pregnancy.

The results of the study by Lamont et al[31] do not concur with those of Kurkinen-Raty et al[39] or Rosenstein et al[28] In the randomized double-blinded study by Lamont et al,[31] 409 women with abnormal genital tract flora on gram stain at 13–20 weeks' gestation received clindamycin vaginal cream or placebo. Those who still had abnormal vaginal flora 3 weeks later received a subsequent course of the original treatment. There was a statistically significant reduction in the incidence of preterm birth in the clindamycin group (4%) compared with placebo (10%) ($p < 0.03$). It was concluded that clindamycin vaginal cream administered to women with abnormal vaginal flora before 20 weeks' gestation can decrease preterm birth by 60% and reduce the need for neonatal intensive care.

Three meta-analyses have evaluated the potential benefit of treating BV in pregnancy. That by Brocklehurst et al[40] included 1504 women. Antibiotics were highly effective in eradicating infection. The effect of treating BV resulted in a trend to fewer births before 37 weeks' gestation, which was most marked in women with a previous preterm birth.

In the meta-analysis by Guise et al[24] seven randomized controlled trials of BV treatment were included. BV treatment was found to be of no benefit for the average-risk woman. In women with previous preterm delivery, three of the studies showed a benefit of BV treatment for preterm delivery before 37 weeks. Two trials of high-risk women found an increase in preterm delivery less than 34 weeks in women who did not have BV but received BV treatment. Both meta-analyses concluded that there is no evidence in favor of screening all pregnant women for BV. For women with a history of previous preterm birth, there is support for diagnosing and treating BV early in pregnancy to prevent a proportion of these women having a further preterm birth.

However, in contrast, screening and treating BV in low-risk pregnancies produced a statistically significant reduction in premature deliveries (relative risk (RR) 0.73) in the meta-analysis by Varma and Gupta,[41] but there was no benefit in high-risk groups. It was hypothesised that premature deliveries in high- and low-risk pregnant women are different entities and not linear extremes of the same syndrome.

There are significant clinical and methodological differences between the above studies that may account for the variation of the results and conclusions. Hay et al[25] recommended that as BV is associated with second-trimester miscarriage and preterm labor, treatment should be given no later than the beginning of the second trimester. Rosenstein et al[28] concluded that earlier diagnosis and treatment may be more effective in preventing abnormal outcome, and they suggested that screening and treating before pregnancy might be advantageous. Some have observed that treatment with topical vaginal antibiotics has proven to be less effective for the prevention of premature delivery than oral antibiotics.[42,43] This would indicate that the microorganisms responsible for premature labor have ascended out of reach of topically administered antibiotics, and the endometrial cavity would be the most likely place for them to initiate contractions.

Some have found reduction of premature delivery only in those with a history of preterm birth.[24,35,37,40] Preterm delivery is the major cause of perinatal mortality and morbidity in the developed world. According to Lamont and Sawant,[44] in up to 40% of cases, infection is a significant cause of spontaneous preterm labour. They recommend clindamycin as the antibiotic of choice.

MISCARRIAGE

ASSOCIATION BETWEEN BV AND EARLY MISCARRIAGE

There have been a few studies linking BV with early first-trimester miscarriage.[45–48] There is stronger evidence, however, that BV is related to late first-trimester and second-trimester loss.[49,50] The relationship between BV and early miscarriage has been assessed mainly in in vitro fertilization (IVF) patients, or threatened miscarriage, rather than recurrent miscarriage.

Miscarriage rates were assessed in 867 consecutive women undergoing IVF.[45] BV was found in 24.6% of the women before egg collection. There were no differences in the conception rates between those women with BV and those with normal vaginal flora. Twenty-two women (31.6%) with BV who conceived had a significantly increased risk of miscarriage in the first trimester compared with 27 women (18.5%) with normal vaginal flora. The increased rate of miscarriage remained significant after adjusting for factors known to increase the risk of miscarriage: maternal age, smoking, a history of recurrent miscarriage, no previous live birth, and polycystic ovary syndrome (PCOS).

In a further study to investigate the effect of vaginal flora and vaginal inflammation on conception and early pregnancy loss, 91 women undergoing IVF were recruited.[46] At the time of embryo transfer, samples were taken for BV. The overall live birth rate was 30% and the rate of early pregnancy loss was 34%. Women with BV, intermediate flora, and normal flora, had early pregnancy loss rates of 33% (1/3), 42% (5/12), and 30% (3/10) ($p = 0.06$), respectively. It was concluded that IVF patients with BV may have increased rates of early pregnancy loss.

French et al[51] reported that in a prospective analysis of 1100 pregnant women, 60% of women with first-trimester bleeding had one or more infections detected, such as BV (RR 1.5), *Trichomonas vaginalis* (RR 2.3) and *C. trachomatis* (RR 2.7). Each of these infections heightened the risk for preterm delivery in women with BV and first-trimester bleeding: RR 4.4 for BV; RR 3.0 for BV with *T. vaginalis*.

ASSOCIATION BETWEEN BV AND LATE MISCARRIAGE

The association with later pregnancy losses has been reported in a number of studies. Llahi-Camp et al[49] found a history of one late miscarriage more than twice as commonly (27/130; 21%) compared with women who had only early miscarriages (31/370; 8%) (*p* <0.001). In this study, BV did not appear to be related to recurrent early miscarriage. Hay et al,[32] in a prospective study, screened 783 women for BV at their first antenatal clinic visit. There were 12 late miscarriages (16–24 weeks' gestation) and a significant association with BV (*p* < 0.001). Oakeshott et al[50] prospectively assessed 1201 women presenting before 10 weeks' gestation. The relative risk of miscarriage associated with BV compared with women who were negative for BV before 16 weeks was 1.2. BV was associated with miscarriage at 13–15 weeks at a relative risk of 3.5. BV was therefore not strongly associated with early miscarriage, but may be a factor for pregnancy loss after 13 weeks' gestation.

Donders et al[52] assessed 228 women at 14 weeks' gestation by culture for BV-associated bacteria, in order to determine whether there is a relationship between BV and pregnancy loss up to 20 weeks. As screening was performed at 14 weeks, only second-trimester losses could be assessed. The relative risk for pregnancy loss between 14 and 20 weeks was 5.4 in the presence of BV. *M. hominis* and *U. urealyticum* were also associated with an increased risk of late miscarriage.

EFFECT OF TREATMENT OF BV ON MISCARRIAGE

There is a general consensus in the literature that antibiotics reduce the incidence of late miscarriages, and preterm labor in the presence of BV. In the study by French et al[51] of 1100 pregnant women, systemic antibiotics reduced the rate of preterm birth for women with BV without first-trimester bleeding (RR 0.37), and treatment of women with BV and first-trimester bleeding reduced preterm birth (RR 0.52). Clindamycin treatment was associated with a reduction in the number of late miscarriages and premature births in Berger and Kane's[53] study of women with asymptomatic BV between 12 and 22 weeks' gestation.

McGregor et al[54] analyzed the effect of systemic treatment to reduce pregnancy loss (<22 weeks), preterm premature rupture of the membranes, and preterm delivery in a prospective controlled treatment trial. The overall presence of BV was 32.5%. BV was associated with pregnancy loss at less than 22 weeks (RR 3.1). The relative risk of preterm premature rupture of the membranes was 3.5 and the relative risk of preterm birth was 1.9. In the treatment phase of the study, women with BV received clindamycin orally. After treatment, there were fever preterm births (RR 0.5) and fever preterm premature ruptures of the membranes (RR 0.5).

Ugwumadu et al[55] prospectively screened 6120 asymptomatic women at the first antenatal visit between 12 and 22 weeks' gestation. The 485 women with abnormal smears were randomly allocated to receive oral clindamycin or placebo. There were significantly fewer midtrimester miscarriages or preterm deliveries in the clindamycin group (13/244) compared with the placebo group (38/241) (*p* = 0.0003).

In a multicenter prospective randomized controlled trial,[56] 4429 low-risk asymptomatic women were screened for BV at their first routine antenatal visit early in the second trimester. In the intervention group, the women received standard antibiotic treatment and follow-up for any detected infection; the number of preterm deliveries was significantly lower (3.0%) than in the control group (5.3%) (*p* = 0.0001). There were 8 late miscarriages in the intervention group and 15 in the control group. It was concluded that introducing a simple infection screening program into routine antenatal care can significantly reduce late miscarriages and preterm births in a low risk-group of pregnant women.

MYCOPLASMAS

Di Bartolomeo et al[57] established the prevalence of microorganisms in 198 pregnant women with vaginal discharge. Endocervical and vaginal samples were assessed using direct methods, culture, immunodetection, and PCR looking for *C. trachomatis*, *Neisseria gonorrhoeae*, *St. agalactiae*, *T. vaginalis*, *Candida*, *M. hominis*, *U. urealyticum*, and BV. In 51 cases (26%), one of the above was detected. BV was diagnosed in 30 cases (15%); *U. urealyticum* was found in 49%, *Candida* in 34%, *M. hominis* in 14.1%, *St. agalactiae* in 5%, *T. vaginalis* in 4%, and *C. trachomatis* in 2.5%; *N. gonorrhoeae* was not detected.

As the evidence suggested that vaginal colonization with genital mycoplasmas plays a role in complications of pregnancy, a study was set up to determine whether antibiotics would reduce spontaneous pregnancy loss.[58] The loss of a pregnancy included spontaneous miscarriage, stillbirths, premature infants who died, or term infants who died from congenital pneumonia due to *U. urealyticum*. Women with spontaneous pregnancy wastage and who were mycoplasma-positive in the genital tract were treated prospectively in 71 pregnancies. There was a significant reduction in pregnancy loss rate among those treated with doxycycline before pregnancy or erythromycin during pregnancy. The pregnancy loss rate in the untreated group was remarkably high, with 22 of the 24 pregnancies being lost. There were 18 out of 37 pregnancies lost in the doxycycline-only group, 3 lost out of 20 pregnancies in the erythromycin group, and 2 of 12 lost after doxycycline and erythromycin. The benefit was independent of maternal age, number of previous miscarriages, or gestational age at miscarriage. It was concluded that antibiotics prescribed for women colonized with mycoplasmas could prevent recurrent spontaneous miscarriage.

The role of *U. urealyticum* in spontaneous and recurrent spontaneous miscarriage has been studied in 633 women.[59] Cervical colonization with *U. urealyticum* was found in 42.6% of 310 normal pregnant women, in 41.6% of 84 patients undergoing pregnancy termination, in 41.5% of normal fertile patients, in 53% of 122 patients with spontaneous miscarriage, and in 64.5% of 76 women with recurrent miscarriage. The cervical colonization rate was significantly higher in patients with spontaneous miscarriage ($p < 0.05$) and recurrent spontaneous miscarriage ($p < 0.005$) compared with normal pregnant women. Endometrial colonization was more frequent in patients with recurrent miscarriage (27.6%) than in normal fertile women (9.7%) ($p < 0.05$). *U. urealyticum* was isolated in five of six women with intact membranes and uncontrollable preterm labor between 20 and 28 weeks' gestation. Ureaplasma was also isolated from the placenta in four patients and the amniotic fluid in two of four patients. It was concluded that *U. urealyticum* is a common commensal of the lower genital tract, but it may play a role in miscarriage and in uncontrollable preterm labor.

However, the role of *U. urealyticum* in adverse pregnancy outcomes is disputed. There was no difference in the incidence of premature rupture of the membranes, preterm labor or low-birth weight infants between women carrying *U. urealyticum* and those who did not in the study by Carey et al.[60] This study assessed whether genital colonization with *U. urealyticum* was associated with adverse pregnancy outcome in 4934 women evaluated between 23 and 26 weeks' gestation.

The prevalence of infection certainly seems to be higher when the abortus is cultured at midtrimester abortion or preterm labor. McDonald et al[61] performed a prospective study of the changes in vaginal flora between midtrimester and labour in 560 women. Forty-five women delivered prematurely. *U. urealyticum* and *G. vaginalis* were both associated with preterm birth when present in the midtrimester. Light and immunofluorescence microscopy were used to investigate 118 late miscarriages at 18–28 weeks' gestation.[62] Intrauterine infections were found in 86 cases, with mycoplasmas being found in 44 (37%). One hundred and twenty-nine spontaneously delivered, non-macerated midgestation placentae and fetuses, between 16 and 26 weeks' gestation, were examined and cultured for aerobic and anaerobic bacteria, genital mycoplasmas, and yeasts.[63] Microorganisms were recovered in 85 (66%). Group B streptococcus was the most significant pathogen, being recovered in 21 cases. *Escherichia coli* (22 cases) and *U. urealyticum* (24 cases) were present mostly as mixed infections. Specimens from 51 spontaneous early miscarriages and 56 pregnancy terminations were investigated by culture for yeasts, gram-positive and gram-negative bacteria, and genital mycoplasmas.[64] Molecular diagnostic tests for DNA sequences were performed for *C. trachomatis*, HSV, adenovirus, and human papilloma virus (HPV). None of these were detected in the pregnancy terminations, whereas spontaneous miscarriage tissues were positive for at least one microorganism in 31.5% of cases.

In the case of first-trimester abortion, an association has not been found with mycoplasmas or ureaplasmas when placental specimens from aborted material were subjected to PCR for karyotyping and detection of bacterial and viral DNA.[65] No evidence of *M. hominis*, *U. urealyticum*, human CMV or adeno-associated virus was found. *C. trachomatis* DNA was detected once. However, Ye et al [66] took endocervical swabs for mycoplasma in 58 women with spontaneous abortion and compared the outcome of pregnancy with a control group of 50 normal pregnant women. In the index cases, positive results for *U. urealyticum* and *M. hominis* were found in 74.1% (43/58) and 27.6% (16/58), respectively. These results were significantly different to those of the controls, the corresponding results being 48% (24/50) (p <0.01) and 10% (5/50) (p <0.05). It was concluded that mycoplasma infection could be one of the causes of early embryonic death.

Microbiological screening of vaginal flora and semen was performed 4 weeks before IVF for 951 couples.[67] Infections were found in 218 women (22.9%) and appropriate treatment was prescribed. There were 69 with *Candida albicans*, 49 with *U. urealyticum*, 43 with *G. vaginalis*, 24 with streptococcus B or D, and 22 with *E. coli*. The implantation rate was significantly reduced in patients with infection: 14.6% versus 19.3% (p <0.02). Positive cultures

from both vagina and semen were found in 77 couples with a spontaneous miscarriage rate of 46.7%, compared with 17.6% with vaginal infection alone (p <0.01). It was concluded that endocervical microorganisms, even when treated, may affect implantation, and this is enhanced when the semen has shown infection.

ANTIBIOTICS IN UNEXPLAINED PREGNANCY LOSSES

Antibiotics have been prescribed in some studies without bacteriological confirmation. The maternal and fetal outcomes of the next pregnancy were recorded in 254 couples attending an infertility clinic following one or more spontaneous miscarriages[20]. One hundred couples requested antibiotics: 96 received doxycycline 100 mg twice daily for 4 weeks or tetracycline 500 mg four times daily for 4 weeks to cover *C. trachomatis* and mycoplasmas. In addition, 49 patients received erythromycin 500 mg four times daily for 2 weeks. Four patients received ampicillin or cephalexin. There was a significantly lower chance of miscarriage in the antibiotic-treated group (10%) compared with the untreated group (38%) (p <0.01). Premature rupture of the membranes occurred in 4% of the treated group, compared with 46% in the control group. The antibiotic group had a higher vaginal delivery rate (69% vs 56%) (p <0.01), lower incidences of fetal distress (6% vs 26%), respiratory distress syndrome, and neonatal infection, a higher birth weight, and better Apgar scores. It was postulated that some spontaneous miscarriages may be caused by bacteria present in the genital tract at the time of conception and that these bacteria may have an adverse effect on the pregnancy.

Antibiotic therapy has been assessed for first-trimester threatened miscarriage in women with previous spontaneous miscarriage.[68] Only those at a gestational age of less than 9 weeks were included. Women with mild abdominal cramping received amoxicillin and erythromycin for 7 days. Severe abdominal pain was treated with amoxicillin and clindamycin for 7 days. Of the 23 pregnancies,

22 were carried to term. It was concluded that antibiotics might prevent pregnancy loss in women with threatened miscarriage and that further clinical trials are warranted.

A randomized placebo-controlled trial was set up to determine whether metronidazole reduces early preterm labour in asymptomatic women with positive vaginal fetal fibronectin in the second trimester of pregnancy.[69] The women had at least one risk factor, including midtrimester loss or preterm delivery, uterine abnormality, cervical surgery, or cervical cerclage. Nine hundred pregnancies were screened for fetal fibronectin at 24 and 27 weeks' gestation, and the positive cases were randomized to receive a 7-day course of oral metronidazole or placebo. The primary outcome was delivery before 30 weeks' gestation, and the secondary outcomes included delivery before 37 weeks. Fetal fibronectin was a good predictor of early preterm birth, with a positive predictive value at 24 weeks' gestation for delivery by 30 weeks of 26% and a negative predictive value of 99%. The trial steering committee stopped the study early; 21% (11/53) of the women receiving metronidazole delivered before 30 weeks, compared with 11% (5/46) of those taking the placebo. Furthermore, there were significantly more preterm deliveries (<37 weeks) in women receiving the metronidazole (33/53; 62%) compared with placebo (18/46; 39%). Treatment was initiated relatively late, and damage would have preceded the metronidazole, as all the patients studied had positive fibronectin tests.

FUTURE DEVELOPMENTS

More than a century ago, Robert Koch devised a scientific standard for determining whether a disease is a result of a specific microorganism. Koch's postulates stated that the pathogen should be isolated from the diseased host, grow in pure culture, and reproduce the disease when inoculated into a susceptible host. Interestingly, Koch accepted that his postulates were not always useful (cited by Fredricks and Relman[2]). In recent years, a previously unexpected infectious etiology has been demonstrated in a variety of clinical conditions. In gynecology, the role of HPV in premalignant and malignant cervical disease has been confirmed, and in obstetrics there appears to be a link between premature delivery and BV. *Helicobacter pylori* has become established as the cause of peptic ulceration. Fredricks and Relman[2] have suggested that there are a number of chronic diseases whose etiology remains obscure but that have characteristics indicating a microbial involvement. These diseases include Crohn's disease, rheumatoid arthritis, systemic lupus erythematosis, atherosclerosis, multiple sclerosis, and diabetes mellitus. Fredricks and Relman[2] have suggested that traditional technology for detecting pathogens is not sufficiently sensitive to identify the microorganisms responsible. Whipple's disease illustrates the limitation of conventional bacteriology. Whipple described the disease that bears his name in 1907. The syndrome consists of polyarthritis, weight loss, diarrhea, malabsorption, and lymphadenopathy. Whipple observed rod-like bacillary structures in mesenteric lymph nodes, raising the possibility of a bacterial etiology. Although Whipple's bacillus could be seen by microscopy, it could not be grown in culture or in animal hosts, and no successful serological test could be devised. It was not until the arrival of molecular biology that the bacillus could be characterized. Fredericks and Relman[2] concluded that failure to cultivate a microorganism does not prove that a disease is not due to a pathogen. Bacteria may cause chronic systemic disease spanning decades. Furthermore, steroids may produce temporary improvement without proving that the disease is inflammatory or autoimmune rather than infectious. Finally, documented improvement or cure associated with antimicrobial agents in a chronic disease suggests a microbial origin.

Bacteria have a remarkable propensity to survive even in the most hostile environments.[70] The vast majority of microorganisms are 'unculturable' or 'fastidious', which means that they cannot be identified by conventional culture techniques. Over the last few years, the development and application of molecular diagnostic techniques has revolutionized the diagnosis and monitoring of infectious diseases.

Molecular biological techniques are increasingly being adopted in clinical laboratories. These molecular methods have made it possible to characterize mixed microflora in their entirety, including unculturables. Molecular studies of the vaginal flora have discovered many unculturable bacteria, including bacteria in the Clostridiales order, which are highly specific indicators of BV. A more complete understanding of vaginal microbial populations resulting from molecular biological techniques may lead to new strategies to maintain healthy vaginal floras, and will provide opportunities to explore the role of novel bacteria in reproductive tract disease.[71]

Biofilms develop by bacteria aggregating in a hydrated polymeric matrix of their own synthesis on moist surfaces. They are inherently resistant to antimicrobial agents and are increasingly recognized as being at the root of many persistent and chronic bacterial infections.[72] Fredricks and Relman[2] have observed that for more than a century bacteriologists have attempted to culture *Treponema pallidum* and *Mycobacterium leprae* without success, although the pathogenicity of these organisms is not in doubt. These authors argue that just as we cannot cultivate known pathogens, we must accept the possibility that other pathogens may exist that resist cultivation. They have provided a set of guidelines to help prove microbial disease causation using molecular biological sequence-based evidence rather than culture.

Some have concluded that the best evidence suggests that infection is an occasional cause of sporadic spontaneous miscarriage and that recurrent miscarriage occurs with a much lower frequency. At the other extreme, mycoplasmas have been found in 74% of spontaneous miscarriages with embryonic death, compared with 48% of controls.[66] Recently, attention has focused on the relationship between periodontal infection and adverse pregnancy outcomes, including late miscarriage.[73] Periodontal disease is one of the most common chronic infections, with a prevalence of 10–60% depending on diagnostic criteria. So far, there have been no reports on any association between first-trimester miscarriage and periodontitis.

The antiphospholipid syndrome (APS) has been linked to recurrent miscarriage and other pregnancy complications. It may respond to thromboprophylaxis, improving the live birth rate.[74] Antiphospholipid antibodies (aPL) may be associated with infection, and one is left to contemplate the possibility that some cases of recurrent miscarriage could be related to underlying treatable infection. In this context, it is of interest that APS disappears when *H. pylori* is eradicated.[75]

While microorganisms can be associated with miscarriage, the question will always arise as to whether they are pathogenic or opportunistic. Ultimately, from a clinical point of view, what really matters is whether treatment can reduce the occurrence of spontaneous miscarriage. A few clinical studies so far have shown encouraging results, and further research is warranted. It is recognized that screening for and treatment of BV in early pregnancy among high-risk women with a previous history of second-trimester miscarriage or spontaneous preterm labor may reduce the risk of recurrent late pregnancy loss and preterm birth. The fundamental question of efficacy of antibiotic treatment for BV before pregnancy in women with recurrent early miscarriage has yet to be addressed in clinical studies. Developments in serological tests and molecular biological techniques are enhancing our capability to detect evidence of infections in obstetrics and gynecology. Ultimately, there is the option of a trial of therapy with a presumptive diagnosis of genital infection being related to recurrent miscarriage without laboratory confirmation. The antibiotics of choice – metronidazole and the macrolides such as erythromycin – are relatively innocuous. Nevertheless, antibiotics should be used with caution, as there is the potential risk of the development of bacterial resistance.

REFERENCES

1. Royal College of Obstetricians and Gynaecologists, Guideline No 17. The Investigation and Treatment of Couples with Recurrent Miscarriage. London: RCOG, 2003.
2. Fredricks DN, Relman DA. Infectious agents and the etiology of chronic idiopathic diseases. Curr Clin Top Infect Dis 1998; 18:180–200.

3. Saracoglu OF, Mungan T, Tanzer F. Pelvic tuberculosis. Int J Gynaecol Obstet 1992; 37:115–20.

4. Figueroa-Damian R, Martinez-Velazco I, Villagrana-Zesati R, et al. Tuberculosis of the female reproductive tract: effect on function. Int J Fertil Menopausal Stud 1996; 41:430–6.

5. Romana C, Salleras L, Sage M. Latent listerosis may cause habitual abortion, intrauterine deaths, fetal malformations. When diagnosed and treated adequately normal children will be born. Acta Microbiol Hung 1989; 36:171–2.

6. Manganiello PD, Yearke RR. A 10-year prospective study of women with a history of recurrent fetal losses fails to identify *Listeria monocytogenes* in the female genital tract. Fertil Steril 1991; 56:781–2.

7. Szkaradkiewicz A, Pieta P, Tulecka T, et al. The diagnostic value of anti-CMV and anti-HPV-B19 antiviral antibodies in studies on causes of recurrent abortions. Ginekol Pol 1997; 68:181–6.

8. Cook SM, Himebaugh KS, Frank TS. Absence of cytomegalovirus in gestational tissue in recurrent spontaneous abortion. Diagn Mol Pathol 1993; 2:116–19.

9. Mezinova NN, Chuchupalov PD, Evdokimova NS, et al. Effect of antichlamydial drugs on the effectiveness of the treatment of habitual abortion. Akush Ginekol (Mosk) 1991; 7:30–2.

10. Mezinova NN, Chuchupalov PD. Endometrial *Chlamydia* infection in women with habitual abortion. Akush Ginekol (Mosk) 1992; 2:25–6.

11. Kishore J, Agarwal J, Agarwal S, et al. Seroanalysis of *Chlamydia trachomatis* and S-TORCH agents in women with recurrent spontaneous abortions. Indian J Pathol Microbiol 2003; 46:684–7.

12. Witkin SS, Ledger WJ. Antibodies to *Chlamydia trachomatis* in sera of women with recurrent spontaneous abortions. Am J Obstet Gynecol 1992; 167:135–9.

13. Olliaro P, Regazzetti A, Gorini G, et al. *Chlamydia trachomatis* infection in 'sine causa' recurrent abortion. Boll Ist Sieroter Milan 1991; 70:467–70.

14. Rae R, Smith IW, Liston WA, et al. Chlamydial serologic studies and recurrent spontaneous abortion. Am J Obstet Gynecol 1994; 170:782–5.

15. Paukku M, Tulppala M, Puolakkainen M, et al. Lack of association between serum antibodies to *Chlamydia trachomatis* and a history of recurrent pregnancy loss. Fertil Steril 1999; 72:427–30.

16. Sugiura-Ogasawara M, Ozaki Y, Nakanishi T, et al, Pregnancy outcome in recurrent aborters is not influenced by *Chlamydiae* IGA and/or G. Am J Reprod Immunol 2005; 53:50–3.

17. Schulz KF, Cates W Jr, O'Mara PR. A synopsis of the problems in Africa in syphilis and gonorrhoea during pregnancy. Afr J Sex Transm Dis 1986; 2:56–7.

18. Amsel R, Totten PA, Spiegel CA, et al. Nonspecific vaginitis. Diagnostic criteria and microbial and epidemiologic associations. Am J Med 1983; 74:14–22.

19. Wilson JD, Ralph SG, Rutherford AJ. Rates of BV in women undergoing in vitro fertilisation for different types of infertility. BJOG 2002; 109:714–17.

20. Toth A, Lesser ML, Brooks-Toth CW, et al. Outcome of subsequent pregnancies following antibiotic therapy after primary or multiple spontaneous abortions. Surg Gynecol Obstet 1986; 163:243–50.

21. Viniker DA. Hypothesis on the role of sub-clinical bacteria of the endometrium (bacteria endometrialis) in gynaecological and obstetric enigmas. Hum Reprod Update 1999; 5:373–85.

22. Lucisano A, Morandotti G, Marana R, et al. Chlamydial genital infections and laparoscopic findings in infertile women. Eur J Epidemiol 1992; 8:645–9.

23. Moller BR, Kristiansen FV, Thorsen P, et al. Sterility of the uterine cavity. Acta Obstet Gynecol Scand 1995; 74:216–19.

24. Guise JM, Mahon SM, Aickin M, et al. Screening for bacterial vaginosis in pregnancy. Am J Prev Med 2001; 20(Suppl 3):62–72.

25. Hay PE, Morgan DJ, Ison CA, et al. A longitudinal study of bacterial vaginosis during pregnancy. Br J Obstet Gynaecol 1994; 101:1048–53.

26. Ugwumadu A, Reid F, Hay P, et al. Natural history of bacterial vaginosis and intermediate flora in pregnancy and effect of oral clindamycin. Obstet Gynecol 2004; 104:114–19.

27. Riduan JM, Hillier SL, Utomo B, et al. Bacterial vaginosis and prematurity in Indonesia: asociation in early and late pregnancy. Am J Obstet Gynecol 1993; 169:175–8.

28. Rosenstein IJ, Morgan DJ, Lamont RF, et al. Effect of intravaginal clindamycin cream on pregnancy outcome and on abnormal vaginal microbial flora of pregnant women. Infect Dis Obstet Gynecol 2000; 8:158–65.

29. McDonald HM, O'Loughlin JA, Jolley P, et al. Vaginal infection and preterm labour. Br J Obstet Gynaecol 1991; 98:427–35.

30. Klebanoff MA, Hillier SL, Nugent RP, et al. Is bacterial vaginosis a stronger risk factor for preterm birth when it is diagnosed earlier in gestation? Am J Obstet Gynecol 2005; 192:470–7.

31. Lamont RF, Duncan SL, Mandal D, et al. Intravaginal clindamycin to reduce preterm birth in women with abnormal genital tract flora. Obstet Gynecol 2003; 101:516–22.

32. Hay PE, Lamont RF, Taylor-Robinson D, et al. Abnormal bacterial colonisation of the genital tract and subsequent preterm delivery and late miscarriage. BMJ 1994; 308:295–8.

33. Goffinet F, Maillard F, Mihoubi N, et al. Bacterial vaginosis: prevalence and predictive value for premature delivery and neonatal infection in women with preterm labour and intact membranes. Eur J Obstet Gynecol Reprod Biol 2003; 108:146–51.

34. Borisov I, Dimitrova V, Mazneikova V, et al. Therapeutic regimens for treating bacterial vaginosis in pregnant women. Akush Ginekol (Sofiia) 1999; 38:14–16.

35. Morales WJ, Schorr S, Albritton J. Effect of metronidazole in patients with preterm birth in preceding pregnancy and bacterial vaginosis: a placebo-controlled, double-blind study. Am J Obstet Gynecol 1994; 171:345–7.

36. Hauth JC, Goldenberg RL, Andrews WW, et al. Reduced incidence of preterm delivery with metronidazole and erythromycin in women with bacterial vaginosis. N Engl J Med 1995; 333:1732–6.

37. McDonald HM, O'Loughlin JA, Vigneswaran R, et al. Impact of metronidazole therapy on preterm birth in women with bacterial vaginosis flora (*Gardnerella vaginalis*): a randomised, placebo controlled trial. Br J Obstet Gynaecol 1997; 104:1391–7.

38. Camargo RP, Simoes JA, Cecatti JG, et al. Impact of treatment for bacterial vaginosis on prematurity among Brazilian pregnant women: a retrospective cohort study. Sao Paulo Med J 2005; 123:108–12.

39. Kurkinen-Raty M, Vuopala S, Koskela M, et al. A randomised controlled trial of vaginal clindamycin for early pregnancy bacterial vaginosis. BJOG 2000; 107:1427–32.

40. Brocklehurst P, Hanna M, McDonald H. Interventions for treating bacterial vaginosis in pregnancy. Cochrane Database Syst Rev 2000; (2):CD00026.

41. Varma R, Gupta JK. Antibiotic treatment of bacterial vaginosis in pregnancy: multiple meta-analyses and dilemmas in interpretation. Eur J Obstet Gynecol Reprod Biol 2006; 124:10–14.

42. Majeroni BA. Bacterial vaginosis: an update. Am Fam Physician 1998; 57:1285–9.

43. McGregor JA. Evidence based prevention of preterm birth/PROM: infection and inflammation. Paper presented at the Problem with Prematurity II. St Thomas' Hospital, London, 7–9 September, 1998.

44. Lamont RF, Sawant SR. Infection in the prediction and antibiotics in the prevention of spontaneous preterm labour and preterm birth. Minerva Ginecol 2005; 57:423–33.

45. Ralph SG, Rutherford AJ, Wilson JD. Influence of bacterial vaginosis on conception and miscarriage in the first trimester: cohort study. BMJ 1999; 319:220–3.

46. Eckert LO, Moore DE, Patton DL, et al. Relationship of vaginal bacteria and inflammation with conception and early pregnancy loss following in-vitro fertilization. Infect Dis Obstet Gynecol 2003; 11:11–17.

47. Ugwumadu AH. Bacterial vaginosis in pregnancy. Curr Opin Obstet Gynecol 2002; 14:115–18.

48. Leitich H, Bodner-Adler B, Brunbauer M, et al. Bacterial vaginosis as a risk factor for preterm delivery: a meta-analysis. Am J Obstet Gynecol 2003; 189:139–47.

49. Llahi-Camp JM, Rai R, Ison C, et al. Association of bacterial vaginosis with a history of second trimester miscarriage. Hum Reprod 1996; 11:1575–8.

50. Oakeshott P, Hay P, Hay S, et al. Association between bacterial vaginosis or chlamydial infection and miscarriage before 16 weeks' gestation: prospective community based cohort study. BMJ 2002; 325:1334–7.

51. French JI, McGregor JA, Draper D, et al. Gestational bleeding, bacterial vaginosis and common reproductive tract infections: risk for preterm birth and benefit of treatment. Obstet Gynecol 1999; 93:715–24.

52. Donders GG, Van Bulck B, Caudron J, et al. Relationship of bacterial vaginosis and mycoplasmas to the risk of spontaneous abortion. Am J Obstet Gynecol 2000; 183:431–7.

53. Berger A, Kane KY. Clindamycin for vaginosis reduces prematurity and late miscarriage. J Fam Pract 2003; 52:603–4.

54. McGregor JA, French JI, Parker R, et al. Prevention of premature birth by screening and treatment for common genital tract infections: results of a prospective controlled evaluation. Am J Obstet Gynecol 1995; 173:157–67.

55. Ugwumadu A, Manyonda I, Reid F, et al. Effect of early oral clindamycin on late miscarriage and preterm delivery in asymptomatic women with abnormal vaginal flora and bacterial vaginosis: a randomised controlled trial. Lancet 2003; 361:983–8.

56. Kiss H, Petricevic L, Husslein P. Prospective randomised controlled trial of an infection screening programme to reduce the rate of preterm delivery. BMJ 2004; 329:371.

57. Di Bartolomeo S, Rodriguez M, Sauka D, et al. Microbiologic profile in symptomatic pregnant women's genital secretions in Gran Buenos Aires, Argentina. Enferm Infecc Microbiol Clin 2001; 19:99–102.

58. Quinn PA, Shewchuk AB, Shuber J, et al. Efficacy of antibiotic therapy in preventing spontaneous pregnancy loss among couples colonized with genital mycoplasmas. Am J Obstet Gynecol 1983; 145:239–44.

59. Naessens A, Foulon W, Cammu H, et al. Epidemiology and pathogenesis of U. urealyticum in spontaneous abortion and early preterm labor. Acta Obstet Gynecol Scand 1987; 66:513–16.

60. Carey JC, Blackwelder WC, Nugent RP, et al. Antepartum cultures for Ureaplasma urealyticum are not useful in predicting pregnancy outcome. The Vaginal Infections and Prematurity Study Group. Am J Obstet Gynecol 1991; 164:728–33.

61. McDonald HM, O'Loughlin JA, Jolley, PT, et al. Changes in vaginal flora during pregnancy and association with preterm birth. J Infect Dis 1994; 170:724–8.

62. Fedotova EP, Shastina GV. Intrauterine mycoplasmosis in late miscarriage. Arkh Patol 1994; 56:61–5.

63. McDonald HM, Chambers HM. Intrauterine infection and spontaneous midgestation abortion: Is the spectrum of microorganisms similar to that in preterm labor? Infect Dis Obstet Gynecol 2000; 8:220–7.

64. Penta M, Lukic A, Conte MP, et al. Infectious agents in tissues from spontaneous abortions in the first trimester of pregnancy. New Microbiol 2003; 26:329–37.

65. Matovina M, Husnjak K, Milutin N, et al. Possible role of bacterial and viral infections in miscarriages. Fertil Steril 2004; 81:662–9.

66. Ye LL, Zhang BY, Cao WL. Relationship between the endocervical mycoplasma infection and spontaneous abortion due to early embryonic death. Zhonghua Fu Chan Ke Za Zhi 2004; 39:83–5.

67. Wittemer C, Bettahar-Lebugle K, Ohl J, et al. Abnormal bacterial colonisation of the vagina and implantation during assisted reproduction. Gynecol Obstet Fertil 2004; 32:135–9.

68. Ou MC, Pang CC, Chen FM, et al. Antibiotic treatment for threatened abortion during the early first trimester in women with previous spontaneous abortion. Acta Obstet Gynecol Scand 2001; 80:753–6.

69. Shennan A, Crawshaw S, Briley A. A randomised controlled trial of metronidazole for the prevention of preterm birth in women positive for cervicovaginal fetal fibronectin: The PREMET Study. BJOG 2006; 113:65–74.

70. Nichols CA, Guezennec J, Bowman JP. Bacterial exopolysaccharides from extreme marine environments with special consideration of the southern ocean, sea ice, and deep-sea hydrothermal vents: a review. Mar Biotechnol (NY) 2005; 7:253–71.

71. Fredricks DN, Marrazzo JM. Molecular methodology in determining vaginal flora in health and disease: its time has come. Curr Infect Dis Rep 2005; 7:463–70.

72. Costerton JW, Stewart PS, Greenberg EP. Bacterial biofilms; A common cause of persistent infections. Science 1999; 284:1318–22.

73. Farrell Nee Moore S, Ide M, Wilson RF. The relationship between maternal periodontitis, adverse pregnancy outcome and miscarriage in never smokers. J Clin Periodontol 2006; 33:115–20.

74. Rai R, Regan L. Antiphospholipid syndrome and pregnancy loss. Hosp Med 1998; 59:637–9.

75. Cicconi V, Carloni E, Franceschi F, et al. Disappearance of antiphospholipid antibodies syndrome after Helicobacter pylori eradication. Am J Med 2001; 111:163–4.

14. Midtrimester loss – the role of cerclage

Israel Hendler and Howard JA Carp

INTRODUCTION

Cervical incompetence or (preferably named) cervical insufficiency is defined as 'the inability of the uterine cervix to retain a pregnancy in the absence of contractions or labor'. It is a clinical diagnosis characterized by recurrent painless cervical dilatation and spontaneous midtrimester loss, generally in the absence of obvious predisposing conditions such as spontaneous membrane rupture, bleeding, or infection, which may indicate other causes of preterm birth rather than cervical insufficiency. Although cervical incompetence was first described in the English language literature in 1678, and great strides have been made in the understanding of this condition, the clinical diagnosis is usually made in retrospect, after a poor obstetric outcome. The diagnosis is difficult to make, and usually depends on a careful history and review of the medical records, rather than accurate diagnostic means or laboratory tests. True cervical insufficiency is probably an uncommon diagnosis; however, the lack of clear diagnostic criteria make the incidence difficult to ascertain objectively. The condition is important, as midtrimester pregnancy loss will ensue or the condition can be part of a spectrum leading to preterm delivery in all stages of the third trimester, with its attendant risks to the infant.

Cervical cerclage has been the classical treatment for cervical incompetence since its introduction by Shirodkar[1] in 1955. However, the indications for cerclage are still far from clear, as are the optimal method and timing. This chapter focuses on the diagnosis of cervical insufficiency, the obstetric management of women at high risk for preterm delivery by ultrasonographic follow-up of cervical length, the particular problems of cerclage in recurrent pregnancy loss (RPL), the role of transvaginal and transabdominal cervical cerclage, and the optimal method of performing the technique.

PATHOPHYSIOLOGY

The pathophysiology of cervical insufficiency is still poorly understood. The cervix of a woman with cervical incompetence contains a higher proportion of smooth muscle cells compared with the cervix of a pregnant woman without cervical incompetence.[2,3] Deficiencies of cervical collagen,[4,5] cervical elastin,[6] or other structural, mechanical components of cervical connective tissue have been postulated as etiological factors. These factors normally resist softening, effacement, and dilatation caused by the gravitational effect of the fetus and amniotic fluid. It has been difficult to confirm any theory of pathophysiology due to the difficulty in obtaining biopsy samples from the human cervix before, during, and after term and preterm deliveries. A different model has been suggested by more recent studies using serial endovaginal ultrasound measurements of cervical length, dilatation, and funneling of the membranes into the cervical canal. This tentative model is based on both the sequential measurements and on individual observations that the pregnant cervix is a dynamic structure, occasionally opening and closing with no apparent relation to uterine contractions. Iams[7] has proposed the model of a continuum of cervical compliance ('competence') similar to the natural biological variation in other physical traits, such as height, tendon strength, and long bone length. According to this model, cervical compliance and cervical length are qualities that vary from woman to woman, and these qualities are just some of the components of uterine function that affect the timing of delivery. At present, we have empirical data about how cervical length and dilatation occur in advancing pregnancy, but not why those changes occur before term in some women and at term in most women. Although the predictive value of these measurements remains controversial, their progressive nature has been employed to develop the concept of varying degrees of functional cervical insufficiency.

DIAGNOSIS OF CERVICAL INSUFFICIENCY

There are essentially no proven objective criteria to diagnose cervical insufficiency (other than those few cases with gross cervical malformations). Shirodkar[1] stated that 95% of cases of cervical insufficiency were due to a weak cervical sphincter and the other few to an underdeveloped or malformed uterus. Shirodkar claimed to diagnose the condition by 'repeated internal examinations'. Since 1955, many physicians have searched for diagnostic tools. The Hegar test is still used to measure the diameter of the endocervical canal. A cut-off of 6–8 mm is usually taken to make the diagnosis of cervical insufficiency.[8,9] However, in RPL, the patient usually presents in the interval between pregnancies, when the endocervical canal is not subject to the forces present in pregnancy, but in a grossly incompetent cervix the Hegar test may give obvious information about the diagnosis. In order to overcome the disadvantage of the lack of pressure from inside the uterus in the Hegar test, the traction test was devised. A catheter is inserted into the uterine cavity, and the balloon is filled with 1 ml of fluid. The catheter is then pulled through the cervical canal. If the balloon can be removed by a force of less than 600 g, then the diagnosis of cervical insufficiency is made.[10] Hysterosalpingography provides information about the diameter and the shape of the cervical canal.[9,11] A funnel-shaped isthmus is taken to be diagnostic for cervical insufficiency.

It may also be necessary to diagnose insufficiency in pregnancy, as the cervix may dilate despite the above tests indicating that there is no cervical insufficiency in the non-pregnant state. The Hegar test has been adapted by Fournil et al.[12] In this technique, an 8 mm Hegar dilator is inserted into the endocervical canal twice weekly until 19 weeks of gestation. However, this technique is not really different to that of Shirodkar. Indeed, Shirodkar's method of digital examination has been used to detect preterm delivery by many other authors.[13,14] We use digital examination on a routine basis when following patients up in pregnancy after RPL. This method is simple and non-invasive, and has picked up a number of patients with impending second-trimester loss and preterm labor. In some cases, it has indicated the need for late cerclage. However, digital examination leads to a diagnosis after cervical dilatation has reached the external os. At this stage, it may be impossible to prevent second-trimester loss or preterm delivery. Therefore, none of the above methods is entirely satisfactory.

Sarti et al[15] introduced abdominal ultrasound to detect cervical dilatation of the cervix. However, transabdominal ultrasonography requires a full bladder in order to visualize the cervix. The full bladder can press on the dilated cervix and cause a false-negative result, as the bladder can cause lengthening of the canal.[16,17] This problem can be overcome if a vaginal probe is used. Funneling and shortening can be identified. The relationship between cervical length and the risk of preterm delivery has been described.[18,19] Figure 14.1(a) shows the sonogram of a normal cervix on ultrasound. As shortening of cervical length seems to be a continuous process, ultrasound can detect dilatation of the internal os before the external os is affected. Figure 14.1(b) shows shortening of the cervical canal. Transvaginal ultrasound can theoretically detect midterm loss and preterm delivery earlier than other methods of detection. Figure 14.2 shows funneling of the internal os and shortening of the cervical canal. However, transcervical ultrasonography has a number of drawbacks. Figure 14.3 shows an apparently normal-looking cervix. However, the application of light fundal pressure allows the insufficiency to become apparent. It is impractical to screen the

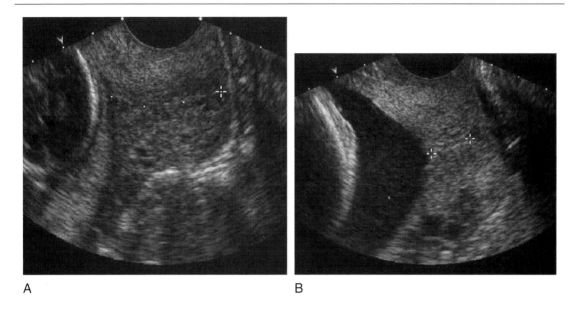

A   B

Figure 14.1 Ultrasound of cervical length: (a) normal cervix of 35 mm length; (b) shortened cervix of 14 mm length. These sonograms show normal cervices. The cervix in (a) is completely closed, with a length of 35 mm (as seen between the calipers). The cervix in (b) is 14 mm in length, but can still be competent.

entire obstetric population, and grand multipara can have wide open cervices without insufficiency. Hence, transcervical ultrasound is not always selective, as Figure 14.1(b) shows. In patients with recurrent first-trimester losses, it is also not practical to screen all patients. Although the incidences of cervical incompetence,[20] midtrimester loss, and preterm labor are higher after RPL,[20,21] (see Figure 11.4 in Chapter 11), this higher incidence is probably not high enough to justify screening

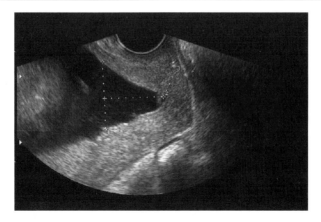

Figure 14.2 Sonogram of cervical incompetence. This shows funneling of the cervix, with a dilatation of the internal os. The remaining cervical canal from the funneling to the external os is extremely shortened.

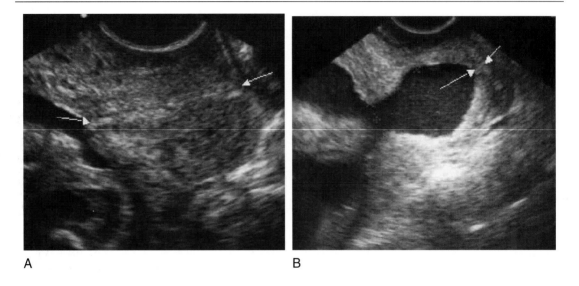

A   B

Figure 14.3 A dynamic cervix: (a) cervix with no fundal pressure;. (b) cervix with fundal pressure. The cervix was shortened from 28 mm to 0 mm during the examination by light fundal pressure.

the entire population on a regular basis. However, transvaginal ultrasonography is warranted to detect short cervical length and funneling in women at high risk for preterm delivery due to cervical incompetence.[22,23] In RPL, we tend to screen pregnant patients by transvaginal ultrasound if there is a high risk of midtrimester loss or preterm labor, as shown by a past history, cervical tears, a previous hysteroscopic diagnosis, or when digital examination indicates cervical insufficiency. In women with midtrimester loss, transvaginal ultrasound measurement of cervical length can be used as a screening tool indicating the need for cerclage, as will be shown later in this chapter.

DIFFERENTIAL DIAGNOSIS

There are various conditions predisposing to midtrimester loss and preterm labor. These include uterine anomalies (see Chapter 11) and exposure to diethylstilbestol (DES) in utero.[24,25] There is also a group of women with an inherently short cervix (below the 5th percentile) who have an increased

risk of preterm labor.[26] Patients with multifetal pregnancies also have a higher risk of preterm labor, possibly due to the additional uterine distension and additional pressure of the uterine contents on the cervix.[27] Spontaneous membrane rupture, bleeding, or infection also lead the uterus to contract, leading to midtrimester loss or preterm labor. As there are essentially no proven objective criteria for diagnosing cervical insufficiency (other than perhaps the rare gross cervical malformation), the diagnosis is usually made by a history of midtrimester loss of a live fetus, after painless dilatation of the cervix. There may be a history of trauma to the cervix from surgical procedures such as conization,[28] or previous dilatation and curettage.[29] Alternately there may be a traumatic delivery, such as precipitated labor with forceful expulsion of the fetus before full dilatation, leading to cervical tearing, or a traumatic instrumental delivery with cervical tearing. However, diagnosis of cervical insufficiency based on exclusion of other factors is flawed, as an appreciable proportion of women who have apparent cervical insufficiency have evidence of subclinical intrauterine infection on amniotic fluid analysis obtained by transabdominal amniocentesis.

CERVICAL CERCLAGE

Cerclage was first introduced by Shirodkar[1] in 1955 for the treatment of cervical insufficiency. Shirodkar described a group of 30 women who had at least 4 (and up to 11) previous abortions. Shirodkar stated that, in his opinion, '95% of cases of cervical incompetence were due to a weak cervical sphincter and the other few to an underdeveloped or malformed uterus, etc.' Shirodkar emphasized that his work was confined to women in whom he could prove the existence of weakness of the internal os by 'repeated internal examinations'. Fifty years later, cerclage is performed in 1:54–220 deliveries worldwide, although there is still confusion about the diagnostic criteria and uncertainty about its benefits. Before describing its benefits and indications, the next section will describe the techniques for performing cerclage.

TECHNIQUES OF CERCLAGE

The McDonald technique[30] is the simplest procedure to perform technically. The procedure consists of suturing of the cervix as high as possible, by a pursestring suture in five or six bites. The knot is positioned on the anterior aspect of the cervix. The advantage of McDonald's technique is that it can be performed by relatively junior staff, and there are few complications. In McDonald's original report, 70 women presented with second-trimester dilatation of the cervix and bulging membranes between 20 and 24 weeks of gestation. Thirty-three women (47%) gave birth to infants that survived. In a subsequent publication,[31] McDonald reported that the proportion of success had increased, due to better selection of patients and the use of a prophylactic cerclage at 14 weeks of gestation before cervical dilatation. We often use a modified McDonald technique in which the cervix is grasped in three or four bites, the knot tied at 10–11 o' clock,

and the free ends of the threads are tied to leave a loop, in order to facilitate early removal. However, the disadvantage of the McDonald technique is that in cases of high cervical tears, it may not be possible to place the suture high enough. Ideally, the suture should be at the level of the internal os, but ultrasound often shows the suture to lay halfway along the cervical canal.

In the Shirodkar technique, a transverse incision is made on the anterior side of the cervix and the bladder is pushed up above the internal cervical os. A vertical incision is then made in the posterior vaginal wall. The stitch is placed in two bites, penetrating the cervical tissue laterally. In this way, the cervix is encircled without affecting the more laterally placed uterine vessels. The mucosal incisions are then closed. The Shirodkar technique has the advantage of reaching up to 3 cm higher than the McDonald technique. If there are cervical tears, the reflection of the bladder and the pouch of Douglas can be continued until above the level of the tear. However, there is the possibility of injury to surrounding tissues. If the uterus contracts and dilates, there may be tearing of the uterus on the stitch. We tend to use a modified Shirodkar technique, in which the bladder is reflected from the cervix, but not the pouch of Douglas. Additionally, we tend to use the modified Shirodkar technique after failure of the McDonald procedure.

If the suture needs to be placed still higher, or in cases with severe cervical scarring after multiple failures of vaginal cerclage,[32] an abdominal approach can be used. This technique can be performed by laparotomy, or more recently by laparoscopy.[33] In the technique of Anthony et al,[34] the bladder is mobilized, the uterine arteries are identified, and tunnels are created medial to the uterine arteries. A 5 mm mersilene tape is then passed through the tunnels, and the stitch is tied anteriorly. In the method of Topper and Farquharson,[35] a 2-gauge ethilon suture is passed through the muscle of the uterus medial to the uterine vessels at the height of the isthmus above the cardinal ligaments, and the stitch is tied anteriorly. The problem with this technique is that laparotomy or laparoscopy are required for insertion. If the technique fails, laparotomy or laparoscopy may be required for removal. However, techniques have been developed for leaving the knot so that it can be accessed without invasive techniques. In patients with badly scarred cervices, the abdominal approach may be the only approach that is possible. However, the vast majority of patients can still be treated with the less invasive vaginal approach.

VALUE OF CERCLAGE

The clinical value of cervical cerclage has been subject of many observational and randomized clinical trials, and the studies have been subject to several systematic reviews. In this section, we will try to summarize the evidence regarding the benefit of cerclage for midtrimester loss. The studies should be classified into those performed prior to or subsequent to the era of transvaginal ultrasound measurement of the cervical length.

Beginning in 1982, three randomized clinical trials of elective cerclage were performed, based on a history of midtrimester loss. Rush et al[36] recruited women who were referred to a reproductive failure clinic, and evaluated whether the policy of performing cerclage prolongs gestation in women with a history of late miscarriage. A total of 194 women were randomized to cerclage or no cerclage. The study population had a very high rate of preterm birth, as expected (33% delivered prior to 37 weeks). The proportion of preterm delivery was 34% in the cerclage group and 32% in the patients who did not undergo cerclage. Women with cerclage had more hospitalizations during pregnancy, a lower birthweight and a higher rate of maternal puerperal fever. Due to the small number of patients in the trial, a subanalysis restricted to women with a history of second-trimester loss was not performed. Lazar et al[37] also failed to show any benefit from cerclage in a larger cohort of 506 women.

The largest randomized study was performed by the Medical Research Council/Royal College of Obstetricians and Gynaecologists (MRC/RCOG).[38]

This was an international multicenter study of women who were considered to be at risk for second-trimester pregnancy loss or preterm delivery by history or previous cervical surgery. However, the treating obstetrician was uncertain of the diagnosis of cervical insufficiency. A total of 1292 women were randomized to cerclage or no cerclage. This was a heterogeneous group of women with one or more risk factors for preterm birth. The 28% overall rate of spontaneous preterm birth prior to 37 weeks was high. The intention-to-treat analysis showed a trend to a lower incidence of preterm labor in the cerclage group compared with the non-cerclage group (26% and 31%, respectively; $p = 0.07$), but this trend did not quite reach statistical significance. However, the trend to a lower preterm labor rate after cerclage did reach statistical significance if 33 weeks was taken as the cut-off point (13% after cerclage vs 17% after no cerclage; $p = 0.03$). In a secondary analysis, stratified by primary risk factor for inclusion in the study, cerclage offered a significant benefit only to women with a history of three or more spontaneous preterm births or second-trimester miscarriages (15% after cerclage vs 32% with no cerclage; $p = 0.015$). There was no advantage from cerclage in women with a history of one or two second-trimester losses. Women who were assigned to cerclage received more tocolytic medications (34% vs to 27% in women without cerclage), and had a higher rate of antepartum hospital admissions (37% vs 29%). Puerperal fever was also more common after cerclage (6% vs 3%; $p = 0.03$). However, it must be noted that women with a definite indication for cerclage (in the opinion of their healthcare provider) were excluded from the study – and this is a major caveat.

A meta-analysis by Drakley et al[39] pooled the results of four trials that together summarized 2062 women. There was no difference in the total pregnancy loss and early (<24 weeks) pregnancy loss rates (relative risk (RR) 0.86; 95% confidence interval (CI) 0.59–1.25). Two trials reported on delivery rates prior to 28 weeks of gestation, and three trials reported on deliveries before 32 weeks. There was no beneficial effect of cerclage (RR 1.29;

95% CI 0.67–2.49). There was also no difference in perinatal deaths (RR 0.8; 95% CI 0.48–1.36) or mean gestational age between the two groups. All four studies reported on preterm delivery at less than 37 weeks of gestation, with no overall significant difference between the two groups (RR 1.04; 95% CI 0.99–1.10). In summary, it appears that the use of cerclage in women with various risk factors for spontaneous preterm birth has little clinical benefit, but is associated with more medical complications and interventions. Women with recurrent preterm birth, including midtrimester losses, represent a population in need of further study.

In 1996, Iams et al[26] described the length of the cervix as measured by transvaginal ultrasound in almost 3000 low-risk women, and found a bell-shaped distribution curve of cervical length among the population, with an inverse relationship between cervical length and the risk of preterm birth. This led to the assumption that cervical length can be used as an indicator of cervical insufficiency. Subsequently, the demonstration of a short cervical length on ultrasound was widely used as an indication for prophylactic cerclage. There have been four recently published randomized clinical trials analyzing the benefit of cerclage in high- and low-risk women based on cervical length. These trials have produced conflicting results. Althuisius et al[40] enrolled 35 women who had risk factors for or symptoms of cervical incompetence and a sonographic cervical length less than 25 mm. This population included women with a clinical history of painless dilatation or early chorioamnion rupture in their previous pregnancies. If painless dilatation or early chorioamnion rupture had occurred in a prior, but not the most recent, gestation, the patient remained eligible for enrollment in the trial if the subsequent pregnancies were managed with cerclage, bed rest or both. Of the 35 women enrolled in the study, the 19 women who were randomly assigned to cerclage and modified bed rest had no preterm births prior to 34 weeks, compared with a 44% preterm birth rate in the 16 women treated by rest alone. Both groups received a 6-day course of broad-spectrum antibiotics, whereas only the cerclage group received preoperative and postoperative indomethacin. Rust et al[41] randomly assigned 138 at-risk women who were found to have a sonographic cervical length of less than 25 mm or more than 25% funneling at 16–24 weeks of gestation to cerclage or to a control group. There was no statistical difference between the cerclage and non-cerclage groups with regard to previous second-trimester loss (12.1% and 27.3%, respectively; $p = 0.07$). The eligible patient population (12% of whom had multifetal gestations) underwent transabdominal amniocentesis before cerclage to rule out intrauterine infection, and both groups were admitted to hospital to receive a 24–48-hour course of antibiotics and indomethacin before discharge home to modified bed rest. Preterm births occurred in 35% of the cerclage group and 36% of the controls. Berghella et al[42] studied women with one or more high-risk factors for preterm birth (one or more preterm births at less than 35 weeks, two or more curettages, DES exposure, cone biopsy, müllerian anomaly, or twin gestation). These women were screened with transvaginal ultrasonography every 2 weeks from 14 weeks up to 24 weeks of gestation. Both asymptomatic women who were at high risk and those who were identified to have a short cervix (< 25 mm) or significant funneling (>25%) were enrolled, but no screened women who were at low risk and who were identified incidentally. Sixty-one women were randomly assigned to receive either McDonald cerclage or bed rest only. Forty-seven pregnancies (77%) were high-risk singleton gestations. Thirty-one women (51%) were allocated to cerclage and 30 women (49%) were allocated to bed rest. Preterm birth (< 35 weeks of gestation) occurred in 14 women (45%) in the cerclage group and in 14 women (47%) in the bed rest group (RR 0.94; 95% CI 0.34–2.58). There was no difference in any obstetric or neonatal outcome. The largest randomized trial to date has been performed by To et al.[43] Cervical length was measured in 47 123 women. The cervix was 15 mm or less in 470 women, 253 (54%) of whom participated in the study. One hundred and twenty-seven women were randomized to undergo cervical cerclage and

126 received expectant management Twenty-two percent (28 of 127 women) in the cerclage group and 26% (33 of 126) of women in the control group had preterm birth prior to 33 weeks (RR 0.84; 95% CI 0.54–1.31; $p = 0.44$). There were no significant differences in perinatal or maternal morbidity or mortality.

Berghella et al[44] have performed a meta-analysis of the four randomized controlled trials described above. The meta-analysis had the support of the authors of each of the trials, and additional data were added for patients whose results were not available at the time of completion of the original reports. In the total population, preterm birth (< 35 weeks) occurred in 29.2% (89/305) of the cerclage group, compared with 34.8% (105/302) of the non-cerclage group (RR 0.84; 95% CI 0.67–1.06). However, there was a significant reduction in preterm births (<35 weeks) in the cerclage group compared with the non-cerclage group in singleton gestations (RR 0.74, CI 0.57–0.96), singleton gestations with prior preterm birth (RR 0.61; 95% CI 0.40–0.92), and singleton gestations with prior second-trimester loss (RR 0.57; 95% CI 0.33–0.99). Berghella et al[44] concluded that cerclage does not prevent preterm birth in all women with a short cervical length on transvaginal ultrasonography, but may reduce the number of preterm births in singleton gestations with a short cervical length, especially in those patients with a prior preterm birth or prior second-trimester loss. Berghella et al,[44] recommended that a sufficiently powered trial should be carried out in this group of patients.

In summary, current evidence suggests the following:

- Cervical cerclage does not reduce the rate of spontaneous preterm birth in women with a sonographically short cervix (≤15 mm) and at low risk for preterm delivery by their history.
- However, recent evidence suggests that cerclage may reduce the incidence of preterm birth prior to 35 weeks in women with a short cervix (≤25 mm) and a history of prior second-trimester loss.

OPTIMAL TIME FOR PLACEMENT OF CERCLAGE

It is debatable whether cerclage should be performed prophylactically at 13–15 weeks of gestation, or whether the procedure should be performed on an emergent basis later in pregnancy when it is found to be definitely indicated by changes in the cervix. Prophylactic cerclage has usually been considered to be preferable, as it is performed when the cervix is closed, before dilatation, before vaginal bacteria can ascend to the membranes, and before the release of cytokines and prostaglandins, all of which occur with cervical dilatation. However, if prophylactic cerclage is performed, a large number of unnecessary procedures will be carried out. Cerclage is not an innocent procedure: it is associated with an increased risk of premature preterm rupture of the membranes, bleeding, and intrauterine infection. Cerclage may also cause severe pain and inconvenience throughout pregnancy. If late cerclage is performed, fewer procedures will be performed, thus reducing the incidence of side-effects. However, effective placement of an 'emergent' cerclage depends on an accurate diagnosis, so that the cerclage is inserted prior to the membranes becoming exposed to the vagina, and prior to dilatation of the external os, and subsequent contractions. Cerclage becomes much less effective if the diagnosis of funneling is missed, and the membranes are exposed to the vagina (leading to infection) and if the external os is dilated.

In order to accept the conclusion of Berghella et al[44] that cerclage may reduce the number of preterm births in singleton gestations with a short cervical length, it is necessary to validate the efficacy of a cerclage that is introduced after the cervix has shortened. Berghella et al[45] have summarized the results of 177 American women with prior second-trimester spontaneous losses between 14 and 24 weeks of gestation. Patients were managed with prophylactic cerclage or serial transvaginal sonograms of the cervix, starting at 14 weeks at the obstetricians' discretion. Cerclage was only performed if the cervical length was less than 25 mm or funneling was greater than 25% of the cervical length prior to 24 weeks of gestation. All cerclages were performed by the McDonald method. Of the 177 patients, 66 received prophylactic cerclage and 111 were followed up with transvaginal sonography, of whom 36% (40/111) had a therapeutic cerclage due to cervical changes. The obstetric outcome, including preterm delivery, was similar whether prophylactic cerclage or late emergent cerclage had been performed. The preterm delivery rates (<35 weeks) were 23% and 21% after prophylactic and late cerclage, respectively ($p = 0.3$). If 33 weeks was taken as the cut-off point, the preterm delivery rate was 21% and 26%, respectively ($p = 0.5$). Nor was there any difference in the gestational age at delivery whether prophylactic (34.6 ± 6.8 weeks) or emergent (34.4 ± 6.8 weeks; $p = 0.8$) cerclage had been performed. Groom et al[46] found similar results in a British population. Thirty-nine women undergoing elective cervical cerclage were matched with women undergoing serial ultrasound surveillance of cervical length with regard to maternal age, ethnic group, previous cervical surgery, previous second-trimester loss and early preterm delivery. Cerclage was performed in 14 (36%) of the 'ultrasound surveillance' patients due to cervical changes. There was no significant difference in median gestation at delivery (266 days after elective cerclage and 260 days after emergent cerclage, $p = 0.9$), number of women delivering before 24 weeks (15% and 13%, respectively; $p = 0.9$), number at 24–32 weeks (7.5% and 15%, respectively; $p = 0.6$), and number at 32–37 weeks (15% and 13%, respectively; $p = 0.9$). Based on these two studies, it appears that in women at high risk of preterm delivery, serial transvaginal ultrasound surveillance of cervical length appears to reduce the number of cerclage procedures performed, without compromising pregnancy outcome.

EMERGENCY CERCLAGE

As stated above, cerclage becomes less effective once the external os is dilated, and the membranes are exposed to the vagina (leading to infection). Two trials have compared cerclage with expectant management with bed rest after cervical dilatation.[47,48]

Both of these studies reported a beneficial effect from cerclage. In the CIPRACT trial,[47] 23 women were randomized to have an emergency cerclage or bed rest. The inclusion criteria were prolapsed membranes through the dilated cervix. Thirteen women were randomized to have a cerclage, and 10 women to bed rest alone. One woman in the cerclage group had a known complication of cerclage in these conditions – rupture of the membranes during the procedure. Cerclage was therefore abandoned. Delivery was delayed by a mean of 54 days in the cerclage group, compared with 24 days in the bed rest group ($p = 0.046$). The prevalence of preterm delivery before 34 weeks of gestation was significantly lower in the cerclage group (7 of 13 women), compared with all of the 10 women in the bed rest group ($p = 0.02$).

The inclusion criteria for the study by Olatunbosun et al[48] were slightly different, requiring a cervical dilatation of at least 4 cm at 20–27 weeks of gestation. The study was prospective and included 43 women. However, the trial was not randomized, and management was chosen by the attending obstetrician. Twenty-three women received a cerclage, whereas 20 women were treated with bed rest. The cerclage failed in one patient, and five of the women due to have bed rest were eventually given a cerclage. The mean gestational age at delivery was 33 ± 4.4 weeks after cerclage, which was significantly later than the 28.8 ± 4.4 weeks in the bed rest group ($p = 0.001$).

The results of both these studies suggest that emergency cerclage should be performed, if possible, in an attempt to delay labor. However, clinical judgment is necessary in order to select patients who may benefit. The presence of infection, frequent contractions, etc. make the procedure less likely to succeed, and increases the possibility of side-effects such as tearing of the cervix if cervical dilatation continues. The addition of tocolytic agents and prophylactic antibiotics at the time of cerclage may increase the efficacy of the procedure. In cases of emergency cerclage, a modified McDonald procedure is usually performed, as there is often little tissue to grasp and this is often the only procedure possible.

SUMMARY

Patients with RPL are at a high risk for midtrimester loss and preterm labor. The increased risk is present even if all previous pregnancy losses have been in the first trimester. Cervical incompetence may be more common in women with RPL due to the large number of previous curettages. Additionally, there may be cervical tears from previous labors that may cause recurrent second-trimester losses in a secondary aborter (one or more labors followed by a string of pregnancy losses). If there are obvious tears of the cervix and a typical history of painless dilatation of the cervix in the second trimester, prophylactic cerclage is indicated, and the suture should be placed high enough to prevent cervical dilatation. This may require the use of the Shirodkar technique or an abdominal approach. If there are no apparent tears but the patient is at a high risk for second-trimester loss or preterm labor, ultrasound should be performed serially, probably on a weekly basis, in order to detect cervical shortening. Cervical shortening is not in itself an indication for cerclage. However, women with the combination of prior second-trimester loss and a cervical length of less than 25 mm or funneling of greater than 25% of the cervical length before 24 weeks may have a reduced rate of preterm birth with cerclage. There is no benefit to be gained from prophylactic cerclage compared with cerclage performed due to cervical changes. In the low-risk patient with RPL, clinical follow-up may be sufficient, and ultrasound can be reserved for those patients in whom it is clinically indicated.

In imminent preterm delivery with a dilated external os and prolapse of the membranes, emergency cerclage seems to be beneficial if technically possible, and if there are no complicating factors such as infection or uterine contractions.

REFERENCES

1. Shirodkar VN. A new method of operative treatment for habitual abortions in the second trimester of pregnancy. Antiseptic 1955; 52:299–300.
2. Buckingham JC, Buethe RA, Danforth DN. Collagen–muscle ratio in clinically normal and clinically incompetent cervices. Am J Obstet Gynecol 1965; 92:232–7.
3. Roddick JW, Buckingham JC, Danforth DN. The muscular cervix – a cause of incompetency in pregnancy. Obstet Gynecol 1961; 17:562–5.
4. Rechberger T, Uldbjerg N, Oxlund H. Connective tissue changes in the cervix during normal pregnancy and pregnancy complicated by cervical incompetence. Obstet Gynecol 1988; 71:563–7.
5. Petersen LK, Uldbjerg N. Cervical collagen in non-pregnant women with previous cervical incompetence. Eur J Obstet Gynecol Reprod Biol 1996; 67:41–5.
6. Leppert PC, Yu SY, Keller S, et al. Decreased elastic fibers and desmosine content in incompetent cervix. Am J Obstet Gynecol 1987; 157:1134–9.
7. Iams JD. Prediction and early detection of preterm labor. Obstet Gynecol 2003; 101:402–12.
8. Page EW. Incompetent internal os of the cervix causing late abortion and premature labor. Technique for surgical repair. Obstet Gynecol 1958; 12:509–15.
9. Toaff R, Toaff ME, Ballas S, et al. Cervical incompetence: diagnostic and therapeutic aspects. Isr J Med Sci 1977; 13:39–49.
10. Bergman P, Svennerud S. Traction test for demonstrating incompetence of the internal os of the cervix. Int J Fertil 1957; 2:163–7.
11. Jeffcoate TNA, Wilson JK. Uterine causes of abortion and premature labor. NY State J Med 1956; 56:680–90.
12. Fournil C, Hidden J, Lajoux P. Evaluation du calibre de l'isthme utérin en début de grossesse. Intérêt dans l'indication du cerclage du col. Nouv Presse Med 1977; 6:523–4, 531–3.
13. Bouyer J, Papiernik E, Dreyfus J, et al. Maturation signs of the cervix and prediction of preterm birth. Obstet Gynecol 1986; 68:209–14.
14. Catalano PM, Ashikaga T, Mann LI. Cervical change and uterine activity as predictors of preterm delivery. Am J Perinatol 1989; 6:185–90.
15. Sarti DA, Sample WF, Hobel CJ, et al. Ultrasonic visualization of a dilated cervix during pregnancy. Radiology 1979; 130:417–20.
16. Andersen HF. Transvaginal and transabdominal ultrasonography of the uterine cervix during pregnancy. J Clin Ultrasound 1991; 19:77–83.
17. Confino E, Mayden KL, Giglia RV, et al. Pitfalls in sonographic imaging of the incompetent uterine cervix. Acta Obstet Gynecol Scand 1986; 65:593–7.
18. Andersen HF, Nugent CE, Wanty SD, et al. Prediction of risk for preterm delivery by ultrasonographic measurement of cervical length. Am J Obstet Gynecol 1990; 163:859–67.
19. Berghella V, Kuhlman K, Weiner S, et al. Cervical funneling: sonographic criteria predictive of preterm delivery. Ultrasound Obstet Gynecol 1997; 10:161–6.
20. Sheiner E, Levy A, Katz M, et al. Pregnancy outcome following recurrent spontaneous abortions. Eur J Obst Gynecol Reprod Biol 2005; 118:61–5.
21. Hughes N, Hamilton EF, Tulandi T. Obstetric outcome in women after multiple spontaneous abortions. J Reprod Med 1991; 36:165–6.
22. Guzman ER, Vintzileos AM, McLean DA, et al. The natural history of a positive response to transfundal pressure in women at risk for cervical incompetence. Am J Obstet Gynecol 1997; 176:634–8.
23. Althuisius SM, Dekker GA, van Geijn HP, et al. Cervical Incompetence Prevention Randomized Cerclage Trial (CIPRACT): study design and preliminary results. Am J Obstet Gynecol 2000; 183:823–9.
24. Ludmir J, Landon MB, Gabbe SG, et al. Management of the diethylstilbestrol-exposed pregnant patient: a prospective study. Am J Obstet Gynecol 1987; 157:665–9.
25. Mangan CE, Borow L, Burtnett-Rubin MM, et al. Pregnancy outcome in 98 women exposed to diethylstilbestrol in utero, their mothers, and unexposed siblings. Obstet Gynecol 1982; 59:315–19.

26. Iams JD, Goldenberg RL, Meis PJ, et al. The length of the cervix and the risk of spontaneous premature delivery. N Engl J Med 1996; 334: 567–72.

27. Michaels WH, Schreiber FR, Padgett RJ, et al. Ultrasound surveillance of the cervix in twin gestations: management of cervical incompetency. Obstet Gynecol 1991; 78:739–44.

28. Kristensen J, Langhoff-Roos J, Wittrup M, et al. Cervical conization and preterm delivery/low birth weight. A systematic review of the literature. Acta Obstet Gynecol Scand 1993; 72:640–4.

29. Wright CSW, Campbell S, Beazley J. Second-trimester abortion after vaginal termination of pregnancy. Lancet 1972; i:1278–9.

30. McDonald IA. Suture of the cervix for inevitable miscarriage. J Obstet Gynaecol Br Emp 1957; 146:346–50.

31. McDonald IA. Incompetent cervix as a cause of recurrent abortion. J Obstet Gynaecol Br Commonw 1963; 70:105–9.

32. Davis G, Berghella V, Talucci M, et al. Patients with a prior failed transvaginal cerclage: a comparison of obstetric outcomes with either transabdominal or transvaginal cerclage. Am J Obstet Gynecol 2000; 183:836–9.

33. Scibetta JJ, Sanko SR, Phipps WR. Laparoscopic transabdominal cervicoisthmic cerclage. Fertil Steril 1998; 69:161–3.

34. Anthony GS, Walker RG, Cameron AD, et al. Transabdominal cervicoisthmic cerclage in the management of cervical incompetence. Eur J Obstet Gynecol Reprod Biol 1997; 72:127–30.

35. Topping J, Farquharson RG. Transabdominal cervical cerclage. Br J Hosp Med 1995; 54:510–12.

36. Rush RW, Isaacs S, McPherson K, et al. A randomized controlled trial of cervical cerclage in women at high risk of spontaneous preterm delivery. Br J Obstet Gynaecol 1984; 91:724–30.

37. Lazar P, Gueguen S, Dreyfus J, et al. Multicentred controlled trial of cervical cerclage in women at moderate risk of preterm delivery. Br J Obstet Gynaecol 1984; 91:731–5.

38. Quinn M. Final report of the MRC/RCOG randomised controlled trial of cervical cerclage. Br J Obstet Gynaecol 1993; 100:1154–5.

39. Drakeley AJ, Roberts D, Alfirevic Z. Cervical cerclage for prevention of preterm delivery: meta-analysis of randomized trials. Obstet Gynecol 2003; 102:621–7.

40. Althuisius SM, Dekker GA, Hummel P, et al. Final results of the Cervical Incompetence Prevention Randomized Cerclage Trial (CIPRACT): therapeutic cerclage with bed rest versus bed rest alone. Am J Obstet Gynecol 2001; 185:1106–12.

41. Rust OA, Atlas RO, Reed J, et al. Revisiting the short cervix detected by transvaginal ultrasound in the second trimester: why cerclage therapy may not help. Am J Obstet Gynecol 2001; 185:1098–105.

42. Berghella V, Odibo AO, Tolosa JE. Cerclage for prevention of preterm birth in women with a short cervix found on transvaginal examination: a randomized trial. Am J Obstet Gynecol 2004; 191:1311–17.

43. To MS, Alfirevic Z, Heath VCF, et al. Cervical cerclage for prevention of preterm delivery in women with short cervix: randomized controlled trial. Lancet 2004; 363:1849–53.

44. Berghella V, Odibo OA, To MS, et al. Cervix on ultrasonography: meta-analysis of trials using individual patient-level data. Obstet Gynecol 2005; 106:181–9.

45. Berghella V, Haas S, Chervoneva I, et al. Patients with prior second-trimester loss: prophylactic cerclage or serial transvaginal sonograms? Am J Obstet Gynecol 2002; 187:747–51.

46. Groom KM, Bennett PR, Golara M, et al. Elective cervical cerclage versus serial ultrasound surveillance of cervical length in a population at high risk for preterm delivery. Eur J Obstet Gynecol Reprod Biol 2004; 112:158–61.

47. Althuisius SM, Dekker GA, Hummel P, et al. Cervical Incompetence Prevention Randomized Cerclage Trial (CIPRACT): emergency cerclage with bed rest versus bed rest alone. Am J Obstet Gynecol 2003; 189:907–10.

48. Olatunbosun OA, al-Nuaim L, Turnell RW. Emergency cerclage compared with bed rest for advanced cervical dilatation in pregnancy. Int Surg 1995; 80:170–4.

15. Midtrimester loss and viability

Victor YH Yu

INTRODUCTION

In Chapter 16 it is shown that women with recurrent miscarriage have a higher incidence of preterm labor. In addition, uterine anomalies and cervical incompetence are two causes of recurrent pregnancy loss (RPL) that predispose to second-trimester fetal loss. Women with recurrent second-trimester fetal loss contribute disproportionately to the stillbirth rate, and second-trimester delivery of live births contributes disproportionately to the neonatal mortality rate, thus significantly increasing the overall perinatal mortality rate. However, a proactive policy of transfer in utero of high-risk pregnancies in danger of extremely preterm delivery to a tertiary perinatal centre for management by maternal–fetal medicine specialists, together with competent resuscitation at birth and prompt initiation of neonatal intensive care by neonatologists, has been found to improve survival and quality-adjusted survival for extremely low-birthweight (ELBW) infants born under 1000 g, including those born in the second trimester between 23 and 26 weeks' gestation. Clinical protocols have been established for the management of those infants born alive at borderline viability, but continued advances made in the knowledge and technology in neonatal intensive care will result in ongoing revisions of current medicolegal and ethical guidelines. Principles behind decision-making on initiating and withdrawing intensive care will, however, remain interpersonal and intimate, respectful to the infants' lives and their parents' autonomy, and sensitive to the emotional concerns of parents and staff.

CONTRIBUTION OF EXTREME PREMATURITY TO PERINATAL MORTALITY

The State of Victoria in Australia has a population of about 6 million and a birth rate of about 15 per 1000. The legal requirements for birth registrations in the State are that a stillbirth must be registered if the gestation was 20 weeks or above or, if the period of gestation was not known, the birthweight was 400 g or more. Any infant, regardless of maturity or birthweight, who shows any sign of life after being born must be registered as a live birth (and if death subsequently occurred within 28 days, as a neonatal death). Regional statewide perinatal mortality figures are generated from the information thus collected.[1] For the purpose of perinatal statistics, a stillbirth is defined as a stillborn infant weighing at least 500 g or, if the weight is not known, born after at least 22 weeks' gestation. A neonatal death is defined as a death occurring within 28 days of birth in an infant whose birthweight is at least 500 g or, if the weight is not known, an infant born after at least 22 weeks.

For the year 2002, there were a total of 62 622 births (of which 267 were stillbirths) in Victoria. The perinatal mortality rate, based on the above definitions, was 6.9 per 1000 births (stillbirth rate 4.2 per 1000, neonatal death rate 2.7 per 1000). For the purpose of international comparison, the World Health Organization (WHO) recommends the publication of a standard mortality rate in which the numerator and denominator are restricted to heavier and more mature infants. A stillbirth is thus defined as a stillborn infant weighing at least 1000 g

Table 15.1 Contribution of low-birthweight and preterm births to perinatal deaths in the State of Victoria

	Percentage of births	Percentage of perinatal deaths
Birthweight		
<2500 g	5.9	66
<1500 g	1.1	44
<1000 g	0.5	35
Gestation		
<37 weeks	6.0	67
<32 weeks	1.1	43
<28 weeks	0.4	29

or, if the weight is not known, born after at least 28 weeks' gestation. A neonatal death is defined as a death occurring within 7 days of birth in an infant whose birthweight is at least 1000 g or, if the weight is not known, in an infant born after at least 28 weeks. In Victoria, the perinatal mortality rate, in accordance with these WHO definitions, was 3.2 per 1000 births (stillbirth rate 2.4 per 1000, neonatal death rate 0.8 per 1000). Table 15.1 shows that ELBW infants have a major impact on perinatal mortality statistics that is disproportional to their numbers.

CHANGING VIABILITY IN EXTREMELY
PRETERM INFANTS

Population-based studies from a designated geographical region, rather than from a single institution, are essential for the assessment of the true impact of maternal–fetal and neonatal intensive care practices on the survival and long-term neurodevelopmental outcome of extremely preterm live births. Significant numbers of preterm infants born outside perinatal centers might not be transferred by a neonatal emergency transport service (NETS) to institutions with a neonatal intensive care unit (NICU), and they would die at their hospital of birth. Our research group, the Victorian Infant Collaborative Study (VICS), has been reporting

on the long-term outcome of a population-based ELBW cohort born in the State of Victoria since 1979–80 and up to 14 years of age.[2–7] Within the State, there are three level III perinatal centers, each with its NICU, and a fourth stand-alone NICU in a children's hospital. There are 20 level II special-care units and 150 level I maternity units with small neonatal nurseries attached.

PLACE OF BIRTH AND OUTCOME

The three perinatal centers deliver only about one-quarter of births in the State of Victoria. However, 70% of ELBW births were being delivered in the three hospitals even during these early years, indicating that there was already an effective effort being made to identify women with high-risk pregnancies who might deliver an ELBW infant, and they were being referred in utero by midwives and obstetricians in the community for consultation by maternal–fetal medicine specialists within our perinatal centers. For the remaining 30% ELBW infants who were born outside the perinatal centers, less than half (42%) were transferred for neonatal intensive care after birth; those not referred, with very few exceptions, died. The perinatal mortality rate of ELBW infants was significantly lower in those born in the perinatal centers compared with those born elsewhere (72% vs 93%), as were the stillbirth rate (36% vs 59%) and neonatal death rate (56% vs 82%).[8,9]

The VICS study defined long-term disability as severe if the child had cerebral palsy and was unable to walk, low IQ defined as a psychological test score of more than two standard deviations (SD) below the mean, or bilateral blindness. Not only did our inborn ELBW infants have a significantly higher survival rate compared with those who were outborn, but the inborn survivors also had a significantly lower severe disability rate: 15% versus 50% at 2 years, 15% versus 38% at 5 years, 13% versus 39% at 8 years, and 10% versus 30% at 14 years. Their high disability rate was attributable to suboptimal perinatal care, which was identified in 72% of outborn survivors, secondary to a failure or a delay in initiating intensive care among these outborn infants.

TRANSFER IN UTERO IMPROVES OUTCOME

The benefits of a more proactive transfer-in-utero policy to level III perinatal centers for management were established when this early VICS regional cohort was compared with later VICS regional cohorts born in 1985–87. Not only was there a significant 50% improvement in ELBW survival rate in 1985–87 compared with 1979–80, but there was also a significant reduction in the disability rate among ELBW survivors at our 2-year assessment: severe from 18% to 11%, moderate from 5% to 1%, and mild from 28% to 18%.[10] In this study, severe disability was defined as cerebral palsy in children unlikely ever to walk, Bayley Mental Developmental Index (MDI) below 69, or bilateral blindness; moderate disability was defined as cerebral palsy in non-ambulant children who were likely to walk or sensorineural deafness requiring amplification; and mild disability was defined as cerebral palsy in ambulant children and Bayley MDI of 69–84.

The VICS study identified that the primary factor in the improved outcome was the significant increase in the proportion of the State's ELBW infants born within the three perinatal centers (from 70% to 77%). A secondary factor was a greater number of outborn ELBW live births who received resuscitation and prompt intensive care even at the level II hospitals prior to the arrival of NETS.[11] At 5 years of age, severe cerebral palsy was reduced from 3% to 1%, blindness from 7% to 3%, deafness from 6% to 0.5%, IQ score <2 SD from 21% to 7%, and IQ score <3 SD from 9% to 4%.[12] However, these figures still show a large number of disabilities.

FURTHER IMPROVEMENT IN OUTCOME IN RECENT ERAS

The VICS study reported that the proportion of ELBW infants who were inborn at the level III perinatal centers continued to increase to 84% in 1991–92 and to 91% in 1997.[13,14] As a result, a greater number had the benefit of proactive resuscitation and prompt intensive care initiated after birth.[15,16] Table 15.2 shows that this has resulted in a progressively improved survival rate, as well as an

Table 15.2 Improving survival and quality-adjusted (QA) survival in a population-based study of extremely low-birthweight (ELBW) infants

Birthweight	Percentage of ELBW infants in the time period			
	1979–80 (n = 351)	1985–87 (n = 560)	1991–92 (n = 429)	1997 (n = 233)
500–599 g:				
Survival	0	0	16	52
QA survival	0	0	13	35
600–699 g:				
Survival	7	12	38	56
QA survival	5	10	27	43
700–799 g:				
Survival	22	33	48	83
QA survival	14	29	43	64
800–899 g:				
Survival	35	51	72	73
QA survival	28	44	60	63
900–999 g:				
Survival	43	65	79	87
QA survival	33	53	70	76
Total:				
Survival	25	38	56	73
QA survival	19	32	48	59

improved adjusted survival rate, secondary to a reduction in the proportion of survivors with disability.[17] Another benefit that has been identified is that, in spite of an increase in the consumption of hospital resources that inevitably results from a proactive treatment policy, economic evaluation of efficiency in terms of cost–effectiveness and cost–utility has remained unchanged.[18–20]

RISK OF RECURRENT PREGNANCY LOSS AND PREMATURITY

Women with a history of pregnancy loss, when compared with those who have delivered a live birth, are known to have a higher risk of pregnancy loss in previous and subsequent pregnancies. In our study of women who had delivered an ELBW infant, the frequency of pregnancy loss in previous pregnancies was 41% and that in subsequent pregnancies was 31%.[21] These rates are higher than that of 10–20% reported for our general population. The perinatal mortality rate is also known to increase more than threefold among women with one prior preterm birth and at least one prior pregnancy loss. In our study of women who had delivered an ELBW infant, the perinatal mortality rate of their subsequent pregnancies was 51.7 per 1000 births. This was four times higher than that reported for our general population in the same time period (12.8 per 1000 births of at least 20 weeks' gestation and 400 g birthweight). We also know that significantly more infants are born preterm when there is a previous history of perinatal loss or prematurity. In our study of women who had delivered an ELBW infant, the prematurity rate was 28% and the low-birthweight rate was 34% in subsequent pregnancies, which was about six times higher than that of the general population. Those women who had a diagnosis of cervical incompetence were at the highest risk of a subsequent preterm birth. The low-birthweight rates among live births subsequent to the birth of an ELBW infant in our study were 36% less than 2500 g, 11% less than 1500 g, and 5% less than 1000 g.

OUTCOME ACCORDING TO GESTATIONAL AGE

The use of birthweight as a framework for the reporting of outcome data is a convenient system for neonatologists, who have an accurate measurement on which to base the study. However, gestational age, not birthweight, is the parameter used by obstetricians as a guide to critical decisions on the management of the mother and fetus. A proactive attitude among physicians in recent years has improved the survival prospects even among extremely preterm births of less than 26 weeks' gestation.[22] There is a tendency to underestimate birthweight in preterm infants before birth, and the perinatal mortality of those with clinical underestimation of birthweight is known to be higher than that of those with correctly estimated birthweight. Therefore, studies with gestation as an independent variable in determining outcome are necessary to assist obstetricians, neonatologists, and parents in their decision-making process, especially prior to an extreme preterm birth.[23–25]

The first VICS regional cohort based on a gestational age cohort consisted of 316 infants consecutively born in the three years 1985–87, at 24–26 weeks' gestation.[26] Gestational age was calculated from dates obtained by menstrual history, usually confirmed by ultrasound before 20 weeks' gestation. Of the 95 five-year-old survivors, one was untraced but was assessed at two years to be free of disability. The overall survival rate to 5 years was 30% and the severe disability rate among survivors was 11% (Table 15.3). There was no trend toward increasing disability with lower gestational age. Cerebral palsy was diagnosed in 13%, bilateral blindness in 5%, deafness requiring hearing aids in 2%, and IQ more than 2 SD below the mean in 7%. These outcome data were mostly favorable, and better than those reported in other contemporaneous regional cohorts born in other parts of the world.

Postnatal surfactant replacement therapy was introduced for routine clinical use in 1991 in Victoria. It has been proven to reduce mortality in randomized controlled trials within NICUs, but regional data are vital to assess the impact of such a therapeutic innovation on a whole population. Therefore, in our post-surfactant era (1991–92), VICS studied 401 infants consecutively born at 23–27 weeks' gestation in Victoria.[27] Of the 225 two-year extremely preterm survivors, 219 (97%) were assessed, in addition to 242 contemporaneous normal-birthweight

Table 15.3 Extremely preterm infants: survival and disability rates among survivors in three eras

	1985–87	1991–92	1997
Survival rate	($n = 316$)	($n = 401$)	($n = 208$)
23 weeks	0%	10%	41%
24 weeks	12%	33%	41%
25 weeks	28%	58%	73%
26 weeks	45%	72%	88%
27 weeks	—	77%	86%
Degree of disability	($n = 95$)	($n = 219$)	($n = 148$)
Severe	11%	8%	16%
Moderate	7%	13%	12%
Mild	25%	25%	24%
None	61%	54%	49%

controls, in whom 2% were found to have severe disability. Compared with our regional 1985–1987 cohort from the pre-surfactant era, the survival rate had improved significantly (Table 15.3) with no significant change in their severe disability rate (20% at 23 weeks 14% at 24 weeks, 6% at 25 weeks, 9% at 26 weeks, and 1% at 27 weeks). The rate of blindness was, however, significantly lower in 1991–92 (from 5% to 2%).

When parents are counseled at different time periods before and after the birth of their extremely preterm infant, they wish to know not only whether their child will survive but also whether their child will survive with or without disability. The 1991–92 VICS regional cohort of infants born at 23–27 weeks' gestation was assessed again at 5 years of age to allow a more certain estimate of disability, and to determine how the prognosis offered to parents changed with increasing postnatal age and when different perinatal variables were taken into account.[28] Of the 401 extremely preterm infants 67 (17%) were born outside level III perinatal centers. Their place of birth was a significant factor for survival: 62% for inborn infants and 28% for outborn infants. The attitude of the attending physician determined whether or not intensive care was offered. Overall, 16% of live births at 23–27 weeks were not offered intensive care and died on the first day: 69% at 23 weeks, 35% at 24 weeks, 6% at 25 weeks, 2% at 26 weeks, and 1% at 27 weeks. Of inborn infants, 9% were not offered intensive care, compared with 54% of outborn infants. Variables that were associated positively with survival on day 1 were increasing maturity, antenatal corticosteroid therapy, multiple births, female sex, and not being small for gestational age, and on day 7, grade 3 or 4 cerebroventricular hemorrhage. Outcome data were available for 221 (98%) survivors (and 245 contemporaneous normal-birthweight controls): non-ambulatory cerebral palsy was diagnosed in 7%, bilateral blindness in 2%, deafness requiring hearing aids in 1%, and IQ score more than 2 SD below the mean for the normal-birthweight controls in 15%. Variables that were associated positively with survival free of major disability on day 1 were postnatal

surfactant therapy plus the other factors associated with survival per se. On day 28 and at hospital discharge, variables significantly associated with a lower rate of survival free of major disability were grade 3 or 4 cerebroventricular hemorrhage, cystic periventricular leukomalacia, postnatal dexamethasone therapy, and surgery. Almost half (47%) of the extremely preterm survivors had none of these adverse prognostic variables, and their major disability rate was 7%, which was not significantly different from the rate of 3% for normal-birthweight children. The risks of major disability increased to 17% with one adverse variable, 47% with two variables, and 67% with three variables.

The most recent VICS regional cohort based on gestational age consisted of 208 consecutive live births at 23–27 weeks' gestation and 188 contemporaneous normal-birthweight controls born in Victoria during 1997.[29] Compared with our regional 1991–92 cohort, the survival rate to 2 years of age had improved at each week of gestation, with no significant changes in the disability rate (Table 15.3). Since the gain from a significant increase in survival was greater than the loss from a marginal increase in disability among survivors, the rate of survival free of disability was higher in 1997 compared with 1991–92, both overall and in all gestational age subgroups. There was no gestational age below which most survivors were disabled.

COMPARISON WITH OTHER REGIONAL STUDIES

In a review of survival rates for extremely preterm infants born in North America, none of the studies had regional or population-based cohorts that could be directly compared with our VICS study.[30] Two regional cohorts reported from the UK had survival rates at individual weeks' of gestation lower than that in our study. In the Trent region of England, with an annual birth rate similar to that Victoria (60 000), the survival rates to discharge home in a cohort from 1994 to 1997 were 14% at 23 weeks, 26% at 24 weeks, 41% at 25 weeks, 61% at 25 weeks, 75% at 27 weeks, and 85% at 28 weeks.[31] For the same time period, survival rates from our VICS cohort

Table 15.4 Comparison between the population-based VICS and EPICure data for infants born at 23–25 weeks' gestation

	VICS 1991–92	EPICure 1995	VICS 1997
Survival rate	38%	29%	69%
23 weeks	10%	10%	41%
24 weeks	33%	26%	41%
25 weeks	58%	43%	73%
Disability rate	8%	15%	13%

were 25% at 23 weeks, 46% at 24 weeks, 79% at 25 weeks, 85% at 26 weeks, 82% at 27 weeks, and 91% at 28 weeks. The EPICure study reported the outcome at 2½ years of 23–25-week gestation live births born in the UK in 1995.[32] Comparative data from the VICS study of cohorts born both prior to the EPICure cohort (1991–92) and after the EPICure cohort (1997) are shown in Table 15.4. The 1991–92 Australian cohort, which was 3 years before the 1995 UK cohort, already had better survival, and the survival rate of the infants born at 23–25 weeks' gestation in the 1997 Australian cohort was more than double that of the UK cohort (69% vs 29%). Hospital survival rates reported from a regional cohort from the Netherlands relating to infants born in 1995 were extremely poor. The majority of deaths in that study at 23 and 24 weeks occurred before admission to the NICU: 2% at 23 weeks, 3% at 24 weeks, 29% at 25 weeks, and 54% at 26 weeks.[33] Disability rates in regional cohorts of infants born at 23–25 weeks' gestation were 15% in the EPICure study,[32] 35% in the Trent region,[34] and 45% in the Netherlands.[35] In comparison, the rates reported in the VICS study were 8% in our 1991–92 cohort and 13% in our 1997 cohort, despite a significantly higher survival rate, especially in the 1997 cohort (Table 15.4).

ETHICAL DILEMMAS FOLLOWING EXTREMELY PRETERM BIRTH

Ethical problems of selective non-treatment arise in caring for extremely preterm infants when clinical decisions have to be made after the birth of a live-born infant to either withhold or withdraw intensive care.[36] Studies have shown great variability in doctors' attitudes and their management policies for extreme prematurity. There is a tendency for both obstetricians and neonatologists to underestimate the potential for survival and overestimate the risks of disability for extremely preterm infants.[37–39] Many neonatologists continue to selectively resuscitatd extremely preterm infants at birth, which means that liveborn infants are left to die through withholding of intensive care. If doctors believe that the infant has little prospect for survival or survival without disability, it is probable that their clinical management would be delayed or less than optimal, and may in fact be creating a self-fulfilling prophecy.[40] An Australian survey in the 1980s had shown at that time that a great number of neonatologists selectively resuscitated extremely preterm infants at birth, suggesting that many of these live births were left to die through withholding of neonatal intensive care.[37] More recent national surveys conducted in 2000 showed a more proactive resuscitation policy among Australian obstetricians and neonatologists (Table 15.5).[38,39]

DECISION TO WITHHOLD INTENSIVE CARE

In the majority of level III perinatal centers within developed countries, all infants with a birthweight of more than 500 g or a gestation of 24 weeks or more are offered intensive care. At Monash Medical Centre (MMC) in Australia, we have reported that 10% of 442 extremely preterm live births born at 23–28 weeks' gestation over the 10-year period 1977–86, were not offered intensive care, 4% had

Table 15.5 Percentage of Australian doctors who would recommend to parents that their extremely preterm infants be resuscitated at the time of birth

	22 weeks	23 weeks	24 weeks	25 weeks
Obstetricians	9%	33%	59%	79%
Neonatologists	13%	48%	92%	100%

obvious major malformations, and 6% were considered 'non-viable', for which resuscitation at birth was not offered or was not successful.[41] The proportion of live births in which treatment was withheld at the time of delivery was 37% at 23 weeks, 17% at 24 weeks, 8% at 25 weeks, 1% at 26 weeks, 1% at 27 weeks, and 0% at 28 weeks. This approach to offering intensive care was considered ahead of its time, even in developed countries 20–30 years ago.[42] During an identical period, 1977–86, in another level III perinatal center within a few kilometers of MMC, 42% of similar live births born at 24–26 weeks' gestation were not offered intensive care, all of whom died.[41] This accounted for a lower survival rate among their infants born at 23–28 weeks' gestation compared with those in MMC (29% vs 44%), as the survival rate among those who were offered intensive care was similar. Our practice during the 1990s was consistent with what the Royal College of Paediatrics and Child Health in the UK published in 1997, which stated that it would not be unreasonable to consider withholding treatment in an infant born at 23 weeks' weighing little more than 500 g.[43] There is a general consensus in developed countries, even to this day, that parents of a 22-week infant should be discouraged from seeking active treatment, whereas those of a 25–26-week infant should be encouraged to consent to intensive care.[44] It is reasonable not to offer resuscitation for all 23–24-week infants, who should be assessed on an individual basis at the time of birth.

DECISION TO WITHDRAW INTENSIVE CARE

However, a proactive policy to initiate intensive care must take into consideration that a decision to withdraw such care might have to be made in selective infants at a later stage in the course of the treatment. In the event that the infant's subsequent clinical course indicates that further curative efforts are futile or lack compensating benefit, intensive care should be discontinued and palliative care, which provides symptomatic relief and comfort, should be introduced. This approach, termed 'individualized prognostic strategy' has been advocated as an acceptable and preferred mode of operation in the NICU, one that has been endorsed by the Canadian Pediatric Society and the American Academy of Pediatrics.[45,46] The attending neonatologist has the primary role as an advocate for the infant and medical advisor to the parents, whereas the parents act as surrogates for their infant. The shift in emphasis from curative to palliative treatment requires consensus among all those involved in the care of the infant, both medical and nursing staff, as well as consent from the parents, who should be closely involved in this widely shared decision-making process. At MMC, over the 8-year period 1981–87, intensive care was withdrawn prior to death in 65% of 316 deaths.[47] Among these infants, death was considered to be inevitable in the short term, even with the continuation of neonatal intensive care in 70% of the cases. In the remainder, the risk of severe brain damage was considered to be so great that death was considered preferable to a life with major disability. Therefore, in our NICU, full treatment until death is uncommon and occurred in only one-third of cases. This experience was not unique, as studies from the UK and New Zealand have shown that 30–80% of deaths in their NICUs follow a deliberate withdrawal of life-sustaining treatment.[48,49]

There are three clinical situations in which selective withdrawal of intensive care is appropriate.

- Firstly, there are few who would disagree that withdrawal of intensive care is morally and ethically acceptable when death is considered to be inevitable and the infant is in the process of dying, whatever treatment is provided. Intensive care would be considered in these cases a futile exercise and not in the best interest of the infant. Examples in this category include those infants with severe respiratory failure or fulminating sepsis who have persistent or worsening hypoxemia, acidosis, and hypotension unresponsive to ventilatory and inotropic support. There is no obligation to provide futile medical care in such cases, as no infant with progressive multiple organ failure survives even with the provision of cardiopulmonary resuscitation.

- Secondly, it is appropriate also to consider withdrawal of intensive care even when death is not inevitable with continued treatment, but where there is a significantly high risk of severe physical and mental disability should the infant survive. Such a decision should not raise too many moral and ethical problems if the infant's development of self-awareness and intentional action is believed to be virtually impossible or there is no prospect of the infant ever being able to act on his or her own behalf. One scenario is that of an extremely preterm infant with large bilateral parenchymal hemorrhages, infarcts, and/or leukomalacia in the brain.
- Thirdly, a more controversial issue is when survival with moderate disability is possible with treatment, but the infant is likely to suffer persistent pain, require recurrent hospitalization and invasive treatment throughout life, and to experience early death in childhood or early adulthood. This situation may arise with a preterm infant with severe chronic lung disease non-responsive to dexamethasone and with no prospect of being weaned from mechanical ventilation, but for whom lung transplant is still considered an experimental option.

The one principle shared by all the guidelines proposed in the UK, Canada, USA, and Australia is that if continued life for the infant with treatment is a worse outcome than death, then the principle of *primum non nocere* imposes a professional, moral, and humanitarian duty upon neonatologists to withhold or withdraw life-sustaining treatment. Infants cannot benefit from such treatment, and death is not the worst outcome for them if they cannot be rescued from irreversible medical deterioration and death, cannot have life prolonged without major sensorineural sequelae, and cannot be relieved of ongoing pain and suffering. When the process of dying is being artificially prolonged, most would agree that the harm of continued treatment exceeds any potential benefit. However, decisions based on quality-of-life considerations are more difficult, as there is inevitably imprecision in predicting the risk of intolerable disability or suffering.

MEDICOLEGAL PERSPECTIVE

Very few cases of selective non-treatment have reached the courts. It is considered appropriate for these difficult decisions to be made within the context of the infant/neonatologist/parent relationship, and experience has shown that there is no excessive abuse in such private decision-making processes. The legal position appears to recognize the importance of respecting parental decisions, but emphasizes that the law court has the right to intervene and overrule a decision if that is necessary to protect the best interests of the infant. The British legal system, for example, had upheld selective non-treatment in the three categories of neonatal conditions referred to previously. Firstly, selective non-treatment was ruled to be legally acceptable when death was inevitable in the case of a hydrocephalic preterm infant on the verge of death. Secondly, legal precedence for selective non-treatment for an infant with severe brain damage, who was neither dying nor in severe pain, was found in a case presenting to court with a high risk of multiple sensorineural disabilities. Thirdly, selective non-treatment was considered lawful in an infant where the benefits of life with treatment failed to outweigh the burdens of a 'demonstrably awful life' of pain and suffering.

THE DECISION-MAKING PROCESS

The importance of less medical paternalism and more informed parental involvement in the decision-making process of selective non-treatment must be emphasized. The neonatologist should never make unilateral decisions regarding the right to die. Adequate and consistent parental communication carried out by medical and nursing staff must begin with the admission of all infants into the NICU so that trust can be developed between the parents and staff, irrespective of outcome.[50] An open-visiting policy for families is essential to promote such parental contact.[51] A realistic assessment of the infant's clinical condition should be given by the neonatologist to the parents as soon as possible. The medical facts should be presented with an honest, sympathetic, and caring attitude. Often, the information has to be repeated and reinforced by the entire staff. Otherwise, misunderstandings and unrealistic expectations can lead to confusion, suspicions, bitterness, and frank hostility. As with most medical decisions made by neonatologists that require parental informed consent, much of the discussion on selective non-treatment depends on trust in the knowledge, judgment, and integrity of the doctor. When a consensus has been reached by the NICU staff that selective non-treatment is an appropriate option to raise with the parents, one or more intense and intimate meetings will be required so that the crucial set of discussions can take place and in which a decision can be reached on the matter. These meetings usually involve both of the parents, the attending neonatologist, a nurse representative, and a non-medical staff member who can act as the parents' advocate, such as a medical social worker. Ways of minimizing the chances of unresolved disagreements and of maximizing the chances of a just and ethical conclusion have recently been reviewed.[52]

The principles underlining clinical practice and the decision-making process should be the same for developed and developing countries, but there must be less medical paternalism and more informed parental involvement in developing countries. Compared with developed countries, communications between the medical and nursing staff and the parents are less adequate in developing countries. In most developed countries, intensive care is routinely offered to all who have reached 24 weeks' gestation. Limited resources in developing countries, however, necessitate a different intervention point, which may be 26 weeks or even 28 weeks.[53] In RPL, additional factors need to be taken into consideration, as the parents may have undergone numerous losses before reaching this stage. They may be subject to further early losses, and may not reach this stage again.

PALLIATIVE CARE

The neonatologist's duty does not end with the decision for selective non-treatment. The principles and guidelines for palliative care demand that basic nursing care should continue, with the emphasis on providing comfort to the infant. Electronic monitoring of physiological parameters, diagnostic investigations (such as X-rays and blood tests), medications (including oxygen and antibiotics), and therapeutic procedures (including resuscitation, all forms of assisted ventilation, and intravenous infusion) that might prolong the dying process should be discontinued. Prolonged terminal weaning, defined as a stepwise or gradual decreasing of ventilator support over a period of hours, is considered inappropriate. Dragging out the withdrawal serves only to prolong the dying process and any attendant suffering. The argument that the sudden withdrawal of ventilator support resembles an intentional killing does not hold merit, as in both cases a treatment on which the infant depends for life is being discontinued and death is the expected outcome. The infant should be nursed in a normal cot and warmth provided by light clothing. If the infant has apparent distress, symptomatic relief should be provided, such as suctioning to remove oropharyngeal secretions and sedation with normal therapeutic doses of morphine, on a PRN basis, even if the pain relief measures may inadvertently shorten the dying process.

A controversial issue involves the withdrawal of enteral nutrition and hydration during palliative care. Preterm or sick infants require gavage feeding, and although it has been advocated that this feeding method is part of medical treatment and should therefore be discontinued during palliative care, others consider it as basic nursing care that must not be withheld under any circumstances.[54] A number of court decisions have supported the withdrawal of nutrition, thus equating the administration of artificial nutrition with other medical procedures.[55] Precedence has been set in a British court on the legality of withholding gavage feeding. Nevertheless, most neonatologists would be reluctant not to provide gavage feeding, even when it might be lawful and appears to be in the infant's best interest. There is an obvious perception of a moral difference between withdrawing ventilatory support and withholding fluids or nutrition with selective non-treatment. The underlying principle is that naturally or artificially administered hydration and nutrition may be given or withheld, depending on the infant's comfort.

Parents need a quiet place to be with their infant during the dying process. They may wish that other family members and religious advisors be present. Hospice concepts have been applied to neonatal care by providing a family room that is private yet close to the NICU and by training NICU staff in more supportive approaches towards the families.[56,57] Such a program allows the staff to cope better with the dying infants offered selective non-treatment and facilitates the grieving process in the parents. Under certain circumstances, withdrawal of intensive care may be arranged to take place in the home, so that death can occur in a more comforting environment for the family.

CONCLUSIONS

A proactive policy of resuscitation at birth and prompt initiation of intensive care have been shown to be associated with an improvement in the survival of extremely preterm infants, including those born in the second trimester, in regional population-based studies within the State of Victoria in Australia. As a greater percentage of live births were offered intensive care in our series of studies, which spanned over 20 years, the survival rate rose progressively in all birthweight and gestation subgroups among ELBW infants, including those who were born at borderline viability down to 23 weeks' gestational age. Their quality-adjusted survival rate also rose progressively, since the large gains in survival over time had not been offset by significant increases in survival with disability. Cost–effectiveness and cost–utility ratios remained stable overall, with efficiency gains in the smaller infants over time, as more such infants were being transferred in utero and were born in level III perinatal centers with the regionalization of perinatal/neonatal healthcare programs. Multicentered collaboration to conduct long-term studies of geographically defined cohorts provides unique information not available from institution-based studies. Such data are vital for answering questions such as 'How low should we go?' Quality outcomes depend more on the comprehensive organization of an effective system of networking perinatal/neonatal services within a geographically determined region than on the introduction of expensive high-technology therapies within individual NICUs.

Among the many neonatal ethical problems, the one that neonatologists are faced with on a regular basis involves the issue of selective non-treatment, that is, clinical decisions made after the birth of a liveborn infant to either withhold or withdraw treatment in certain clinical situations. If medical doctors believe that the infant has little prospect for intact survival, their management would be suboptimal and they create a self-fulfilling prophecy. A policy establishing criteria for initiating life-sustaining treatment must be developed with proper consideration of the cultural, social, and economic factors operating in the developed or developing country. There are infants whose subsequent clinical course after initiation of neonatal intensive care will indicate that further curative efforts are futile or lack compensating benefit. A policy establishing criteria for withdrawing life-sustaining treatment must also be developed, to allow the appropriate use of palliative care in these instances. The clinical situations in which selective non-treatment is taking place in the neonatal intensive care unit are (1) when death is considered to be inevitable whatever treatment is provided, (2) even when death is not inevitable, there is a significantly high risk of severe physical and mental disability should the infant survive, and (3) when survival with moderate disability is possible, but the infant is likely to experience ongoing pain and suffering, repeated hospitalization and invasive treatment, and early death in childhood.

REFERENCES

1. Consultative Council on Obstetric and Paediatric Mortality and Morbidity. Annual Report for the Year 2002. Melbourne: Health Department of Victoria, 2004.
2. Kitchen WH, Campbell N, Drew JH, et al. Provision of perinatal services and survival of extremely low birth weight infants in Victoria. Med J Aust 1983; 2:314–18.

3. Kitchen WH, Ford F, Orgill A, et al. Outcome of extremely low birth-weight infants in relation to the hospital of birth. Aust NZ J Obstet Gynaecol 1984; 24:1–5.

4. Kitchen WH, Ford F, Orgill A, et al. Outcome of infants with birth weight 500 to 999 gm: a regional study of 1979 and 1980 births. J Paediatr 1984; 104:921–7.

5. Kitchen WH, Ford F, Orgill A, et al. Outcome of infants of birth weight 500 to 999 g: a continuing regional study of 5-year-old survivors. J Pediatr 1987; 111:761–6.

6. Victorian Infant Collaborative Study Group. Eight-year outcome in infants with birth weight 500 to 999 grams: continued regional study of 1979 and 1980 births. J Pediatr 1991; 118:761–7.

7. Victorian Infant Collaborative Study Group. Outcome at 14 years and birth weight 1000 g – a regional study. Arch Dis Child 2001; 85:F159–64.

8. Lumley J, Kitchen WH, Roy RND, et al. The survival of extremely low birth weight infants in Victoria: 1982–85. Med J Aust 1988; 149:242–6.

9. Lumley J, Kitchen WH, Roy RND, et al. Method of delivery and resuscitation of very low birth weight infants in Victoria: 1982–85. Med J Aust 1990; 152:143–6.

10. Victorian Infant Collaborative Study Group. Impact of improved care for infants of birth weight under 1000 g. Arch Dis Child 1991; 66:765–9.

11. Victorian Infant Collaborative Study Group. Improving the quality of survival for infants of birth weight <1000 g born in non-level III centres in Victoria. Med J Aust 1993; 158:24–7.

12. Victorian Infant Collaborative Study Group. Neurosensory outcome at 5 years and extremely low birth weight. Arch Dis Child 1995; 73:F143–6.

13. Victorian Infant Collaborative Study Group. Improved outcome into the 1990s for infants of birth weight 500–999 g. Arch Dis Child 1997; 77:F91–4.

14. Victorian Infant Collaborative Study Group. Changing outcome for infants of birth weight 500–999 g born outside level III centres in Victoria. Aust NZ J Obstet Gynaecol 1997; 37:253–7.

15. Victorian Infant Collaborative Study Group. Changing availability of neonatal intensive care for extremely low birth weight infants in Victoria over two decades. Med J Aust 2004; 81:136–9.

16. Victorian Infant Collaborative Study Group. Evaluation of neonatal intensive care for extremely low birth weight infants in Victoria over two decades: I. Effectiveness. Pediatrics 2004; 113:505–9.

17. Yu VYH, Doyle LW. Regionalised long-term follow-up. Semin Neonatol 2004; 9:135–44.

18. Victorian Infant Collaborative Study Group. The cost of improving the outcome for infants of birth weight 500 to 999 g in Victoria. J Paediatr Child Health 1993; 29:56–62.

19. Victorian Infant Collaborative Study Group. Economic outcome for intensive care of infants of birth weight 500–999 g born in Victoria in the post-surfactant era. J Paediatr Child Health 1997; 33:202–8.

20. Victorian Infant Collaborative Study Group. Evaluation of neonatal intensive care for extremely low birth weight infants in Victoria over two decades: II. Efficiency. Pediatrics 2004; 113:510–14.

21. Yu VYH, Davis NG, Mercado MF, et al. Subsequent pregnancy following the birth of an extremely low birth-weight infant. Aust NZ J Obstet Gynaecol 1986; 26:115–19.

22. Yu VYH, Doyle LW. Survival and disabilities in extremely tiny babies. Semin Neonatol 1996; 1:257–66.

23. Yu VYH, Wood EC, eds. Prematurity. Edinburgh: Churchill Livingstone, 1987.

24. Yu VYH, Carse EA, Charlton MP. Outcome of infants born at less than 26 weeks' gestation. In: McIntosh N, Hansen T, eds. Current Topics in Neonatal Care. Philadelphia: WB Saunders, 1996:67–84.

25. Yu VYH, ed. The Extremely Tiny Baby. London: WB Saunders, 1996.

26. Victorian Infant Collaborative Study Group. Outcome to five years of age of children 24–26 weeks' gestational age born in the State of Victoria. Med J Aust 1995; 163:11–14.

27. Victorian Infant Collaborative Study Group. Outcome at 2 years of children 23–27 weeks' gestation born in Victoria in 1991–92. J Paediatr Child Health 1997; 33:161–5.

28. Victorian Infant Collaborative Study Group. Outcome at 5 years of age of children 23–27 weeks' gestation: refining the prognosis. Pediatrics 2001; 108:134–41.

29. Victorian Infant Collaborative Study Group. Neonatal intensive care at borderline viability – Is it worth it? Early Hum Dev 2004; 80:103–13.

30. Lorenz JM. The outcome of extreme prematurity. Semin Perinatol 2001; 25:348–59.

31. Draper ES, Manktelow B, Field DJ, et al. Prediction of survival for preterm births by weight and gestational age: retrospective population based study. BMJ 1999; 319:1093–7.

32. Wood NS, Marlow N, Costeloe K, et al. Neurologic and developmental disability after extremely preterm birth. EPICure Study Group. N Engl J Med 2000; 343:378–84.

33. den Ouden AL, van Baar AL, Dorrepaal CA, et al. Overlevingskans van zeer immature pasgeborenen in Nederland. Tijdschr Kindergeneeskd 2000; 142:241–6.

34. Bohin S, Draper ES, Field DJ. Health status of a population of infants born before 26 weeks' gestation derived from routine data collected between 21 and 27 months post-delivery. Early Hum Dev 1999; 55:9–18.

35. Rijken M, Stoelhorst GMSJ, Martens SE, et al. Mortality and neurologic, mental, and psychomotor development at 2 years in infants born less than 27 weeks' gestation: the Leiden Follow-Up Project on Prematurity. Pediatrics 2003; 112:351–8.

36. Yu VYH. The extremely low birth weight infant: an ethical approach to treatment. Aust Paediatr J 1987; 23:97–103.

37. deGaris C, Kuhse H, Singer P, et al. Attitudes of Australian neonatal paediatricians to the treatment of extremely preterm infants. Aust Paediatr J 1987; 23:223–6.

38. Mulvey S, Partridge JC, Martinez AM, et al. The management of extremely premature infants and the perceptions of viability and parental counselling practices of Australian paediatricians. Aust NZ J Obstet Gynaecol 2001; 41:269–73.

39. Munro M, Yu VYH, Partridge JC, et al. Antenatal counselling, resuscitation practices and attitudes among Australian neonatologists towards life support in extreme prematurity. Aust NZ J Obstet Gynaecol 2001; 44:275–80.

40. Martinez AM, Partridge JC, Yu VYH, et al. Physician counseling practices and decision-making for extremely low birth weight infants in the Pacific Rim. J Paediatr Child Health 2005; 41:209–14.

41. Yu VYH, Gomez JM, Shah V, et al. Survival prospects of extremely preterm infants: a 10-year experience in a single perinatal centre. Am J Perinatol 1992; 9:164–9.

42. Yu VYH. Selective non-treatment of newborn infants. Med J Aust 1994; 161:627–9.

43. RCPCH Ethic Advisory Committee. Withholding or Withdrawing Life Saving Treatment in Children. A Framework for Practice. London: Royal College of Paediatrics and Child Health, 1997.

44. Rennie JM. Perinatal management at the lower margin of viability. Arch Dis Child 1996; 74:F214–18.

45. Fetus and Newborn Committee, Canadian Pediatric Society; Maternal–Fetal Medicine Committee, Society of Obstetricians and Gynecologists of Canada. Management of the woman with threatened

birth of an infant of extremely low gestational age. CMAJ 1994; 151:547–53.

46. AAP Committee on Bioethics. Ethics and the care of critically ill infants and children. Pediatrics 1996; 98:149–52.

47. Carse EA, Yu VYH. Deaths following withdrawal of treatment in a neonatal intensive care unit. In: Wiknjosastro GK, ed. Proceedings of the 5th Congress of the Federation of Asia–Oceania Perinatal Societies. Denpasar: Perinatal Society of Indonesia, 1988:55.

48. Whitelaw A. Death as an option in neonatal intensive care. Lancet 1986; ii:328–31.

49. Kelly NP, Rowley SR, Harding JE. Death in neonatal intensive care. J Paediatr Child Health 1994; 30:419–22.

50. Yu VYH. Caring for parents of high-risk infants. Med J Aust 1977; 2:534–7.

51. Yu VYH, Jamieson J, Astbury J. Parents' reactions to unrestricted parental contact with infants in the intensive care nursery. Med J Aust 1981; 1:294–6.

52. Tripp J, McGregor D. Withholding and withdrawing of life sustaining treatment in the newborn. *Arch* Dis Child 2006; 91:F67–71.

53. Partridge JC, Martinez AM, Nishida H, et al. International comparison of care for very low birth weight infants: parents' perception of counseling and decision-making. Pediatrics 2005; 116:263–71.

54. Doyal L, Wilsher D. Towards guidelines for withholding and withdrawal of life prolonging treatment in neonatal medicine. Arch Dis Child 1994; 70:F66–70.

55. Mirale ED, Mahowald MB. Withholding nutrition from seriously ill newborn infants: a parent's perspective. J Pediatr 1988; 113:262–5.

56. Yu VYH. Death as an option in the neonatal intensive care unit. The ethics of withdrawal of life-support. In: Burrows GD, Petrucco OM, Llewellyn-Jones D, eds. Psychosomatic Aspects of Reproductive Medicine and Family Planning. Melbourne: York Press, 1987:112–19.

57. Whitfield JM, Siegel RE, Glicken AD, et al. The application of hospice concepts to neonatal care. Am J Dis Child 1982; 136:421–4.

16. Obstetric outcomes after recurrent pregnancy loss

Howard JA Carp

INTRODUCTION

Most work on recurrent pregnancy loss (RPL) has concentrated on the causes, prognosis, treatment, and subsequent live birth rate. However, a question arises as to whether this group of patients is at a higher risk for obstetric complications such as bleeding, fetal anomalies, preeclampsia, intrauterine growth restriction (IUGR), preterm labor, and perinatal mortality, and whether prenatal care has to be modified to seek these complications. The question then arises as to whether these complications are associated with specific conditions associated with RPL. Antiphospholipid syndrome (APS) and hereditary thrombophilias are two such conditions that have been described to be associated with recurrent pregnancy loss and late obstetric complications. Various interventions have also been reported to affect the incidence of later obstetric complications. These interventions include paternal leukocyte immunization and intravenous immunoglobulin (IVIG) for unexplained RPL, anticoagulants and aspirin or IVIG for APS, and anticoagulants for hereditary thrombophilias. This chapter assesses some of the obstetric complications associated with different forms of RPL and the treatment modalities that have been used.

METHOD OF STUDY

Publications describing the obstetric complications in RPL were sought by a thorough literature search including online databases, MEDLINE and EMBASE. The original database of the Recurrent Miscarriage Trialists Group is held by the author as one of the data contributors to that database. Figures were also obtained from one of the author's own databases, which contains information on 1800 patients attending the Recurrent Miscarriage Clinic of the Sheba Medical Center, Tel Hashomer, Israel. The figures were entered into a computerized database (SPSS, Chicago, Ill) and analyzed.

STATISTICAL ANALYSIS

Odds ratios (OR) with 95% confidence intervals (CI) were calculated for developing obstetric complications such as vaginal bleeding, anomalies, preeclampsia, IUGR, and perinatal mortality. When true incidences were available from cohort studies, the relative risks (RR) were calculated. These figures were also compared in subgroups of patients and after various treatment interventions.

INCIDENCE OF OBSTETRIC COMPLICATIONS AFTER RPL

Most of the literature on obstetric complications comes from an era after APS had been defined but before hereditary thrombophilias had been defined. Reginald et al,[1] in a retrospective observational cohort study, assessed the results of 175 pregnancies in 97 recurrently miscarrying women whose subsequent pregnancy progressed beyond 28 weeks. However, the underlying causes of RPL in this group of women were not documented. The results were not compared with a control group attending the same hospital, but with standard figures from Scotland between 1973 and 1979. A significantly higher incidence of preterm deliveries, perinatal deaths, and IUGR was found. In contrast, Hughes et al[2] examined the obstetric outcome in 88 women with a past history of three or more consecutive pregnancy losses and compared the results with a control group drawn from their local obstetric population. The incidences of small-for-gestational-age infants (3.4%), preterm delivery (12.5%), and perinatal mortality (0%) were no different to those in the control group. As in the study by Reginald et al,[1] there was no mention of APS. However, an increased incidence of gestational diabetes and pregnancy-induced hypertension was found. Tulppala et al[3] conducted a prospective study of 32 deliveries in 63 women with RPL and presented the results of a detailed investigative protocol, including APS. The incidences of IUGR (20%), preterm delivery (9.7%), and impaired glucose tolerance (22.8%) appeared to be increased. Unfortunately, the results were not compared with any control population. Jivraj et al[4] studied a cohort of 162 women with RPL compared with local controls, and found an increased incidence of the same complications as Reginald et al,[1] but also an increased incidence of cesarean sections, which were performed for the above obstetric conditions. Although that study did define the causes of pregnancy loss in the control group, the figures were too small to allow comparisons to be drawn between different groups of patients. Seidman et al[5] reported the same complications in 338 women with pregnancy losses compared with 13 338 parous women in a multicenter study in four large hospitals in Jerusalem. In the survey by Seidman et al,[5] there was a statistically significant 14% prevalence of preterm labor, compared with 7.5% in control women (OR 2.32; 95% CI 1.67–3.22). The different prevalence of IUGR was even more significant: 14% in aborting women, compared with 5% in control women (OR 3.02; 95% CI 2.17–4.18). However, the study by Seidman et al[5] included patients with one pregnancy loss and was not restricted to patients with RPL. A more recent population-based study has been reported by Sheiner et al,[6] in which all singleton pregnancies were assessed in women with and without two or more consecutive recurrent abortions. Between 1988 and 2002, 154 294 singleton deliveries occurred. Of these deliveries, 7503 occurred in patients with RPL. The following complications were found to be associated with RPL: advanced maternal age, cervical incompetence, diabetes mellitus, hypertensive disorders, placenta praevia and abruptio placentae, malpresentations, and premature rupture of the membranes (PROM). A higher rate of cesarean section was also found in patients with previous RPL compared with controls: 15.9% and 10.9%, respectively (OR 1.6; 95% CI 1.5–1.7).

An attempt was made to determine the common OR for various late complications of pregnancy after RPL compared with controls. The series of Reginald et al[1] could not be included as there was no relevant control group. The series of Seidman et al[5] was not included as it only described patients with one previous miscarriage. The series of Tulppala et al[3] could not be included as there was no control group. The other three publications were combined in a meta-analysis.

VAGINAL BLEEDING

The incidence of bleeding was only described in the series of Reginald et al quoted by Beard,[7] and in that of Seidman et al.[5] Hence no common OR could be calculated. Vaginal bleeding seems to be increased in pregnancies that develop. Vaginal bleeding is a common complication, occurring in 50 of 162 women in the series of Reginald et al[7] and in 50 of 102 patients in the author's series.[8] The reason for this bleeding remains unclear. Seventy-five percent of habitual abortions are blighted ova.[8] However, when the pregnancy succeeds and there is a live embryo within the uterus, bleeding still occurs in 40–50% of patients. Seidman et al[5] also reported a 13.7% incidence of first-trimester bleeding, compared with a 13.8% incidence in the standard population.

ANOMALIES

Little information is available on anomalies. The study by Sheiner et al[6] reports 2 anomalies in 29 patients. Although this is a very small series, the figures are higher than expected. Analysis of the figures in the RMITG trial[9] showed an anomaly rate

Study	Statistics for each study				OR and 95% CI
	OR	Lower limit	Upper limit	p	
Hughes et al[2]	7.001	3.977	12.323	0.000	
Jivraj et al[4]	2.335	0.739	7.379	0.149	
Sheiner et al[6]	2.233	2.073	2.406	0.000	
Common OR	2.277	2.116	2.451	0.000	

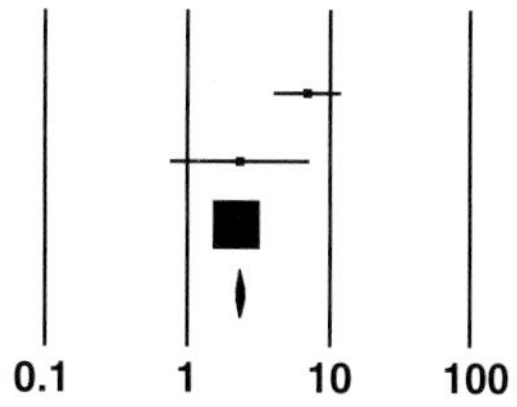

Figure 16.1 Odds ratio (OR) for gestational diabetes in recurrent pregnancy loss.

of 4%. In the author's series, there were three anomalies in 99 developing pregnancies in non-treated patients. However, in the RMITG series and the author's series, no control group is available.

DIABETES

Three papers have described the prevalence of diabetes: Hughes et al,[2] Jivraj et al,[4] and Sheiner et al.[6] As a control group was available, their common OR could be determined for 7753 patients with RPL and 172 490 control patients. The prevalence of diabetes was 11.75% and 4.95% in recurrently miscarrying and control patients, respectively. The OR are summarized in Figure 16.1. As can be seen, there was a common OR of 2.27 for gestational diabetes in RPL. This figure was statistically significant (95% CI 2.1–2.45). Tulppala et al[3] also found a prevalence of 22.6% (7 of 31 patients tested).

PREGNANCY-INDUCED HYPERTENSION

Hughes et al,[2] Jivraj et al,[4] and Sheiner et al[6] quoted the incidence of pregnancy-induced hypertension (PIH). The figures are summarized in Figure 16.2. In order to obtain significant numbers, the figures for preeclampsia and other forms of PIH were analyzed as a whole. The common OR was 1.89 (95% CI 1.74–2.06), which was statistically significant. The total number of patients was identical to those with gestational diabetes. The prevalence of PIH was 671 of 7753 patients (8.6%) of recurrently miscarrying patients, compared with 5.7% of control women (9921 of 172 490 control patients).

Study	Statistics for each study				OR and 95% CI
	OR	Lower limit	Upper limit	p	
Hughes et al[2]	1.941	0.783	4.814	0.152	
Jivraj et al[4]	0.728	0.412	1.285	0.274	
Sheiner et al[6]	1.933	1.778	2.102	0.000	
Common OR	1.894	1.743	2.057	0.000	

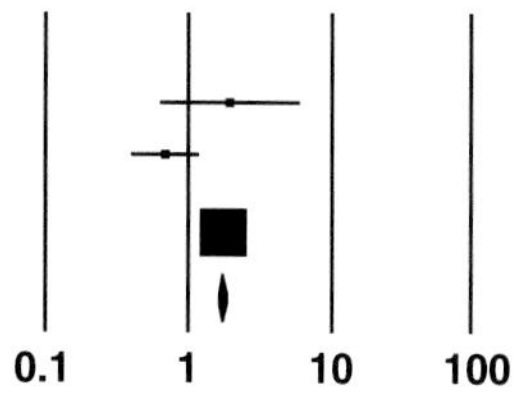

Figure 16.2 Odds ratio (OR) for pregnancy-induced hypertension in recurrent pregnancy loss.

Study	Statistics for each study				OR and 95% CI
	OR	Lower limit	Upper limit	p	
Hughes et al[2]	2.433	0.762	7.768	0.133	
Jivraj et al[4]	6.885	4.318	10.978	0.000	
Sheiner et al[6]	1.000	0.847	1.181	0.998	
Common OR	1.257	1.076	1.467	0.004	

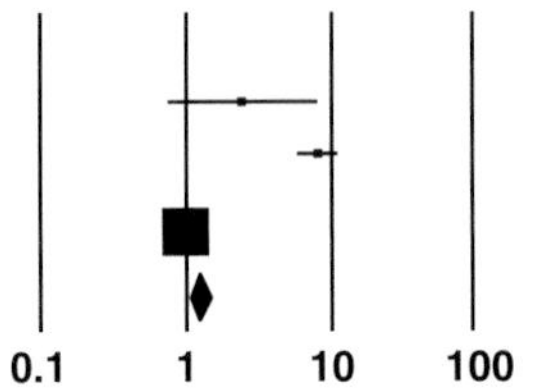

Figure 16.3 Odds ratio (OR) for intrauterine growth restriction in recurrent pregnancy loss.

Neither Reginald et al[1] nor Tulppala et al[3] quoted figures for PIH.

INTRAUTERINE GROWTH RESTRICTION

The same three papers as above give figures for IUGR. The common OR for developing IUGR is 1.25 (95% CI 1.08–1.47) (Figure 16.3). Reginald et al[1] reported a 33% incidence in 344 pregnancies prospectively followed up, and reported that this showed a relative risk of 3 compared with the standard Scottish population. Tulppala et al[3] also reported a 20% incidence (6 out of 30 pregnancies).

PRETERM LABOR

Comparative figures are only available for preterm labor from the series of Hughes et al[2] and Jivraj et al.[4]

Figure 16.4 summarizes the results. Again, there was a statistically significant association between preterm labor and RPL. The common OR was 2.84 (95% CI 1.96–4.1). In the series of Reginald et al,[1] there was a 28% incidence of preterm labor. The relative risk was 3.3 when compared with the Scottish data for the equivalent period. Tulppala et al[3] quoted a 9.7% incidence in their series.

PERINATAL MORTALITY

Again, there was an increased tendency for mortality after RPL, loss with a common OR of 1.25 (95% CI 1.05–1.49). This is summarized in Figure 16.5. However, the perinatal mortality may be artificially low due to obstetric intervention for other complications in pregnancy. Reginald et al[1] reported 19 perinatal deaths in 118 infants (16.1%), which

Study	Statistics for each study				OR and 95% CI
	OR	Lower limit	Upper limit	p	
Hughes et al[2]	1.530	0.811	2.887	0.189	
Jivraj et al[4]	3.890	2.470	6.126	0.000	
Common OR	2.837	1.961	4.104	0.000	

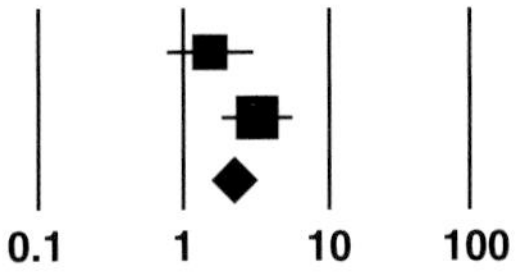

Figure 16.4 Odds ratio (OR) for preterm labor in recurrent pregnancy loss.

Study	Statistics for each study				OR and 95% CI
	OR	Lower limit	Upper limit	p	
Hughes et al[2]	1.103	0.060	20.305	0.947	
Jivraj et al[4]	2.506	0.922	6.814	0.072	
Sheiner et al[6]	1.222	1.021	1.464	0.029	
Common OR	1.250	1.047	1.492	0.014	

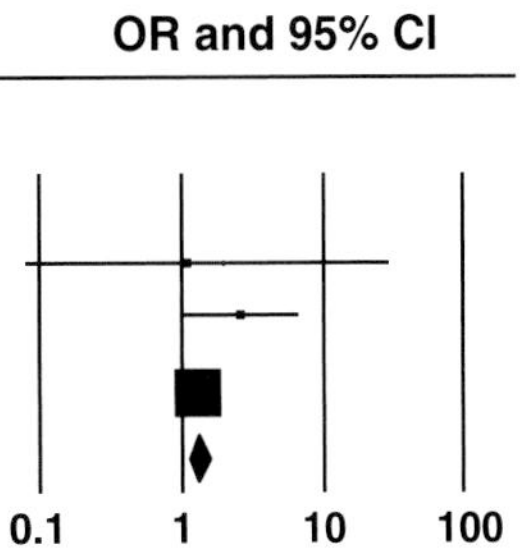

Figure 16.5 Odds ratio (OR) for perinatal mortality in recurrent pregnancy loss.

was considerably higher than the standard figures for England and Wales in the same period of time, when the perinatal mortality was 10.1/1000. Tulppala et al[3] did not quote perinatal mortality.

It seems, therefore, that the currently available literature on the obstetric and neonatal outcome of pregnancies from women with a history of RPL shows a consistently worse prognosis. However, it is unclear whether the worse prognosis is only found in patients with predisposing causes such as APS and hereditary thrombophilias or is also present in patients with unexplained pregnancy losses.

ANTIPHOSPHOLIPID SYNDROME

Most series on APS have concentrated on the subsequent live birth rate and ignored the late obstetric complications. The present author published a series[10] in which the outcome of 24 pregnancies in patients with lupus anticoagulant (LA) and five or more first-trimester abortions was compared with 22 pregnancies in women with no antiphospholipid antibodies (aPL), and 5 or more miscarriages. Although the subsequent number of first-trimester miscarriages and the live birth rate were similar in both groups of patients, the incidences of second- or third-trimester fetal deaths, IUGR, and need for premature induction of labor or preterm cesarean section were significantly higher in the APS patients. The similar live birth

rate was only obtained by early obstetric intervention to prevent intrauterine fetal deaths. A number of other publications have attested that the risk of obstetric complications is high in APS.[11,12] The incidence of preeclampsia is particularly high in APS.[13,14] IUGR has been reported with a frequency ranging from 30% to 12% in different series. Some series show a significant increase in the incidence of IUGR,[15,16] whereas others have not confirmed the increased incidence.[17,18] The different results on the association of obstetric complications with aPL might have various explanations. None of the results has been correlated with β_2-glycoprotein I(β_2GPI)-dependent antibodies. None has corrected for fetal chromosomal aberrations, in which the aPL may just be an epiphenomenon. Alternatively, the obstetric complications may be dependent on other factors associated with RPL rather than aPL. No series has compared the incidence of obstetric complications in RPL due to APS and in RPL without APS. The incidence of preterm labor is increased in APS patients,[16] but again has not been compared with patients with RPL and no APS.

The currently accepted optimal treatment regimen for APS is heparin or low-molecular-weight heparin (LMWH) with the addition of low-dose aspirin. However, anticoagulants do not seem to lower the incidence of obstetric complications associated with this syndrome.[19] IVIG may have a beneficial effect in APS, as the action and production of aPL are inhibited by IVIG. The F(ab') fragment of IVIG inhibits binding of anticardiolipin antibody (aCL) to cardiolipin in a dose-dependent manner.[20] The F(ab′) fragment of IVIG inhibits LA activity.[21] IVIG lowers levels of aCL after each infusion.[22] IVIG may contain anti-idiotypic antibodies to aPL, or may inactivate B-cell clones, leading to decreased autoantibody production.[23] In the late 1980s and early 1990s, IVIG was used to improve the live birth rate in APS.[24-27] However, these were small series, and showed IVIG to have no apparent benefit over anticoagulants in terms of live births. However, when the obstetric complications are considered, a different clinical picture emerges. Vaquero et al[28] compared IVIG with prednisone and aspirin. The prevalence of IUGR and pre-term labor was similar in both groups, but the prevalences of PIH and gestational diabetes were significantly lower ($p<0.05$) after IVIG (5% of 41 patients and 14% of 22 patients, respectively). Branch et al[29] compared IVIG with placebo: there were fewer cases of IUGR after IVIG (14% of 7 patients, compared with 33% of 9 patients, respectively), and fewer admissions to the neonatal intensive care unit (14% of 7 patients after IVIG, compared with 44% of 9, respectively). Harris and Pierangelli[30] reported that preeclampsia, IUGR and prematurity were reduced when IVIG was compared with prednisone and aspirin or heparin and aspirin.

HEREDITARY THROMBOPHILIAS

There have recently been numerous publications associating genetic predispositions (hereditary thrombophilias) to thrombosis with pregnancy loss. The hereditary thrombophilias include protein C, protein S, and antithrombin III deficiencies, activated protein C resistance (APCR), factor V Leiden mutation, methylenetetrahydrofolate reductase (MTHFR) mutation, the prothrombin gene mutation (G20210A) and excessive factor VIII. The features of hereditary thrombophilias and the effects on obstetric complications are discussed in Chapter 10. Suffice it to say here that Kuperminc et al[31] have reported an association between

thrombophilias and severe preeclampsia, placental abruption, IUGR, and stillbirth. However, theirs was a case–control study looking at the prevalence of hereditary thrombophilias in women with obstetric complications. Additionally, these findings have beeen disputed by Infante-Rivarde et al,[32] who also performed a case–control study. Alfirevic et al[33] have published a systematic review of the various reports and have described the strengths of association between hereditary thrombophilias and preeclampsia, placental abruption, stillbirth, and IUGR. Sheiner et al[6] have drawn attention to the fact that the other publications on obstetric complications in RPL were written at a time when the hereditary thrombophilias had not yet been recognized. In their series, higher rates of IUGR, cesarean section, low Apgar scores and perinatal mortality were found among the 22 patients with known thrombophilia as compared with the controls, although the differences did not reach statistical significance. There are no cohort studies assessing the true incidence of obstetric complications in the presence of thrombophilia and RPL. In the present author's series of 21 pregnancies with factor V Leiden which were followed up prospectively, there was one case of HELLP syndrome (hemolysis, elevated liver enzymes, and low platelet count), but no other obstetric complications, and no deep vein thrombosis or pulmonary embolus.

The LMWH enoxaparin has been shown to be associated with a significantly increased chance of a live birth, both overall and when corrected for the number of miscarriages[34] (RR 0.53; 95% CI 1.07–3.28), in women with RPL and hereditary thrombophilia. There are isolated reports[35–37] of the use of anticoagulants in the presence of thrombophilias to reduce the late obstetric complications, and this approach has been endorsed by the American College of Chest Physicians.[38] However, there is as yet insufficient evidence that anticoagulants actually reduce the incidence of late obstetric complications. Further trials need to be performed in order to determine whether anticoagulants do indeed reduce the incidence of obstetric complications.

OBSTETRIC COMPLICATIONS AFTER ALLOIMMUNIZATION

Some 20 years ago, alloimmunization had become the treatment of choice for patients with RPL. Two methods of alloimmunization had been used in order to improve the subsequent live birth rate in recurrently aborting women: active immunization with paternal leukocytes and passive immunization using IVIG.[39] Paternal leukocyte immunization became standard management after the double-blinded randomized trial by Mowbray et al[40] and a subsequent meta-analysis by the Recurrent Miscarriage Immunization Trialists Group,[9] but fell out of favor due to the paper by Ober et al,[41] which claimed lack of efficacy. As with treatment for APS and hereditary thrombophilias, most publications on immunomodulation have assessed the subsequent live birth rate as the primary outcome measure, and have ignored the late obstetric complications of pregnancy occurring in women with a subsequent live birth.

In order to summarize the obstetric complications with or without immunotherapy, the various series in the literature have been pooled to obtain a sufficient number of patients available for meaningful analysis. The databases of Beard et al,[7] the RMITG meta-analysis[9] and the present author's series have been combined in order to compare the obstetric complications after paternal leukocyte immunization: 979 immunized patients were available for analysis, compared with 483 non-immunized patients. The prevalence of IUGR, perinatal mortality, and the incidence of anomalies were assessed. These figures are summarized in Table 16.1. As can be seen, there was a significantly lower incidence of preterm labor, perinatal mortality, and IUGR after paternal leukocyte immunization than in controls. The incidence of fetal anomalies was not significantly different in the two groups of patients. As the RMITG meta-analysis[9] did not assess bleeding and preeclampsia, data could only be obtained from Beard's[7] series and the present author's series. Two hundred and sixteen immunized patients and 191 control patients are available for analysis.

Table 16.1 Preterm labor, IUGR, perinatal mortality, and anomalies with paternal leukocyte immunization compared with controls[a]

	Immunized ($n = 979$)[b]	Controls ($n = 483$)[b]	Relative risk[c]
Preterm labor	39 (3.9%)	52 (10.8%)	0.63 (0.49–0.79)
IUGR	17 (1.7%)	59 (12.2%)	0.32 (0.21–0.49)
Perinatal mortality	9 (0.9%)	21 (4.3%)	0.44 (0.26–0.47)
Anomalies	25 (2.6%)	19 (3.9%)	0.84 (0.65–1.10)

[a]Figures include 92 immunized and 175 non-immunized patients from Beard's series[7], 759 immunized patients and 279 non-immunized patients from the RMITG register,[9] and 128 immunized patients and 29 non-immunized patients from the present author's series.
[b]Incidences in parentheses.
[c]95% confidence intervals in parentheses.

These figures are summarised in Table 16.2. As can be seen, the incidence of preeclampsia was lower in immunized women. However, there was no significant difference in the incidence of vaginal bleeding, which remained high: 38% and 34% in immunized and control women, respectively.

Table 16.3 shows the obstetric complications after IVIG in the 136 women in the present author's series. There is no relevant control group, as some of the patients were administered IVIG after failure of paternal leukocyte immunization. The figures were compared with those for non-immunized patients in the registers above and those in control patients in other series on IVIG in the literature. The incidences of IUGR, perinatal mortality, bleeding,

Table 16.2 Bleeding and preeclampsia with paternal leukocyte immunization compared with controls[a]

	Immunized ($n = 216$)[b]	Controls ($n = 191$)[b]	Relative risk[c]
Bleeding	83 (38%)	64 (34%)	1.10 (0.92–1.33)
Preeclampsia	27 (13%)	57 (30%)	0.55 (0.40–0.76)

[a]Figures include 88 immunized and 162 non-immunized patients from Beard's series[7] and 128 immunized patients and 29 non-immunized patients from the present author's series.
[b]Incidences in parentheses.
[c]95% confidence intervals in parentheses.

Table 16.3 Obstetric complications after IVIG compared with controls[a]

	IVIG[b]	Controls[b]	Relative risk[c]
Preterm labor	15/136 (11%)	52/483 (10.8%)	1.02 (0.53–1.96)
IUGR	6/136 (4%)	59/483 (12.2%)	0.39 (0.18–0.86)
Perinatal mortality	2/136 (1.5%)	21/483 (4.3%)	0.39 (0.10–0.47)
Bleeding	5/136 (3.7%)	64/191 (34%)	0.14 (0.06–0.33)
Preeclampsia	4/136 (2.9%)	57/191 (30%)	0.13 (0.05–0.34)
Anomalies	1/136 (0.7%)	19/483 (3.9%)	0.22 (0.03–1.51)

[a]Figures show the incidence of anomalies as a function of the total number of patients in the sample. IVIG figures are from the present author's series. The control figures are pooled data from the literature.
[b]Incidences in parentheses.
[c]95% confidence intervals in parentheses.

and preeclampsia were all lower after IVIG, but the incidences of preterm labor and anomalies did not seem to be affected. However, these results should be interpreted with caution due to the nature of the control group.

CYTOKINES AS MEDIATORS OF PREGNANCY LOSS AND OBSTETRIC COMPLICATIONS

Cytokines are low-molecular-weight peptides or glycopeptides, which are produced by lymphocytes, monocytes/macrophages, mast cells, eosinophils, and blood vessel endothelial cells. Cytokines seem to influence all stages of pregnancy. Cytokines such as interleukin-3 (IL-3), granulocyte-macrophage colony-stimulating factor (GM-CSF), and epidermal growth factor (EGF) stimulate placental cell proliferation[42] in vitro, and may enable the trophoblast to secrete human chorionic gonadotropin(hCG) and human placental lactogen (hPL). Cytokines such as transforming growth factor β2 (TGF-β2) can inhibit lymphokine activation of natural killer (NK) cells (which may attack the trophoblast). Although cytokines can have pleiotropic actions, these actions of the above cytokines are classified as T-helper 2 (Th2) or anti-inflammatory in nature, and they seem to benefit the development of pregnancy. Other cytokines can have actions that are known as Th1 or proinflammatory, and these may be detrimental to pregnancy; for example, tumor necrosis factor α (TNF-α) can activate NK cells at the fetomaternal interface,[43] leading to apoptosis and trophoblast cell death.[44] Wegman[23] suggested that appropriate cytokines are necessary in order to confer benefits on the developing fetoplacental unit. In early pregnancy, the conceptus and placental tissues produce a variety of Th1-type cytokines, including interferons, interleukins and TNF.[45] In normal pregnancy, the maternal immune system seems to modulate the cytokine pattern to preferential expression of Th2 cytokines, including GM-CSF, IL-3, IL-4, IL-5, IL-10, and IL-13, that may enhance fetal survival.[46] Preferential expression of Th1 cytokines (TNF-α, interferon-γ (IFN-γ), and IL-2) may result in abnormal placental and embryonic growth and subsequent fetal demise.

An inappropriate cytokine balance has been reported to act in early pregnancy, causing NK-cell activation,[43] placental apoptosis,[44] teratogenesis,[47] and excessive coagulation, particularly TNF-α and IL-6.[48] Hence, cytokine imbalance is among the mechanisms that have been proposed to underlie RPL. The effect of cytokine imbalance on coagulation may explain some of the effects of hereditary thrombophilias. Additionally, APS and most of the late complications of pregnancy have also been shown to have an underlying cytokine basis.

Although it is generally accepted that aPL may act by causing blood coagulation in decidual vessels, cytokines may also be responsible for the action of aPL early in the pathogenesis of the condition. Serum TNF-α is increased in women with APS.[49] IL-3 is decreased in APS,[50] and fetal loss can be prevented in experimental APS by in vivo administration of recombinant IL-3.[51] Alteration of the Th1/Th2 balance may also be involved in the effect of anti-idiotypic antibodies on APS.[52]

Late obstetric complications have also been shown to be associated with altered cytokine levels. Preeclampsia is associated with reduced IL-10 and higher IL-2 production from peripheral blood mononuclear cells (PBMC),[53,54] and high serum IL-8 and TNF-α.[55] In preterm births, cytokine involvement has been reported,[56] particularly increased amniotic IL-6, IL-8, and TNF-α.[57–60]

In IUGR, TGF-β in cord blood and mRNA for IL-10 are significantly reduced, whereas IL-8 mRNA is significantly higher[61,62] and placental TNF-α secretion is enhanced.[62]

The various interventions used for improving the live birth rate in RPL may exert their effects by modulating cytokine balance, and this modulation may also influence the incidence of later obstetric complications. As stated in Chapter 10 it is possible that heparin or enoxaparin may work by anti-inflammatory mechanisms rather than anticoagulation. Heparin increases serum TNF-binding protein, hence protecting against systemic harmful manifestations.[63] LMWH inhibit TNF-α production.[64] Thrombosis results in an inflammatory response of the vein wall. Both heparin and LMWH limit the anti-inflammatory response, but in the series of Downing et al,[65] LMWH was more effective than heparin in limiting neutrophil extravasation and was the only intervention to decrease vein wall permeability. In addition, heparin has been shown to prevent the accumulation of proliferating vascular smooth muscle cells encroaching on the lumen of arteries injured at angioplasty, hence enlarging the lumen.[66]

The mode of action of paternal leukocyte immunization (PLI) is unclear. The two most plausible explanations seem to be that PLI may downregulate the numbers and killing activity of NK cells,[67] which may attack the trophoblast when activated by cytokines. PLI may also alter the balance between Th1 and Th2 cytokines. (PLI has been reported to reduce IFN-γ and increase the secretion of IL-10 and TGF-β,[68] and has also been shown to lower the serum IL-6 and soluble IL-6 receptor (sIL-6R) levels to the values observed in normal pregnancy.[69])

IVIG has numerous actions. The actions of IVIG in pregnancy, including its effects on APS, have been summarized elsewhere.[70] In addition to various other mechanisms, IVIG, like PLI, depresses NK-cell function[71] and enhances the action of Th2 cytokines.[72]

CONCLUSIONS

Patients with RPL seem to comprise a high-risk group for later obstetric complications. Late obstetric complications have been described in APS and hereditary thrombophilias. However, there is insufficient evidence at present to determine whether the late obstetric complications occur exclusively in these two conditions, or whether they are associated with RPL per se. Immunomodulation seems to reduce the incidence of some of these complications. The role of anticoagulants in reducing obstetric complications is more doubtful. However, careful surveillance is required in pregnancies following RPL, in order to detect obstetric complications. Further prospective cohort studies are necessary in order more accurately define the patient at risk, the role of APS and hereditary thrombophilia, and the effect of treatment modalities.

REFERENCES

1. Reginald PW, Beard RW, Chapple J, et al. Outcome of pregnancies progressing beyond 28 weeks gestation in women with a history of recurrent miscarriage. Br J Obstet Gynaecol 1987; 94:643–8.
2. Hughes N, Hamilton EF, Tulandi T. Obstetric outcome in women after multiple spontaneous abortions. J Reprod Med 1991; 36:165–6.
3. Tulppala M, Palosuo T, Ramsay T, et al. A prospective study of 63 couples with a history of recurrent spontaneous abortion: contributing factors and outcome of subsequent pregnancies. Hum Reprod 1993; 8:764–70.
4. Jivraj S, Anstie B, Cheong YC, et al. Obstetric and neonatal outcome in women with a history of recurrent miscarriage: a cohort study. Hum Reprod 2001; 16:102–6.
5. Seidman DS, Gale R, Ever-Hadani P, et al. Reproductive complications after previous spontaneous abortions. Pediatr Rev Commun 1990; 5:1–10.
6. Sheiner E, Levy A, Katz M, et al. Pregnancy outcome following recurrent spontaneous abortions. Eur J Obstet Gynecol Reprod Biol 2005; 118:61–5.
7. Beard RW. Clinical associations of recurrent miscarriage. In: Beard RW, Sharp F, eds. Early Pregnancy Loss: Mechanisms and Treatment. London, UK: RCOG, 1988:3–8.
8. Carp HJA, Toder V, Mashiach S, et al. Recurrent miscarriage: a review of current concepts, immune mechanisms, and results of treatment. Obstet Gynecol Surv 1990; 45:657–69.
9. Recurrent Miscarriage Immunotherapy Trialists Group. Worldwide collaborative observational study and metaanalysis on allogenic leucocyte immunotherapy for recurrent spontaneous abortion. Am J Reprod Immunol 1994; 32:55–72.
10. Carp HJA, Menashe Y, Frenkel Y, et al. Lupus anticoagulant: significance in first trimester habitual abortion. J Reprod Med 1993; 38:549–52.
11. Tincani A, Balestrieri G, Danieli E, et al. Pregnancy complications of the antiphospholipid syndrome. Autoimmunity 2003; 36:27–32.
12. Brewster JA, Shaw NJ, Farquharson RG. Neonatal and pediatric outcome of infants born to mothers with antiphospholipid syndrome. J Perinat Med 1999; 27:183–7.
13. Branch DW, Dudley DJ, Scott JR, et al. Antiphospholipid antibodies and fetal loss. N Engl J Med 1992; 326:952.

14. Lima F, Khamashta MA, Buchanan NM, et al. A study of sixty pregnancies in patients with the antiphospholipid syndrome. Clin Exp Rheumatol 1996; 14:1316.

15. Branch DW, Silver RM, Blackwell JL, et al. Outcome of treated pregnancies in women with antiphospholipid syndrome: an update of the Utah experience. Obstet Gynecol 1992; 80:614–20.

16. Kutteh WH, Ermel LD. A clinical trial for the treatment of antiphospholipid antibody-associated recurrent pregnancy loss with lower dose heparin and aspirin. Am J Reprod Immunol 1996; 35:4027.

17. Pattison NS, Chamley LW, McKay EJ, et al. Antiphospholipid antibodies in pregnancy: prevalence and clinical associations. Br J Obstet Gynaecol 1993; 100: 909–13.

18. Lynch A, Marlar R, Murphy J, et al. Antiphospholipid antibodies in predicting adverse pregnancy outcome. A prospective study. Ann Intern Med 1994; 120:470–5.

19. Shehata HA, Nelson-Piercy C, Khamashta MA. Management of pregnancy in antiphospholipid syndrome. Rheum Dis Clin North Am 2001; 27:643–59.

20. Caccavo D, Vaccaro F, Ferri GM, et al. Anti-idiotypes against antiphospholipid antibodies are present in normal polyspecific immunoglobulins for therapeutic use. J Autoimmun 1994; 7:537–48.

21. Galli M, Cortelazzo S, Barbui T. In vivo efficacy of intravenous gammaglobulins in patients with lupus anticoagulant is not mediated by anti-idiotypic mechanisms. Am J Hematol 1991; 38:184–8.

22. Kwak JY, Quilty EA, Gilman-Sachs A, et al. Intravenous immunoglobulin infusion therapy in women with recurrent spontaneous abortions of immune etiologies. J Reprod Immunol 1995; 28:175–88.

23. Wegmann TG. The cytokine basis for cross-talk between the maternal immune and reproductive systems. Curr Opin Immunol 1990; 2:765–9.

24. Carreras LD, Perez GN, Vega HR, et al. Lupus anticoagulant and recurrent fetal loss: successful treatment with gammaglobulin. Lancet 1988; ii:393–4.

25. Cowchock FS, Wapner RJ, Needleman L, et al. A comparison of pregnancy outcome after two treatments for antibodies to cardiolipin (ACA). Clin Exp Rheumatol 1988; 6:200–6.

26. Triplett DA. Antiphospholipid antibodies and recurrent pregnancy loss. Am J Reprod Immunol 1989; 20:52–67.

27. Wapner RJ, Cowchock FS, Shapiro SS. Successful treatment in two women with antiphospholipid antibodies and refractory pregnancy losses with intravenous immunoglobulin infusions. Am J Obstet Gynecol 1989; 161:1271–2.

28. Vaquero E, Lazzarin N, Valensie H, et al. Pregnancy outcome in recurrent spontaneous abortion associated with antiphospholipid antibodies: a comparative study of intravenous immunoglobulin versus prednisone plus low-dose aspirin. Am J Reprod Immunol 2001; 45:174–9.

29. Branch DW, Peaceman AM, Druzin M, et al. A multicenter, placebo-controlled pilot study of intravenous immune globulin treatment of antiphospholipid syndrome during pregnancy. The Pregnancy Loss Study Group. Am J Obstet Gynecol 2000; 182:122–7.

30. Harris EN, Pierangeli SS. Utilization of intravenous immunoglobulin therapy to treat recurrent pregnancy loss in the antiphospholipid syndrome: a review. Scand J Rheumatol 1998; 107 (Suppl):97–102.

31. Kupferminc MJ, Eldor A, Steinman N, et al. Increased frequency of genetic thrombophilia in women with complications of pregnancy. N Engl J Med 1999; 340:9–13.

32. Infante-Rivard C, Rivard GE, Yotov WV, et al. Absence of association of thrombophilia polymorphisms with intrauterine growth restriction. N Engl J Med 2002; 347:19–25.

33. Alfirevic Z, Roberts D, Martlew V. How strong is the association between maternal thrombophilia and adverse pregnancy outcome? A systematic review. Eur J Obstet Gynecol Reprod Biol 2002; 101:6–14.

34. Carp HJA, Dolitzky M, Inbal A. Thromboprophylaxis improves the live birth rate in women with consecutive recurrent miscarriages and hereditary thrombophilia. J Thromb Hemost 2003; 1:433–8.

35. Younis JS, Ohel G, Brenner B, et al. Familial thrombophilia – the scientific rationale for thrombophylaxis in recurrent pregnancy loss. Hum Reprod 1997; 12:1389–90.

36. Brenner B, Hoffman R, Blumenfeld Z, et al. Gestational outcome in thrombophilic women with recurrent pregnancy loss treated by enoxaparin. Thromb Hemost 2000; 83:693–7.

37. Riyazi N, Leeda M, de Vries JI, et al. Low-molecular-weight heparin combined with aspirin in pregnant women with thrombophilia and a history of preeclampsia or fetal growth restriction: a preliminary study. Eur J Obstet Gynecol Reprod Biol 1998; 80:49–54.

38. Bates SM, Greer IA, Hirsh J, et al. Use of antithrombotic agents during pregnancy: the Seventh ACCP Conference on Antithrombotic and Thrombolytic Therapy. Chest 2004; 126:627S–44S.

39. Coulam CB, Krysa LW, Stern JJ, et al. Intravenous immunoglobulin for treatment of recurrent pregnancy loss. Am J Reprod Immunol 1995; 34:333–7.

40. Mowbray JF, Gibbings CR, Liddell H. et al. Controlled trial of treatment of recurrent spontaneous abortions by immunization with paternal cells. Lancet 1985; i:941–3.

41. Ober C, Karrison T, Odem RR, et al. Mononuclear-cell immunisation in prevention of recurrent miscarriages: a randomised trial. Lancet 1999; 354:365–9.

42. Chaouat G, Menu E, Wegmann TG. Role of lymphokines of the CSF family and of TNF, gamma interferon and IL-2 in placental growth and fetal survival studied in two murine models of spontaneous resorptions. In: Chaouat G, Mowbray JF, eds. Cellular and Molecular Biology of the Maternal–Fetal Relationship. Paris: INSERM/John Libbey Eurotext, 1991:91.

43. King A, Jokhi PP, Burrows TD, et al. Functions of human decidual NK cells. Am J Reprod Immunol 1996; 35:258–60.

44. Baines MG, Duglos AJ, de Fougerolles AR, et al. Immunological prevention of spontaneous early embryo resorption is mediated by non specific immunostimulation. Am J Reprod Immunol 1996; 35:34–42.

45. Schäfer-Somi S. Cytokines during early pregnancy of mammals: a review. Animal Reprod Sci 2003; 75:73–94.

46. Saito S. Cytokine network at the feto–maternal interface. J Reprod Immunol 2000; 47:87–103.

47. Savion S, Brengauz-Breitmann M, Torchinsky A, et al. A possible role for granulocyte macrophage-colony stimulating factor in modulating teratogen-induced effects. Teratog Carcinog Mutagen 1999; 19:171–82.

48. Levi M, Ten Cate H. Disseminated intravascular coagulation. N Engl J Med 1999; 341:586–92.

49. Bertolaccini ML, Atsumi T, Lanchbury JS, et al. Plasma tumor necrosis factor α levels and the 238*A promoter polymorphism in patients with antiphospholipid syndrome. Thromb Haemost 2001; 85:198–203.

50. Shoenfeld Y, Sherer Y, Fishman P. Interleukin-3 and pregnancy loss in antiphospholipid syndrome. Scand J Rheumatol 1998; 107 (Suppl): 19–22.

51. Fishman P, Falach-Vaknine E, Zigelman R, et al. Prevention of fetal loss in experimental antiphospholipid syndrome by in vivo administration of recombinant interleukin-3. J Clin Invest 1993; 91:1834–7.

52. Krause I, Blank M, Levi Y, et al. Anti-idiotype immunomodulation of experimental anti-phospholipid syndrome via effect on Th1/Th2 expression. Clin Exp Immunol 1999; 117:190–7.

53. Darmochwal-Kolarz D, Rolinski J, Leszczynska-Goarzelak B, et al. The expressions of intracellular cytokines in the lymphocytes of preeclamptic patients. Am J Reprod Immunol 2002; 48:381.

54. Orange S, Horvath J, Hennessy A. Preeclampsia is associated with a reduced interleukin-10 production from peripheral blood mononuclear cells. Hypertens Pregnancy 2003; 22:1–8.

55. Velzing-Aarts FV, Muskiet FA, Van der Dijs FP, et al. High serum interleukin-8 levels in Afro-Caribbean women with pre-eclampsia. Relations with tumor necrosis factor-α, Duffy negative phenotype and von Willebrand factor. Am J Reprod Immunol 2002; 48:319–22.

56. Park JS, Park CW, Lockwood CJ, et al. Role of cytokines in preterm labor and birth. Minerva Ginecol 2005; 57:349–66.

57. Fortunato SJ, Menon R, Lombardi SJ. Role of tumor necrosis factor-α in the premature rupture of membranes and preterm labor pathways. Am J Obstet Gynecol 2002; 187:1159–62.

58. Jacobsson B, Mattsby-Baltzer I, Andersch B, et al. Microbial invasion and cytokine response in amniotic fluid in a Swedish population of women in preterm labor. Acta Obstet Gynecol Scand 2003; 82:120–8.

59. Maymon E, Ghezzi F, Edwin SS, et al. The tumor necrosis factor-α and its soluble receptor profile in term and preterm parturition. Am J Obstet Gynecol 1999; 181:1142–8.

60. Ognjanovic S, Bryant-Greenwood GD. Pre-B-cell colony-enhancing factor, a novel cytokine of human fetal membranes. Am J Obstet Gynecol 2002; 187:1051–8.

61. Hahn-Zoric M, Hagberg H, Kjellmer I, et al. Aberrations in placental cytokine mRNA related to intrauterine growth retardation. Pediatr Res 2002; 51:201–6.

62. Holcberg G, Huleihel M, Sapir O, et al. Increased production of tumor necrosis factor-α (TNF-α) by IUGR human placentae. Eur J Obstet Gynecol Reprod Biol 2001; 94:69–72.

63. Lantz M, Thysell H, Nilsson E, et al. On the binding of tumor necrosis factor (TNF) to heparin and the release in vivo of the TNF-binding protein I by heparin. J Clin Invest 1991; 88:2026–31.

64. Baram D, Rashkovsky M, Hershkoviz R, et al. Inhibitory effects of low molecular weight heparin on mediator release by mast cells: preferential inhibition of cytokine production and mast cell-dependent cutaneous inflammation. Clin Exp Immunol 1997; 110:485–91.

65. Downing LJ, Strieter RM, Kadell AM, et al. Low-dose low-molecular-weight heparin is anti-inflammatory during venous thrombosis. J Vasc Surg 1998; 28:848–54.

66. San Antonio JD, Verrecchio A, Pukac LA. Heparin sensitive and resistant vascular smooth muscle cells: biology and role in restenosis. Conn Tiss Res 1998; 37:87–103.

67. Kwak JY, Gilman-Sachs A, Moretti M, et al. Natural killer cell cytotoxicity and paternal lymphocyte immunization in women with recurrent spontaneous abortions. Am J Reprod Immunol 1998; 40:352–8.

68. Gafter U, Sredni B, Segal J, et al. Suppressed cell-mediated immunity and monocyte and natural killer cell activity following allogeneic immunization of women with spontaneous recurrent abortion. J Clin Immunol 1997; 17:408–19.

69. Zenclussen AC, Kortebani G, Mazzolli A, et al. Interleukin-6 and soluble interleukin-6 receptor serum levels in recurrent spontaneous abortion women immunized with paternal white cells. Am J Reprod Immunol 2000; 44:22–9.

70. Carp HJA, Sapir T, Shoenfeld Y. Intravenous immunoglobulin and recurrent pregnancy loss. Clin Rev Allergy Immunol 2005; 29:327–32.

71. Ruiz JE, Kwak JY, Baum L, et al. Effect of intravenous immunoglobulin G on natural killer cell cytotoxicity in vitro in women with recurrent spontaneous abortion. J Reprod Immunol 1996; 31:125–41.

72. Graphou O, Chioti A, Pantazi A, et al. Effect of intravenous immunoglobulin treatment on the Th1/Th2 balance in women with recurrent spontaneous abortions. Am J Reprod Immunol 2003; 49:21–9.

17. Coping with recurrent pregnancy loss: Psychological mechanisms

Keren Shakhar

INTRODUCTION

Recurrent pregnancy loss (RPL) is clearly a stressful experience, but very little is known about what sets its emotional effects apart from isolated spontaneous miscarriages and from other forms of infertility. When studying the psychological effects of RPL, it is important not only to examine them through a pathological perspective, i.e., the induction of distress and depression, but also to appreciate how couples cope with this experience in their everyday life. A more general perspective would also examine the effect of RPL on self-esteem and marital and social relations. The degree of emotional anguish couples experience largely depends on the significance they ascribe to RPL. This meaning is influenced not only by the couple's views, but also by the perception of infertility and the view of prenatal life in their specific society. Here I shall describe the psychological aspects of RPL based on a review of the literature and on my assessment of such couples using a focus group, stress questionnaires, and informal interactions in the setting of a clinical study.

PSYCHOLOGICAL REACTIONS TO RECURRENT MISCARRIAGE

RPL is a type of infertility that confronts couples with repeated cycles of hope and despair. Many couples view parenthood as an indispensable component of their marriage and many cases of RPL occur before they have had a child. Young couples often take for granted their ability to conceive and become parents, and are only concerned with the question when to have a child. RPL shatters their basic expectations about family life. What is expected to be a fulfilling experience is instead an experience of loss and disappointment. These miscarriages usually occur at a very sensitive phase in the couple's development: becoming parents is a transitional stage that requires reconstruction of identities and preparation for new roles.

Only a few studies have specifically addressed the psychological difficulties of couples suffering from more than one miscarriage, focusing, as a rule, on the women. These studies suggest that the second miscarriage has harsher emotional impact than the first.[1-3] Although it seems logical, the question as to whether the third and fourth miscarriages further aggravate distress has never been assessed. Surprisingly, no differences in psychological distress were found between women who have had a child and those who have not (primary or secondary aborters).[3-5] Perhaps mothers feel guilty for failing to provide a sibling for their child, and fear that their child feels lonely. It is estimated that around 30% of women with RPL are depressed and that even a higher proportion have high levels of state and trait anxiety.[4,5]

When women with RPL conceive again, they exhibit high levels of anxiety, having difficulty getting through each day.[6] This anxiety is manifested as general tension, despondence, and premonitions of miscarriage, and may be exhibited by weeping, fear of detecting bleeding when going to the toilet or examining underwear, extreme anxiety over any abdominal pain, checking continuously for signs of pregnancy, avoidance of other pregnant women, and reluctance to discuss the pregnancy with anyone, including their husband.[6,7] As a so-called defense mechanism, some women show less emotional attachment to their subsequent pregnancies, and avoid thinking about their future child.[6,8]

Although this type of reaction may alleviate the constant anxiety and may protect women emotionally if eventually they miscarry, it also diminishes the pleasure women can derive from being pregnant, and may prevent grief from being processed and the experience from being integrated. In addition, it is unclear how deep into pregnancy women are less attached to their embryo and whether it complicates the transition to motherhood.

Since the psychological literature on RPL is limited, and since women with RPL must cope with both miscarriages and potential infertility, I will next examine what is known about these two entities. The reaction to a sudden loss of pregnancy varies greatly among different individuals: some exhibit little or no reaction, whereas others demonstrate a significant decline in their coping ability.[9,10] Major themes that describe the experience of miscarriage are emptiness and guilt.[11] Increased anxiety and depressive symptoms are also very common.[9,12,13] These depressive symptoms can include staying in bed and doing nothing, difficulty to perform daily tasks, and a feeling of a physical illness. There is disagreement, however, as to when these symptoms decline. Several studies have found that 4 weeks after miscarriage, about half of the women were still depressed, and 18% of the women feared another miscarriage to the extent that they considered not conceiving again.[3] Others have shown increased levels of depression as long as 6 months after miscarriage.[12,13]

An isolated miscarriage has little prognostic value. Hence, one should be cautious in drawing inferences from a single miscarriage and applying these conclusions to RPL. In RPL, each additional miscarriage reduces the prospects of having children. Consequently, the repeated nature of RPL may exacerbate the experience or teach couples to cope with it. Although never studied, the prognostic meaning the couple associates with the miscarriage can further damage their sense of well-being.

Many couples experiencing miscarriage undergo a process of grieving[10] (to be described later). They mourn the lost child, their failed hopes for the child, and their unaccomplished parenthood. Unlike the grief over the death of a relative, these couples generally do not receive social support, and may also face insensitive attitudes. Sometimes, miscarriage occurs before the couple had shared the news of the pregnancy with anyone, leaving them lonely in the grieving process. It is crucial to understand that even if the embryo was lost at a very early gestational week, many couples already regard their embryo as a baby, name or nickname him, talk to him, ascribe a specific personality to him, and imagine his future.[14]

Unfortunately, family members and friends may not know how to respond to the bereaved couple, and may not grasp what the pregnancy meant to them.[15] The variability in couples' attitudes may make it hard for their friends and family to support them. A break in communications sometimes occurs because of lack of response or because the couple consider the response inappropriate.[16,17] Typical attempts at consolation include 'At least you can get pregnant', 'Maybe it's good you miscarried, the baby was probably abnormal anyway', 'How can you grieve so much, you were barely pregnant' and 'You can always conceive again'. While these perspectives may help some couples, many others do not want to forget their miscarried child at this time, and resist the possibility that someday they would feel as if the loss has never happened.[6,17] Based on studies of general infertility, friends and family may feel guilty of their pregnancies and may sometimes try to hide their pregnancy or talk less about their children, resulting in the couple feeling distanced from their friends, which can result in social withdrawal.[15] In addition, the couple may feel that family and friends expect that they will shortly conceive again to quickly replace their loss.

Couples may also avoid social gatherings, parties, and family occasions to avoid interactions with pregnant women or children. Some of them cannot bear being expected to hold someone else's child or to listen to stories about the pleasures and difficulties others are experiencing when raising children. These often remind them of their loss.

One way to compensate for the lack of social support from family and friends is to seek couples who share similar experiences. However, unlike the experience of an isolated spontaneous miscarriage, where many women have had a similar experience, women suffering from RPL usually do not know other women in their situation and may lack someone to truly share their feelings with. Some of their closest friends may be pregnant or already have children, making it difficult for them to feel their experience can be shared. Support groups are hard to find and there are hardly any internet forums that are specific for RPL.

Apart from being emotionally traumatic, miscarriage can be physically traumatic as well; it may involve sudden pain, loss of blood, rapid hospitalization, and curettage.[16] Some women identify the physical process of miscarriage as the most stressful aspect, and they may find it harder to cope with each time.

There has been considerable research on variables that moderate the influence of miscarriage on well-being, some of which may vary with time since the loss. Identifying these moderators is essential to understand the variability in response to the loss, and, more importantly, it points at potential targets for psychological interventions. Some of these mediators are uncontrollable – for example, young age is associated with lesser well-being,[2] and a later gestational week of miscarriage has harsher psychological consequences. However, other factors can be controlled and are associated with adverse well-being: these include attributing high personal significance to miscarriage, low investment in domains of life other than parenthood, and low satisfaction in other aspects of life, such as work, lack of social support, lower emotional strength, and use of passive coping strategies.[10,18–20] In contrast, women who reported that the recurrent miscarriages taught them to place greater value on their relationship with their spouses and to change priorities or personal goals scored higher on well-being.

Coping with infertility has been much explored over the last 50 years. Many researchers describe infertility as a crisis having psychological effects, including loss of self-esteem, increased anxiety, sexual problems, anger, depression, and self-blame.[21–25] The uncertainty of having biological children evokes a sense that life is unpredictable and that significant events in life are not under control.

Loss of self-esteem, guilt, and self-blame may be even more evident in women suffering from RPL. Unlike many fertility problems, where the cause is either unknown or is attributed to both partners, in RPL, women feel that they are to blame because it was their body that betrayed and could not support the pregnancy. This feeling is reinforced by the medical examinations that couples undergo: most clinical examinations evaluate possible etiologies in the women.

An aspect that is unique to RPL among fertility problems is the period when women are most stressed and anxious. In most fertility problems, getting pregnant is the aim, and, once achieved, the mission has largely been accomplished. In contrast, this period is usually the most stressful for women who have experienced RPL, and the anxiety level may peak around gestational weeks when previous miscarriages occurred.[6] This anxiety is reflected by extreme sensitivity to body signals, and increased fear that miscarriage will happen again. The decision to conceive again is often very hard, because women have to consider whether they can bear another miscarriage. In my interviews with women with RPL, they have often spoken about times that are problematic for them to conceive, such as major holidays when they have to face family members.

THE GRIEVING PROCESS

Couples experiencing RPL will often grieve for their lost children, their lost parenthood, their biological failure, the loss of control over their life, and for the possibility that they would not have biological children.[12,25] Unlike losing a child, the couples do not have memories of the baby, and their loss is often not acknowledged by society.[10] There are no rituals associated with mourning a miscarriage. Couples may feel reluctant to share the experience with others, often cannot take days off from work, and may lack the time they would like to grieve for the loss. Couples may also be torn between their hopes for a successful pregnancy and their grief.

This grief process is often characterized by intense fluctuations in emotions, ranging from crying to laughing to being angry. This grief process may last for months and even years, and often extends into the subsequent pregnancies that serve as reminders for previous losses and can trigger intense emotions. Many couples may be very surprised by their mood swings and the intensity of the emotions that they experience. They may not be aware that this is a normal reaction to their loss. It is very important to reassure them that their reaction is normal and common.

Although there is no single right way to grieve, several stages of grief are commonly experienced by people. There is disagreement whether all people pass through each of these stages, and people differ in the time they spend at each stage. The following list of the stages is mostly based on Menning's experience in his work as a counselor with infertile couples.[26]

1. *Denial, shock and numbness.*[27,28] This stage often begins with the shock that another miscarriage has occurred and is characterized by the feeling that 'this can't be happening to me'. Sometimes, the couples will not even admit to themselves that something may be wrong. This reaction serves as a defense mechanism, and will usually diminish as couples begin to acknowledge their loss, usually within hours to days. This emotional numbness and denial should not be confused with 'lack of caring'.

2. *Anger.*[8,27] During this stage, the couple is preoccupied with the miscarriages that they have had. A feeling of unfairness surrounds these thoughts: 'Why me? Why us?' The couple also experiences an intense yearning for the lost child, for the lost parenthood, pregnancy, and dreams. The anger associated with the unfairness of the entire experience can focus on the pain and inconvenience associated with miscarriage, with the tests and treatments, with the social pressure they feel from their family and friends, and on comments regarding their miscarriages and childlessness. The anger may also include broader targets such as abortion rights advocates, people who easily carry to

term, and the medical team. Social support and respect can help abate this anger.

3. *Isolation.*[27] Many couples exhibit social withdrawal. This often happens because couples try to hide their pregnancies and miscarriages, do not want to be judged or pitied by others, or avoid occasions where they might meet children or pregnant women. They also feel that their experience is unique, and that others whose experience of being pregnant is joyous cannot comprehend what they are going through. Moreover, peers and family members often avoid discussing the recurrent miscarriages with the couples – either because they are embarrassed with the ease of their having children or because they do not want to disrupt the couple's privacy.

4. *Guilt.*[8,27] Women sometimes feel that the recurrent miscarriages represent punishment for something they did. They may regret actions they took or failed to take prior to the miscarriages.

5. *Depression.*[4,8] At this stage, there is full penetration of the distress and facing the loss. Thoughts such as 'My life is over, I can't go on' or 'I don't care any more' are very frequent. Some women may feel a sense of great loss, mood fluctuations, and loneliness.

6. *Rebuilding and healing.* There is disagreement whether complete healing can occur. Still, at this stage, the couple start to deal with the reality of the situation. They restructure the event, organize their activities, and plan to move forward in life, and become more energetic and social.

WHAT DOMAINS OF LIFE ARE AFFECTED?

RPL can affect many domains in a couple's life: from self-esteem to relationship with others, and even to financial costs. Here is a list of the main domains that are affected:

- *Self-esteem.*[21,25] Most people view the ability to conceive and have children as central to their personal identity. Our socialization process teaches girls and women to view motherhood as an integral part of their self-worth and femininity.[29] In several religions, including the Jewish communities where I conducted my research, 'Reproduce and fill the earth' is one of the most important precepts. Consequently, not reproducing is often perceived in traditional societies as a degrading failure – impinging on self-esteem and putting in question the woman's femininity and worth as a spouse.

- *Loss of control*.[6,15,25] For many women, RPL is the first experience of a major loss of control: they lose control over their life, their body, and their ability to plan the future. Some of this planning includes the time of conception (e.g., the best time to be absent from work, when it fits well with their and their spouse's career plans), and plans for adequate housing for an expanding family.
- *Relationship with peers*.[15,25] Couples may feel excluded from friends whose interests focuses on children, and may seek new reference groups to belong to. Difficulties in facing pregnant women and young children also lead couples to avoid peers who are pregnant or already have children. In addition, their friends may feel uncomfortable in disclosing their pregnancies, and this may be misinterpreted by the couple as a sign of alienation. In contrast to many other fertility problems and despite the fact that RPL is not so rare, many women with RPL do not know other women in the same situation to whom they can relate.
- *Marital stress*.[4,15,30] While the experience of infertility can improve marital adjustment for some couples, it may damage the relationships of others and increase marital stress.[24,30,31] This may result from differences between the spouses in the attitude toward the losses, in the grief response, and in their motivation to have children. In addition, women may feel guilty for failing their spouse's expectations, and may feel responsible for his pain. Many women fear that their partner would leave them to find someone else with whom to have children. Pressures to have children from the husband's family can further exacerbate this fear.

- *Sexual life*.[30,32] RPL, like other fertility problems, may increase sexual discontent. Couples may feel a pressure to quickly conceive again, and with it an increased demand to have sex at certain times. Not being in the mood or being absent due to various reasons such as business trips may increase the tension.
- *Financial cost*. In addition, RPL frequently taxes couples with financial costs: visits to a specialist, tests, treatment, and absence from work.

THE MALE PARTNER

Spouses are often very lonely in their experience of RPL. Women are, after all, considered the main patients – they experience the physical miscarriage, their reproductive system is assumed to hold the cause, and they are subject to most diagnostic tests. The idea that the spouse may also experience intense grief is often forgotten by society, by the couple's acquaintances, and by the medical team. Compared with women, the grief of male partners is less active and is expressed for a shorter duration.[33] Men are often ready to carry on with their lives earlier than women, and are also less interested in discussing the miscarriage repeatedly.[9, 21]

Spouses frequently find themselves in a very delicate position: at the same time, they endure a crisis, grieve, and need support, they feel that they ought to be strong to emotionally support their partners. As a result, spouses suppress their feelings of loss instead of sharing it with their partners. Moreover, if the woman is depressed, they often feel that they are not doing a good job of supporting her.[33] They may struggle to say the right words, and fear that what they say would make their partners feel worse. Many of them fail to realize that their female partners want to know that their grief is shared by others. Also, although the spouses may have the best intentions of providing support, there are sex differences in coping strategies with life stressors,[34] and males tend to give instrumental rather than social support, leaving women feeling unsupported and the male partners feeling guilty and unappreciated.

THE PHYSICIAN

Although the physician and the couple share the desire for pregnancy to succeed, the cooperation between them is complex and may be very vulnerable. The challenge with which the physician is confronted when first seeing couples with RPL is almost impossible. Usually, the time that can be devoted to each couple is very limited when the routine components of a medical consultation are considered: taking a history, sorting and interpreting the results of previous investigations, explaining the problem and its possible causes, subsequent prognosis, suggesting additional investigations, answering the couple's questions, and showing sympathy. Often, this is a time when the couple's anxiety and stress are very intense, and they are very attentive and sensitive to every word and gesture. Their first visit to the specialist can evoke many emotions: frustration, anger, stress, and inadequacy. This visit reminds them of past miscarriages, confronts them with their lack of control, clarifies that they should prepare for more miscarriages, and confirms that they have a medical condition that might leave them childless. Physicians are often unaware that the high stress that the couple experiences interferes with their ability to process the information received at the visit. This is a very common experience for many patients undergoing diagnosis: they often cannot recall what the physician said, and tend to misinterpret what has been told to them.

Couples hope to identify a cause for their miscarriages. Understanding the cause, from their point of view, means that a treatment can be offered. It was suggested that women assign a cause to the miscarriage themselves, when one is not assigned by the doctor.[16] Self-diagnoses include stress, certain foods, and too much or too little exercise. This may reflect an attempt to regain a sense of control. It is thought that when the cause is detected, there is less self-blame.[35]

However, there is still no evidence to support this notion in RPL.[36]

VALUE OF PSYCHOLOGICAL SUPPORT IN COUPLES WITH RPL

Clearly, the experience of RPL increases levels of distress, depressive symptoms, and anxiety. To lower the emotional burden, couples often withdraw from friends. RPL can affect almost every aspect of life, and the emotional burden usually becomes heavier during pregnancy. Obviously, these couples could benefit from psychological support. Although there is no one path that fits the needs of all couples, the following are some options.

- *Support groups.* Support is viewed as most credible coming from someone who has previously experienced and successfully managed a similar crisis. In contrast to many other medical conditions, couples with RPL often do not know similarly afflicted people with whom to openly share their feelings, thoughts, and concerns. Internet support groups usually lump together women with one miscarriage and women with several. Forums for infertility are more focused on fertility treatments than on anxieties of women with previous miscarriages. Meeting other couples with RPL (past or present) can decrease the sense of loneliness, and reassure couples that their reactions and feelings are normal.
- *Teaching couples about the grieving process.* This can help them realize that their reaction to the grief process is normal and is experienced by many other couples. It can also help couples accept their grief, and proceed with it in their own way and pace.
- *Activities for reducing anxiety.* Physical activity, art, meditation, relaxation and, yoga can reduce general anxiety in a non-specific manner.
- *Cognitive restructuring.*[37] The individual interpretation of RPL influences the emotions evoked by this experience. Some of the negative thoughts invoked are automatic and erroneous.

Challenging these thoughts and restructuring them into more truthful and positive thinking can improve well-being. Such techniques have been shown to diminish stress, anxiety, depression, and self-blame, and to increase enjoyments in everyday life, in having each other, in work, etc. An example of a common automatic thought in women with RPL may be 'I'll never have any children.' This thought is definitely not true, and should be challenged. Some examples may be 'This process is very painful for me, but there is a chance that I will eventually have children.' In addition, the significance attributed to having biological children can be reframed.

- *Improving dialogue with spouse.* Sometimes, spouses fail to recognize what their partners are going through; this may create a cycle of disrupted communication that decreases a couple's enjoyment in doing things together and increases their marital stress. It is therefore important to encourage couples to have a fruitful dialogue, by learning to listen more to each other, by acknowledging the feelings of each other, by being aware that they may be using different coping strategies, and by recognizing each other's needs.

- *Learning of other parenting options.* Although not all couples feel ready to explore other means to achieve parenthood, many could benefit from meeting couples who have chosen to adopt or use the aid of a surrogate mother. This not only informs them of the procedures and the emotions associated with choosing other paths, but it also confronts them with 'their worst nightmare'. Although they may not decide to follow these paths, couples often realize this is not as bad an option as they have imagined, and some of the fear that is associated with infertility may be relieved.

- *Discussing legitimacy.* Many women with RPL report that they feel it is illegitimate to stop trying to conceive or to choose alternative means for parenthood. Many feel like that they invest a lot of their energy in conceiving and reconceiving, in hurrying to become parents, but at the same time

they need to deal with the pain and grief. They often feel that everyone is expecting them to quickly continue and to try again. They feel that others deny them the legitimacy to say 'I don't want to try again'. Raising the option to take a break or to stop conceiving by the medical team may help relieve some of such pressure from some women.

Since emotional anxiety tends to peak during pregnancy, therapy should also be targeted to that period. Although many of the above strategies can only be realistically offered between pregnancies, many can help to cope better with emotional difficulties in subsequent pregnancies. Relaxation techniques can be employed whenever a woman recognizes an increase in her stress levels, and cognitive restructuring can help maintain positive thoughts and avoid the loop of negative thoughts.

CAN STRESS CONTRIBUTE TO RECURRENT MISCARRIAGE?

A common question that bothers couples is whether excessive stress can adversely affect pregnancy and lead to miscarriage. A belief in such a relationship can increase feelings of guilt and self-blame and further increase stress in a self-perpetuating circle. Although it is a sensitive matter, this is an important question to study. This question is difficult to examine, since retrospective reports of stress are skewed by the already-experienced outcome, since many women in the general population miscarry due to abnormal chromosomes, and since women at a high risk for miscarriage often experience high levels of stress during pregnancy.

Prospective human studies on the effects of stress on miscarriage or IVF success are rare: some have suggested a causative relation, some have indicated correlations, while others have found no association.[38–43] With regard to miscarriage, a distinction is not usually made between unexplained miscarriage and miscarriage due to chromosomal abnormalities. One study that attempted to separate the two groups found a correlation between stress levels and miscarriage only in cases thought not to involve chromosomal abnormalities.[44] This, together with the fact that miscarriage is a dichotomous variable, would necessitate a very large sample to detect a correlation.

Studies in rodents have suggested that stress increases the rates of implantation and resorption. Exposing pregnant rats or mice to stress can result in lower pregnancy rates, higher embryonic death, more resorptions, and smaller litters.[45–48] Adrenocorticotropic hormone (ACTH) treatment for the first 8 days of pregnancy reduced the number of implantation sites in naive/sham operated as well as adrenalectomized mice,[49] suggesting a direct role for this hormone.

Overall, based on animal models and on correlative studies in humans, there is some evidence that stress can adversely affect fertility in general. However, it is unclear whether this effect can be extended to recurrent miscarriage. Two studies in women with RPL found that depressive symptoms and low satisfaction with social support are predictive of subsequent miscarriage.[50,51] Another prospective study, though, has failed to find such an association with regard to perceived stress.[42]

The best support for the contribution of psychological factors to RPL comes from studies that have evaluated the effect of psychological support or therapy in women suffering from RPL.[7,52–55] Interventions ranged from basic 'tender loving care' to relaxation workshops and audiocassettes, weekly ultrasound examinations (to assure the woman that the embryo develops appropriately), and other psychological interventions. Remarkably, all four studies reported that women who received psychological support had two- to fourfold lower miscarriage rates than those who did not (Table 17.1). Although these studies suffer from methodological problems, it is doubtful whether these flaws can account for such a marked reduction in miscarriage rates (on average from 62% to 23%).

If stress does indeed contributes to miscarriage in women with RPL, it could lead couples into a vicious circle. The first miscarriage could be due to some biological cause such as abnormal karyotype.

Table 17.1 Pregnancy outcome in women with recurrent pregnancy loss after supportive care

Study	Success rates	
	Control group	Supportive care group
Stray-Pedersen and Stray-Pedersen[52]	8/24 (33%)	32/37 (86%)
Clifford et al[53]	20/41 (49%)	118/160 (74%)
Liddel et al[7]	3/9 (33%)	38/44 (86%)
Tupper and Weil[54]	5/19 (26%)	16/19 (84%)
Brigham et al[55]		167/222 (75%)
Total	36/93 (38%)	371/482 (77%)

During the second pregnancy, these women are more stressed, which boosts the risk of another miscarriage. If another miscarriage occurs, this increases their stress, and their chances of another miscarriage.

PSYCHONEUROIMMUNOLOGY AND ITS RELEVANCE

There are several potential neuroendocrinological pathways through which stress might promote miscarriage. However, an interesting pathway that has captured the attention of several investigators is the psychoneuroimmunologic (PNI) path.[56,57] Over the past 30 years, it has become clear that the immune system is not autonomous but has bidirectional connections with the central nervous system.[58–60] It has been shown that the immune responses can be behaviorally conditioned, that various emotional and cognitive states can influence both cellular and humoral immunity, and that cytokines can affect neural function.

The effects of psychological stress on various immune measures have been extensively studied. In most cases, stress interferes with the normal function of the immune system rather than assisting it. It has also been demonstrated that this perturbation can result in actual consequences to health, for example lowering resistance to infections and slowing wound healing.[60,61] This is especially the case with chronic and severe stress.

Interestingly, the subset of immune cells that seem to be most affected by stress are natural killer (NK) cells,[61] the cells thought to be involved in the etiology of RPL. NK cells seem to carry the greatest density of adrenergic receptors, and are thus more susceptible to the influence of the sympathetic nervous system.[62] These receptors contribute to direct suppression of NK-cell activity, detachment from endothelial cells, and redistribution after exposure to stress. The number and activity of circulating NK cells were reported to be highly affected by stressors such as academic examination, exposure to disastrous hurricanes, interpersonal stress, first parachuting jumps, and marital disputes.

From the PNI perspective, stress might be promoting miscarriage by interfering with the uterine immunological conditions that protect pregnancy. In several experiments in mice, Arck et al[63] have shown that stress around the fifth day of pregnancy more than tripled the resorption rates in miscarriage-prone mice; depletion of NK cells prevented this effect. Studying women, we have recently shown that the number and activity of peripheral NK cells in RPL, which have previously been shown to predict the outcome of subsequent pregnancy, is a transient response to the blood withdrawal.[64] A cannula was inserted into the veins of women with RPL and controls, and blood was drawn immediately and 20 minutes later. NK-cell activity and cell number were increased in RPL patients in the first blood withdrawal, but declined to a level similar to that of the control in the second blood withdrawal. These levels remained almost unchanged in the control groups. This may suggest that the increased NK-cell activity and numbers often observed in women with RPL reflect hypersensitivity to the stress of blood withdrawal rather than the immunological steady state. It remains to be determined whether such hypersensitivity is also predictive of pregnancy outcome.

SUMMARY

More than any other fertility problem, RPL submits patients to repeated cycles of hope and despair.

Although management of physician's emotions is not considered part of the physician's role, I believe that adopting an inclusive psychosocial perspective would greatly improve the treatment of couples with RPL. The anxiety, depression, anger, and frustration these couples experience are critically influenced by how significant they regard their miscarriages, by how their family, friends, and society perceive these miscarriages, and by how much emotional support they receive. A supportive and empathic approach by the medical team can ease this suffering, and psychological interventions can be used to improve couples' coping and enhance their well-being.

Such interventions may not only relieve the emotional burden of RPL but also lower the risk of another miscarriage. Although some clinicians may dismiss such effects, the evidence for such a possibility exceeds the support for several medical interventions already employed in RPL. Larger randomized studies should examine this possibility more carefully. Until proven, the psychosocial hypothesis should be raised with caution, as it can lead women to blame themselves for the miscarriage.

REFERENCES

1. Aoki K, Furukawa T, Ogasawara M, et al. Psychosocial factors in recurrent miscarriages. Acta Obstet Gynecol Scand 1998; 77:572–3.
2. Neugebauer R. Depressive symptoms at two months after miscarriage: interpreting study findings from an epidemiological versus clinical perspective. Depress Anxiety 2003; 17:152–61.
3. Friedman T, Gath D. The psychiatric consequences of spontaneous abortion. Br J Psychiatry 1989; 155:810–13.
4. Klock SC, Chang G, Hiley A, et al. Psychological distress among women with recurrent spontaneous abortion. Psychosomatics 1997; 38:503–7.
5. Craig M, Tata P, Regan L. Psychiatric morbidity among patients with recurrent miscarriage. J Psychosom Obstet Gynaecol 2002; 23:157–64.
6. Cote-Arsenault D, Morrison-Beedy D. Women's voices reflecting changed expectations for pregnancy after perinatal loss. J Nurs Scholarsh 2001; 33:239–44.
7. Liddell HS, Pattison NS, Zanderigo A. Recurrent miscarriage – outcome after supportive care in early pregnancy. Aust NZ J Obstet Gynaecol 1991; 31:320–2.
8. Madden ME. The variety of emotional reactions to miscarriage. Women Health 1994; 21:85–104.
9. Athey J, Spielvogel AM. Risk factors and interventions for psychological sequelae in women after miscarriage. Prim Care Update Ob/Gyns 2000; 7:64–9.
10. Lee C, Slade P. Miscarriage as a traumatic event: a review of the literature and new implications for intervention. J Psychosom Res 1996; 40:235–44.

11. Adolfsson A, Larsson PG, Wijma B, et al. Guilt and emptiness: women's experiences of miscarriage. Health Care Women Int 2004; 25:543–60.

12. Nikcevic AV, Tunkel SA, Nicolaides KH. Psychological outcomes following missed abortions and provision of follow-up care. Ultrasound Obstet Gynecol 1998; 11:123–8.

13. Janssen HJ, Cuisinier MC, Hoogduin KA, et al. Controlled prospective study on the mental health of women following pregnancy loss. Am J Psychiatry 1996; 153:226–30.

14. Klier CM, Geller PA, Ritsher JB. Affective disorders in the aftermath of miscarriage: a comprehensive review. Arch Womens Ment Health 2002; 5:129–49.

15. Imeson M, McMurray A. Couples' experiences of infertility: a phenomenological study. J Adv Nurs 1996; 24:1014–22.

16. Bansen SS, Stevens HA. Women's experiences of miscarriage in early pregnancy. J Nurse Midwifery 1992; 37:84–90.

17. Cecil R. 'I wouldn't have minded a wee one running about': Miscarriage and the family. Soc Sci Med 1994; 38:1415–22.

18. Mindes EJ, Ingram KM, Kliewer W, et al. Longitudinal analyses of the relationship between unsupportive social interactions and psychological adjustment among women with fertility problems. Soc Sci Med 2003; 56:2165–80.

19. Brier N. Understanding and managing the emotional reactions to a miscarriage. Obstet Gynecol 1999; 93:151–5.

20. Swanson KM. Predicting depressive symptoms after miscarriage: a path analysis based on the Lazarus paradigm. J Womens Health Gend Based Med 2000; 9:191–206.

21. Pasch LA, Dunkel-Schetter C, Christensen A. Differences between husbands' and wives' approach to infertility affect marital communication and adjustment. Fertil Steril 2002; 77:1241–7.

22. Greil AL. Infertility and psychological distress: a critical review of the literature. Soc Sci Med 1997; 45:1679–704.

23. Alesi R. Infertility and its treatment – an emotional roller coaster. Aust Fam Physician 2005; 34:135–8.

24. Schover LR. Recognizing the stress of infertility. Cleve Clin J Med 1997; 64:211–14.

25. Gonzalez LO. Infertility as a transformational process: a framework for psychotherapeutic support of infertile women. Issues Ment Health Nurs 2000; 21:619–33.

26. Menning BE. The emotional needs of infertile couples. Fertil Steril 1980; 34:313–19.

27. Matthews AM, Matthews R. Beyond the mechanics of infertility – perspectives on the social-psychology of infertility and involuntary childlessness. Family Relations 1986; 35:479–87.

28. Lee C, Slade P, Lygo V. The influence of psychological debriefing on emotional adaptation in women following early miscarriage: a preliminary study. Br J Med Psychol 1996; 69:47–58.

29. Becker G, Nachtigall RD. 'Born to be a mother': the cultural construction of risk in infertility treatment in the U.S. Soc Sci Med 1994; 39:507–18.

30. Monga M, Alexandrescu B, Katz SE, et al. Impact of infertility on quality of life, marital adjustment, and sexual function. Urology 2004; 63:126–30.

31. Connolly KJ, Edelmann RJ, Cooke ID, et al. The impact of infertility on psychological functioning. J Psychosom Res 1992; 36:459–68.

32. Seibel MM, Taymor ML. Emotional aspects of infertility. Fertil Steril 1982; 37:137–45.

33. Beutel M, Willner H, Deckardt R, et al. Similarities and differences in couples' grief reactions following a miscarriage: results from a longitudinal study. J Psychosom Res 1996; 40:245–53.

34. Jordan C, Revenson TA. Gender differences in coping with infertility: a meta-analysis. J Behav Med 1999; 22:341–58.

35. Nikcevic AV, Tunkel SA, Kuczmierczyk AR, et al. Investigation of the cause of miscarriage and its influence on women's psychological distress. Br J Obstet Gynaecol 1999; 106:808–13.

36. Rowsell E, Jongman G, Kilby M, et al. The psychological impact of recurrent miscarriage, and the role of counselling at a pre-pregnancy counselling clinic. J Reprod Infant Psychol 2001; 19:33–45.

37. Beck JS. Cognitive Therapy: Basic and Beyond. New York: Guilford Press, 1995.

38. Domar AD, Clapp D, Slawsby EA, et al. Impact of group psychological interventions on pregnancy rates in infertile women. Fertil Steril 2000; 73:805–11.

39. Merari D, Feldberg D, Elizur A, et al. Psychological and hormonal changes in the course of in vitro fertilization. J Assist Reprod Genet 1992; 9:161–9.

40. Boivin J, Takefman JE. Stress level across stages of in vitro fertilization in subsequently pregnant and nonpregnant women. Fertil Steril 1995; 64:802–10.

41. Facchinetti F, Matteo ML, Artini GP, et al. An increased vulnerability to stress is associated with a poor outcome of in vitro fertilization–embryo transfer treatment. Fertil Steril 1997; 67:309–14.

42. Bergant AM, Reinstadler K, Moncayo HE, et al. Spontaneous abortion and psychosomatics. A prospective study on the impact of psychological factors as a cause for recurrent spontaneous abortion. Hum Reprod 1997; 12:1106–10.

43. Boivin J, Andersson L, Skoog-Svanberg A, et al. Psychological reactions during in-vitro fertilization: similar response pattern in husbands and wives. Hum Reprod 1998; 13:3262–7.

44. Boyles SH, Ness RB, Grisso JA, et al. Life event stress and the association with spontaneous abortion in gravid women at an urban emergency department. Health Psychol 2000; 19:510–14.

45. Wiebold JL, Stanfield PH, Becker WC, et al. The effect of restraint stress in early pregnancy in mice. J Reprod Fertil 1986; 78:185–92.

46. Euker JS, Riegle GD. Effects of stress on pregnancy in the rat. J Reprod Fertil 1973; 34:343–6.

47. Arck PC, Merali F, Chaouat G, et al. Inhibition of immunoprotective CD8$^+$ T cells as a basis for stress-triggered substance P-mediated abortion in mice. Cell Immunol 1996; 171:226–30.

48. Arck PC, Merali FS, Manuel J, et al. Stress-triggered abortion: inhibition of protective suppression and promotion of tumor necrosis factor-α (TNF-α) release as a mechanism triggering resorptions in mice. Am J Reprod Immunol 1995; 33:74–80.

49. Kittinger JW, Gutierrez-Cernosek RM, Cernosek SF, Jr, et al. Effects of adrenocorticotropin on pregnancy and prolactin in mice. Endocrinology 1980; 107:616–21.

50. Nakano Y, Oshima M, Sugiura-Ogasawara M, et al. Psychosocial predictors of successful delivery after unexplained recurrent spontaneous abortions: a cohort study. Acta Psychiatr Scand 2004; 109:440–6.

51. Sugiura-Ogasawara M, Furukawa TA, Nakano Y, et al. Depression as a potential causal factor in subsequent miscarriage in recurrent spontaneous aborters. Hum Reprod 2002; 17:2580–4.

52. Stray-Pedersen B, Stray-Pedersen S. Etiologic factors and subsequent reproductive performance in 195 couples with a prior history of habitual abortion. Am J Obstet Gynecol 1984; 148:140–6.

53. Clifford K, Rai R, Regan L. Future pregnancy outcome in unexplained recurrent first trimester miscarriage. Hum Reprod 1997; 12:387–9.

54. Tupper C, Weil RJ. The problem of spontaneous abortion. Am J Obstet Gynecol 1962; 83:421–4.

55. Brigham SA, Conlon C, Farquharson RG. A longitudinal study of pregnancy outcome following idiopathic recurrent miscarriage. Hum Reprod 1999; 14:2868–71.

56. Clark DA, Arck PC, Jalali R, et al. Psycho–neuro–cytokine/endocrine pathways in immunoregulation during pregnancy. Am J Reprod Immunol 1996; 35:330–7.

57. Arck PC. Stress and pregnancy loss: role of immune mediators, hormones and neurotransmitters. Am J Reprod Immunol 2001; 46: 117–23.

58. Ader R. On the development of psychoneuroimmunology. Eur J Pharmacol 2000; 405:167–76.

59. Maier SF, Watkins LR, Fleshner M. Psychoneuroimmunology. The interface between behavior, brain, and immunity. Am Psychol 1994; 49:1004–17.

60. Glaser R, Kiecolt-Glaser JK. Stress-induced immune dysfunction: implications for health. Nat Rev Immunol 2005; 5:243–51.

61. Cohen S, Herbert TB. Health psychology: psychological factors and physical disease from the perspective of human psychoneuroimmunology. Annu Rev Psychol 1996; 47:113–42.

62. Landmann R. Beta-adrenergic receptors in human leukocyte subpopulations. Eur J Clini Invest 1992; 1:30–6.

63. Arck PC, Merali FS, Stanisz AM, et al. Stress-induced murine abortion associated with substance P-dependent alteration in cytokines in maternal uterine decidua. Biol Reprod 1995; 53:814–19.

64. Shakhar K, Rosenne E, Loewenthal R, et al. High NK activity in recurrent miscarriage: What are we really measuring? Hum Reprod 2006; 21:2421–5.

18. Methodological issues in evidence-based evaluation of treatment for recurrent miscarriage

Salim Daya

INTRODUCTION

The philosophy of using evidence from valid and current studies to assist in the clinical decision-making process is now widely acknowledged as desirable for improving the quality of care provided to patients. The underlying principle of this evidence-based approach to healthcare management is having access to reliable and valid evidence that is obtained by either searching the literature for papers that can be critically appraised or designing studies of high methodological rigor. The resulting best available evidence is then used to answer clearly defined and focused questions generated from encounters with patients presenting with their clinical problems. This approach is now guiding management in obstetrics and gynecology, including the subspecialty of infertility dealing with the problem of recurrent miscarriage.

Over the years, increased attention has focused on the evaluation and management of recurrent miscarriage. Protocols have been developed for diagnostic evaluation in couples with recurrent miscarriage so that a plan of care can be outlined based on the findings. However, to date, there is no consensus on the optimal evaluation and management strategy to effectively address the problem of recurrent miscarriage. The situation is made more challenging by the fact that the published literature is generally of poor quality and often has contradictory findings, in part due to sampling variability, but largely due to studies of low validity. The approach of systematically gathering the evidence and pooling outcome data with meta-analyses is an attempt to bring some order to this field, but it too has its pitfalls, leading in some instances to erroneous inferences and misleading recommendations for clinical care.

Recently, the Special Interest Group for Early Pregnancy, under the auspices of the European Society for Human Reproduction and Embryology, updated their guidelines for the investigation and medical treatment of recurrent miscarriage.[1] Unfortunately, the paucity of good-quality evidence led to the conclusion that many of the proposed investigations require further evaluation within research programs. In addition, 'tender loving care' and health advice were the only interventions that did not require further study; most of the other proposed therapies either require more investigation of their efficacy with randomized trials or are associated with more harm than benefit.[1]

Reliable inferences regarding therapeutic interventions can only be drawn from trials that have addressed all the elements necessary for internal validity. The important issues include the folowing:

- definition of recurrent miscarriage and its subgroups
- avoidance of including women with repeated implantation failure
- establishing the baseline risk for miscarriage so that a control event rate can be obtained
- controlling for female age and for male partner status
- formulation of an appropriate research question
- use of randomization
- importance of concealment of treatment allocation and blinding
- avoidance of co-intervention
- requirement for an adequate sample size

- avoidance of using historical controls
- importance of analyzing data using an intention-to-treat approach
- clear identification of the orientation of the study from the perspectives of superiority, equivalence, or non-inferiority of the interventions being compared
- clarity on when treatment should be commenced
- avoiding postrandomization withdrawals
- submitting products of conception for karyotypic analysis in cases of intervention failure.

These requirements will be discussed in this chapter by highlighting the common pitfalls that are encountered. Also, by addressing these issues, it is hoped the reader will become more versed in reviewing the literature on management of recurrent miscarriage so that the judicious and explicit use of the best current evidence can guide clinical management.

METHODOLOGICAL ISSUES IN ASSESSMENT OF
EVIDENCE FROM THERAPEUTIC TRIALS IN
RECURRENT MISCARRIAGE

**DEFINITION OF RECURRENT MISCARRIAGE
(DEFINING THE POPULATION)**

The term 'miscarriage' is used to describe a pregnancy that fails to progress, resulting in death and expulsion of the embryo or fetus. The generally accepted definition stipulates that the fetus or embryo should weigh 500 g or less,[2,3] a stage that corresponds to a gestational age of up to 20 weeks. Unfortunately, this definition is not used consistently, and pregnancy losses at higher gestational ages are also classified as miscarriage in some countries. Additionally, the literature is replete with studies on women with pregnancy loss – a term that includes miscarriage and pregnancies that have ended in stillbirth or preterm neonatal death. Thus, from a definitional perspective, it is important to characterize the population being studied so that comparisons across therapeutic trials can be made more appropriately and reliably. Consensus on this issue is urgently required.

The term 'recurrent miscarriage' has now replaced the original term 'habitual abortion' because it is kinder and does not imply that the woman is deliberately causing her pregnancies to be terminated. Recurrent miscarriage defines a clinical condition in which a woman has had at least three miscarriages. However, because the pregnancy history in women with recurrent miscarriage may include pregnancies that have ended in live birth, three different groups can be identified. The groups should be assessed separately because the risk of subsequent miscarriage within each group varies.[2]

- *Primary recurrent miscarriage group.* This group consists of women with three or more consecutive miscarriages with no pregnancy progressing beyond 20 weeks' gestation.
- *Secondary recurrent miscarriage group.* This group consists of women who have had three or more miscarriages after a pregnancy that, having gone beyond 20 weeks' gestation, may have ended in live birth, stillbirth, or neonatal death.
- *Tertiary recurrent miscarriage group.* This is a group that has not been well characterized or studied, and consists of women who have had at least three miscarriages that are not consecutive but are interspersed with pregnancies that have progressed beyond 20 weeks' gestation (and may have ended in live birth, stillbirth, or neonatal death).

These three groups are mutually exclusive and distinct, and should be evaluated separately because the group being selected will undoubtedly influence the prognosis for a successful outcome. The current approach of combining all three groups together does not allow the effect of the experimental intervention to be detected easily, because the prognosis is determined by the relative contribution of subjects from each of the three groups.

**EXCLUSION OF IMPLANTATION FAILURES
(AVOIDING CLINICAL HETEROGENEITY)**

The widespread availability of treatment with assisted reproduction has created a challenge for the management of women who repeatedly fail to conceive despite undergoing uterine transfer of good-quality embryos. Repeated implantation failure (RIF) is now a recognized entity defined as failure to achieve a pregnancy after at least three cycles of in vitro fertilization (IVF)[4] in which at least 10 high-grade embryos were transferred into the uterus. It is now being suggested that RIF and recurrent miscarriage represent different ends of the same disorder.[5] This position is difficult to accept, because the former is a preimplantation failure that results in no pregnancy whereas the latter is a postimplantation failure that results in no live birth. Although there may be some overlap in the two conditions from the diagnostic protocol perspective, it is evident from the results of these tests that the two entities are distinct and should not be combined. For example, studies of cytokine expression in the endometrium have produced conflicting and sometimes contradictory findings in these two conditions.[6] Similarly, there is no evidence that measuring serum levels of antiphospholipids is of benefit in RIF, in contrast to measurement in women with recurrent miscarriage.[7,8] The results of studies such as these indicate that RIF and recurrent miscarriage are two distinct entities that should not be lumped together under the assumption that they represent different aspects of the spectrum of reproductive failure. By investigating them separately and by conducting efficacy trials in each group separately, the problem of clinical heterogeneity is avoided and the benefit (or lack thereof) of interventions can be evaluated more accurately.

BASELINE RISK OF MISCARRIAGE (ESTABLISHING THE CONTROL EVENT RATE)

Initial estimates of the likelihood of a successful pregnancy in women with previous miscarriages were based on the assumption that the overall miscarriage rate consists of the sum of two independent rates: one resulting from a random factor and the other from a recurrent factor in miscarriage sequences. Such mathematical calculations demonstrated a higher risk of miscarriage in a subsequent pregnancy as the number of previous miscarriages

increased; the chance of a fourth pregnancy going to term in women with three previous miscarriages is considerably lower than that of a third pregnancy going to term with two previous miscarriages.[2] For many years, these mathematical estimates of miscarriage rate were used as control rates against which the efficacy of therapeutic regimens for recurrent miscarriage was assessed. The reliability of these rates was challenged after evidence from a number of clinical studies suggested that the miscarriage rate after three consecutive miscarriages was substantially lower than had been predicted by the earlier mathematical models.[2]

Despite the varied methods of ascertainment, the results of the studies showed remarkable consistency in finding a positive correlation between risk of miscarriage and the number of previous miscarriages. This effect of prior losses on subsequent probability of live birth was confirmed using the data from the placebo arm of studies in unexplained recurrent miscarriage and provided a quantitative estimate of the risk.[9,10] Similar risk estimates were obtained from a longitudinal study of pregnancy outcome in women with idiopathic recurrent miscarriage.[11] It is clear from this evidence that the number of previous miscarriages is an important covariate, which has to be taken into account when planning therapeutic trials: women with a higher number of previous miscarriages constitute a group with a more severe form of recurrent miscarriage than those with relatively lower numbers of previous miscarriages. Consequently, the magnitude of the treatment effect is expected to be much larger in these more severe forms of the disorder (because the control event rate is so much lower) and is likely to be more easily detected if the subjects are grouped by severity.[12] Thus, the ideal trial should have stratification for the number of previous miscarriages, with randomization of subjects to control or experimental interventions being performed within each stratum.

To date, such a study with a priori stratification has not been undertaken. Instead, the general (and incorrect) approach has been to select the study sample from the population of women having three or more miscarriages and ignore the importance of stratification for number of previous miscarriages.

The consequence is a sample that is likely to consist of a higher proportion of women with lower numbers of previous miscarriages, thereby reducing the probability of detecting a significant treatment effect.

CONTROLLING FOR FEMALE AGE (REDUCING SELECTION BIAS)

The risk of miscarriage resulting from fetal chromosomal anomalies increases with maternal age,[13,14] especially after age 35. Additionally, women who have recurrent miscarriages tend to have more pregnancies and have their pregnancies at a later age than those who have successful outcomes. The relationship of gravidity with female age and the relationship of chromosomal anomalies and female age suggest that the increased risk of miscarriage with gravidity, can in part, be ascribed to the effect of maternal age. Thus, clinical trials of treatment efficacy must take female age into consideration during the design phase by using stratification for this covariate. This approach will avoid the possibility of bias that may show the treatment to be less favorable if the experimental group has a higher proportion of older women than the control group.

CONTROLLING FOR MALE PARTNER (REDUCING SELECTION BIAS)

Women who have recurrent miscarriages with one male partner may have successful pregnancies with a different male partner. This issue of partner specificity is an important consideration in avoiding selection bias when evaluating treatment efficacy. To ensure homogeneity of the sample and maximize the probability of detecting a true treatment effect, couples should be chosen for the trial only if the consecutive miscarriages experienced by the subject have occurred with the same male partner.

CLEARLY DEFINED OBJECTIVE (ARTICULATING THE RESEARCH QUESTION)

Before commencing a trial, it is important to articulate the objective clearly and concisely so that the inferences that are drawn from the results can be communicated without ambiguity. To do so requires formulating the research question that is relevant to the problem at hand and is structured in four parts: the population being evaluated, the experimental intervention being tested, the control intervention used as the comparator, and the outcome that has clinical importance. A lack of clarity in the objective formulation becomes evident when the findings are discussed, because often several different outcomes are considered. Attempts are then made at the end of the trial to develop an explanation for the findings that has strayed from the original idea for which the study was commissioned.

RANDOMIZATION (ENSURING SIMILARITY AMONG INTERVENTION GROUPS)

The randomized controlled trial has become the 'gold standard' in evaluating treatment efficacy. Randomization of subjects to receive either experimental or control intervention generates two groups that are generally similar in all respects except for the single factor (the intervention) being studied. This approach ensures that any significant difference in the outcome between the two groups is likely due only to this single factor. Also, by ensuring their equal distribution in the two groups, it guards against differences in factors not known to be important to the outcome of interest.

There are many methods of randomization, including simple coin tossing, drawing straws, and the use of computer-generated random number tables. The use of block randomization is an additional maneuver that produces equal numbers of subjects in each group – a result not usually obtained with the other methods of randomization. Another approach that is not infrequently used is that of quasirandomization, wherein subjects are allocated using either the subject's clinical chart number (even number for the experimental group and odd number for the control group) or the subject's date of birth (first half of the year for the experimental group and second half of the year for the control group), or the day of the week when the subject is seen in the clinic

(Monday, Wednesday, and Friday for the experimental group, and Tuesday, Thursday, and Saturday for the control group). Additionally, alternation is often used to create two intervention groups by alternating the assignment between experimental and control interventions for each successive subject enrolled in the trial (i.e., first subject allocated to the experimental group, second subject to the control group, third subject to the experimental group, and so on). When carried out properly, both quasirandomization and alternation are fairly simple and effective methods for generating experimental and control groups. However, both methods have several pitfalls, including the openness of the process and, in the case of quasirandomization, the allocation of unequal numbers of subjects to each group.

To improve validity of the trial and to minimize postrandomization withdrawals of subjects (for reasons such as change of mind, relocation to another city, and so on), it is important to perform randomization as late as possible, preferably just prior to the intervention being administered.

CONCEALMENT OF GROUP ALLOCATION (AVOIDING SELECTION BIAS)

Selection bias is encountered when potentially eligible subjects are selectively excluded from the trial because of prior knowledge of the group to which they would have been allocated had they participated in the trial. Although randomization is generally effective in creating equally balanced groups, it does not guard against selection bias, because the investigator may have a notion of the efficacy (or lack thereof) of the experimental intervention and may consciously or unknowingly steer subjects towards or away from this intervention. An effective strategy to avoid selection bias is to ensure information regarding the group allocation is concealed from the investigators and care providers until the subject is irreversibly committed to the trial. In the absence of concealment, it has been shown that the effect of an experimental intervention may be overestimated by as much as 40%.[15,16]

There are several methods to conceal group allocation, including (i) covering each consecutive assignment on the random list with opaque tape that is removed to reveal the group only when the next eligible subject is enrolled, (ii) the use of consecutively numbered opaque envelopes containing the group assignment, and (iii) the use of an individual not directly involved with the trial. Although the first two methods are simple and pragmatic, they are not tamperproof and need to be policed to prevent investigators from peeking ahead of time under the tape or in the envelope to determine where their preferred intervention is located in the random sequence of assignments. The use of a third party, such as a telephone operator who is located at a site distant from the study center and who can be contacted at the time of enrolment, or a pharmacist who is responsible for dispensing the treatments, provides the highest level of security because it ensures that the randomization list is kept away from the investigators.

The openness of the quasirandomization and alternation methods makes them less reliable in preventing selection bias unless all eligible subjects are enrolled sequentially. From a methodological perspective, the debate over the validity of using these methods in efficacy trials is still ongoing.

BLINDING OR MASKING (AVOIDING ASCERTAINMENT BIAS)

The response to an intervention may not be entirely due to the active chemical compound administered or the surgical procedure performed, but may be influenced by other factors, such as the subject's expectations, the enthusiasm and reputation of the healthcare provider, and the nature of the intervention. Consequently, the outcome of a trial may be biased (ascertainment bias) if the subject, the investigator, or the outcomes assessor has knowledge of the intervention that the subject is receiving. Blinding (or masking) is a strategy that keeps those involved in the trial unaware of the identity of the intervention and is used to prevent ascertainment bias because it eliminates the influence (either positive or negative) that any knowledge of the intervention being administered may have on the estimation of the treatment effect.

Blinding is not the same as allocation concealment. The role of blinding is in safeguarding the randomization sequence after allocation has been performed. In addition, for subjects enrolled in the trial, blinding enhances their compliance with the treatment protocol and encourages them to complete the trial. A subject who perceives the experimental intervention to be better than the control intervention may be less willing to remain in the trial, comply with the treatment protocol, or adhere to the follow-up procedures if she is aware that she has not received the experimental intervention. In the absence of blinding, the treatment effect is overestimated, leading to incorrect inferences about the value of the experimental intervention.[16] The magnitude of the overestimation is much larger in infertility trials with pregnancy as the outcome measure.[17]

The testing of subjects under conditions of intentional ignorance may include the use of dummy interventions, such as placebo and sham surgery. These methods ensure that none of the subjects and, where possible, the trial personnel, is able to recognize whether the intervention administered is active or inert until the code is broken at the conclusion of the trial. A placebo is designed to be indistinguishable in physical properties from the active intervention. However, when a standard treatment exists, it should be used as the comparator for the new intervention, and every effort should be taken to make the interventions indistinguishable from each other by the trial participant. To do so often requires the use of a double-dummy approach (i.e., two placebos), especially if the routes of administration of the two interventions are different – for example oral versus intravenous, in which case the subject receives both oral and intravenous agents, one of which will be a placebo in the experimental group and vice versa for the control group.

The magnitude of the placebo effect (the response observed in the placebo group) is difficult to quantify, unless the placebo is compared with no treatment. Estimates of the benefit have ranged from none to between 35% and 75% of trial participants showing improved outcome.[18] The observation that the use of 'tender loving care' was more efficacious than when it was not used in women with recurrent miscarriage undergoing another pregnancy[19,20] suggests that in recurrent miscarriage research the placebo effect is likely to be of significant magnitude for which appropriate measures should be taken when designing an efficacy trial.

In trials evaluating surgical procedures, the use of placebo poses a unique challenge.[21] Placebo surgery (also known as a sham operation) requires the subject to undergo all preparations (including anesthesia and surgical incision) essential to the true operation except the surgical procedure itself. The beneficial effect of the sham operation has been attributed to the placebo effect, with estimates that the placebo response in surgery may be of the same magnitude (about 35%) as that observed in medical trials.[22] The placebo effect in surgery may be defined as the difference between the overall effect of surgery and that attributable to the procedure itself.[23] This realization has prompted researchers to reintroduce the sham operation to evaluate surgical interventions so that the high standard required in efficacy studies can be maintained. The risks to subjects undergoing a sham operation are not trivial, and it is important to balance these risks against the potential benefits to society at large if the surgical procedure is proven effective. It is also important that future patients be spared from the risks and cost of an ineffective surgical procedure. However, if there is no proven alternative therapy available, then the sham operation for surgical therapy trials is a desirable and valid approach to evaluate the efficacy of the intervention, provided an appropriate risk assessment has been undertaken.[24]

In management of recurrent miscarriage, there are very few instances when surgical treatment can be considered, except for uterine anomalies, as described in Chapter 11. The use of the sham procedure has not yet been explored in recurrent miscarriage.

CO-INTERVENTION (AVOIDING TREATMENT BIAS)

The appeal of the randomized trial is the assurance that random allocation of the subjects to experimental or control groups will produce groups that have similar characteristics at baseline so the efficacy of the experimental intervention can be tested cleanly and quantified reliably without interference from any extraneous factors. In this context, it is important to ensure that, except for the interventions being compared, the management protocol is held the same for both groups. Co-intervention occurs when one group is provided with additional care (e.g., supplementary treatment, more monitoring, easier access to health care personnel, and so on) that is not offered to the other group. The efficacy of the experimental intervention will be biased by co-intervention, leading to incorrect estimation of the size of the treatment effect. Also, with co-intervention, the research question changes from the original question 'Is the experimental intervention more efficacious than the control interventions?' to the new question 'Is experimental treatment in addition to the co-intervening care more efficacious than the control intervention?'

SAMPLE SIZE ESTIMATION (ENSURING THE ABILITY TO DETECT A DIFFERENCE IN OUTCOME)

In an efficacy trial with comparable groups, any differences observed in the primary outcome event are due either to chance or to the effect of the experimental intervention. The possibility of finding a treatment effect of the magnitude observed in such a trial is expressed by a probability value (p-value) that indicates how likely an ineffective treatment would have been expected to produce the result observed; the lower the p-value, the less likely is the effect due to chance and the more likely is it due to the experimental intervention being evaluated. By convention, the threshold of this likelihood is taken to be a probability value of 0.05, so that when the p-value is less than 0.05, the observed data are inconsistent with the experimental intervention being ineffective (i.e., the experimental intervention is more efficacious than the control intervention).

In clinical trials, it is important to be able to detect with a high level of confidence a clinically meaningful difference between experimental and control interventions. To do so requires conducting a trial with sufficient numbers of subjects to avoid a chance finding (type I error) and to avoid missing the detection of a true difference if one exists (type II error). The ideal situation is to conduct the trial with a sample size just large enough to test the null hypothesis. The goal is to increase the signal-to-noise ratio by recognizing that statistical 'noise' (i.e.,variability) is inversely proportional to the square root of the sample size (i.e., noise decreases as the sample size increases). When the variation within groups gets larger (the louder the noise) or when the difference in outcomes between the groups gets smaller (the fainter the signal), the larger is the sample size needed to detect the signal.

The size of the sample needed to adequately test the hypothesis of treatment efficacy can be calculated using a standard formula or with the use of readily available software programs. The size of the treatment effect (the 'signal') is the difference in magnitude between the outcomes in the experimental and control groups, and is selected by the investigators because it has clinical relevance and importance. This chosen, clinically important, difference is the smallest difference at which the experimental treatment would be expected to alter current clinical management. In addition, an indication of the variability (the 'noise') is obtained from the standard deviation for outcomes that are continuous variables; for proportions, the difference in event rates is all that is needed. It is also necessary to select appropriate values for the probability of making errors of hypothesis testing (typically 0.05 for type I errors and 0.2 for type II). Finally, it should be established whether the statistical test used to compare the difference in outcomes is to be based on a one-tailed (difference in outcomes in one direction; i.e., benefit with experimental intervention) or two-tailed (difference in outcomes in either direction; i.e., benefit or harm with the experimental intervention).

In research into recurrent miscarriage, the outcome events of most clinical relevance are clinical pregnancy and live birth, the rates of which are generally high. The sample size required to test the efficacy of most interventions purported to improve pregnancy rates is often small enough to permit the trial to be undertaken. For example, the control event rate (i.e., success rate with placebo or no treatment) after three miscarriages is expected to be 65%, and any experimental intervention that can improve the outcome to that expected in the normal population (i.e., 85%) would produce an absolute treatment effect of 20% – a difference that is clinically important, implying that for every five women with recurrent miscarriage treated with the experimental intervention, one additional successful outcome would be obtained compared with the control intervention.

To detect this magnitude of difference in clinical pregnancy rates would require a sample size of 162 (81 in each group) using a two-tailed hypothesis test with probabilities for types I and II errors set at 0.05 and 0.2, respectively. Accruing this number of subjects is not difficult in centers specializing in the evaluation and management of recurrent miscarriage, but may require several years to complete a trial in institutions with an average volume of clinical activity. Consequently, in everyday practice, smaller trials are usually conducted, because they are easier to complete in a shorter period of time. Unfortunately, because they are insufficiently powered to test the null hypothesis, the results obtained often lead to erroneous inferences being drawn unless the results from these trials can be pooled with meta-analysis to generate more precise estimates of the treatment effect.

Reviewing the literature on recurrent miscarriage demonstrates an urgent need for trials with adequate power to be carried out so that conclusions about treatment efficacy can be made more reliably. For example, a systematic review of immunotherapy for recurrent miscarriage included 12 trials with an average sample size of 53 (range 22–131).[25] Only 1 of the 12 trials had a sufficiently large sample size, with 131 subjects. Similarly, a systematic review of treatment for recurrent miscarriage in women with antiphospholipid antibody or lupus anticoagulant included 13 trials with an average sample size of 66 (range 16–202).[26] This review contained only one trial with a sufficiently large sample size of 202 subjects. Thus, if progress is to be made in research into recurrent miscarriage, larger trials are needed to test the efficacy of new (and existing) interventions.

AVOIDING HISTORICAL CONTROLS (AVOIDING OVERESTIMATION OF THE EFFECT OF TREATMENT)

Despite the acknowledgement that the randomized trial is the ideal in evaluating therapeutic efficacy,

clinical decisions are often made from evidence derived from non-randomized observational studies, such as cohort, case control, and historical-control. When randomized trials were compared with observational studies to answer the same clinical question, between-study heterogeneity was observed more frequently among observational studies.[27] Some of this variability was reduced after historical-control studies were excluded from the analyses.

A historical-control study is one in which the outcome of an intervention is compared with the outcome observed prior to the administration of the experimental intervention. In research into recurrent miscarriage this design is used fairly frequently to support claims of improved efficacy of new interventions. As an example, a historical-control study was performed to determine whether metformin administered to women with polycystic ovary syndrome to achieve pregnancy and then continued throughout the pregnancy would reduce the likelihood of first-trimester miscarriage.[28] Among the ten women evaluated in the study, their collective history of 22 previous pregnancies without metformin included 16 (73%) miscarriages. In contrast, the current pregnancy on metformin therapy ended in miscarriage in only one woman (10%). The authors statistically (and incorrectly) compared the two rates of miscarriage and concluded that there was a significant benefit with metformin use. This approach is invalid from both design (inappropriate controls) and analytical (lack of independence) perspectives.

There is also evidence demonstrating that historical-control studies are associated with an overestimation of the effect of treatment.[27] Thus, historical-control studies should be avoided in research into recurrent miscarriage because treatment estimates derived from them are less reliable than those from prospectively undertaken controlled studies.[29]

INTENTION-TO-TREAT ANALYSIS (AVOIDING POST-RANDOMIZATION EXCLUSION OF DATA)

In trials of treatment efficacy, the purpose of randomization is to avoid bias in the selection of subjects so that comparable experimental and control groups can be studied to provide a reliable estimate of the size of the treatment effect. Once a subject has been randomized into the trial, she needs to be included in the analyses, even if she never began the treatment or stopped taking the treatment partway through the trial. After randomization, any changes in the composition of the groups (e.g., withdrawing from treatment, being excluded from the analysis for failing to follow protocol, crossing over to the alternative intervention group, and so on) will disturb the balance between them and may affect their comparability. Therefore, it is important to ensure that subjects not only remain in the groups to which they were allocated, but also complete the study.

Unfortunately, despite diligent attention to detail and monitoring of trial progress, the ideal goal of achieving perfect compliance is often not reached. The usual approach to dealing with such postrandomization withdrawals is to analyze the data from only those who completed the assigned treatment (i.e., per-protocol analysis) and ignore those who deviated from the protocol. Although this approach seems sensible, it is not correct from a methodological perspective because the power of the study to detect a clinically meaningful treatment effect is reduced. Also, confining the analysis only to those who are compliant with the protocol will produce an estimate of the treatment effect that is biased because non-compliance is not a random occurrence and may be associated with a poorer (or better) outcome. The correct approach is to perform the analysis according to the original random assignment using an *intention-to-treat* method whereby all subjects allocated to the group at the time of randomization are analyzed together as having received the intervention originally assigned to that group.

In most clinical trials, because it is expected that there will be some degree of non-compliance, the intention-to-treat analysis will tend to underestimate the effect of the experimental intervention. Maintaining group similarity and preserving the balance among prognostic factors in the study groups produce a cautious method for evaluation

and minimizes the likelihood of making a type I error in hypothesis testing.

A good strategy to reduce the numbers of post-randomization withdrawals is to perform the random allocation as late as possible, preferably just prior to the administration of the intervention.

LACK OF SUPERIORITY, EQUIVALENCE, AND NON-INFERIORITY (ENSURING APPROPRIATE TESTING OF NULL HYPOTHESIS)

The placebo-controlled trial is the optimal design for evaluating the efficacy of new treatments. However, once efficacy of a treatment has been established, newer treatments should be compared against these standard active treatments, because the use of placebo for such subsequent evaluations is considered unethical.

In general, efficacy trials of active treatments are designed to determine whether a new (experimental) intervention is superior to the standard (control) intervention. The objective of such superiority trials is to rule out equality of the interventions by rejecting the null hypothesis that there is no difference between the two treatments. Sometimes, such trials are undertaken with the expectation that the new intervention will fare better, and the objective is to demonstrate this fact unequivocally. More commonly, though, the new intervention is only expected to demonstrate similar efficacy to the standard intervention so that healthcare providers can offer their patients a choice of treatment options. The objective in such a trial is to demonstrate equivalent efficacy (equivalence) of the two interventions.

A common mistake, when a superiority trial fails to reject the null hypothesis of no difference, is to conclude that the two interventions are equivalent. For example, consider a trial with a sample size of 50 women with recurrent miscarriage in which the standard intervention produced a live birth rate of 65% and the experimental treatment intervention produced a live birth rate of 85%. After performing the χ^2 test, this difference in pregnancy rates of 20% is found not to be statistically significant and may lead one to conclude that the two interventions are the same (i.e., equivalent). This is an incorrect interpretation, because, although a lack of proof of superiority may be consistent with equivalence, it is not proof that equivalence is present. If the same result were observed in a sample of 200 women, the observed treatment effect would be statistically significant. The current practice of conducting small comparative trials that fail to show superiority of the new intervention should be avoided when the objective is to demonstrate equivalence, because the 'lack of evidence of a difference' is not synonymous with 'evidence of a lack of difference'.

The goal in an equivalence trial is to rule out differences of clinical importance in the primary outcome between two interventions. To calculate a sample size for an equivalence trial requires defining a priori a clinically important difference, starting with the assumption that there is a zero difference in the outcome event rates between the two interventions. The null hypothesis (in contrast to that in a superiority trial) is stated differently as a minimum difference that is acceptable that would render the two interventions interchangeable.[30] By rejecting this null hypothesis in favor of the alternative hypothesis that the difference in outcomes between the two interventions is zero, one can conclude that the interventions are equivalent.

It should be recognized that the outcome event rate with the experimental intervention might be slightly larger or slightly smaller than that with the control intervention. Thus, a range of possible outcome event rates can be generated. By starting with a zero percent difference in outcome event rates, a confidence interval around this value is chosen to represent the clinically important range within which any differences in outcome rates can lie for interventions that are equivalent. If the observed difference in outcome event rates lies entirely within the range selected for clinical importance, when the trial is completed, equivalence can be claimed. The smaller the selected range, the larger the sample size required. Thus, the execution of an equivalence trial is challenging, because it requires a much larger sample size than that for a superiority trial.

An alternative strategy that avoids the need for a very large sample size is to conduct a 'non-inferiority' trial. The objective of the active-controlled, non-inferiority trial is not to demonstrate superiority, but rather to establish that the effect of the experimental intervention, when compared with the control intervention, is not below some prestated non-inferiority margin. In other words, given that it is impossible to prove the null hypothesis of no difference, an operational definition must be considered that allows the experimental intervention to be inferior to the standard (control) intervention by a clinically tolerable amount (i.e., the experimental intervention is 'not much inferior' to the control intervention). Clinicians have to decide on the amount of non-inferiority they are willing to accept as medically insignificant or tolerable as the basis for non-inferiority claims. Such an approach is often used for newer drugs that may have lower side-effects, better tolerance, or lower cost than the standard intervention. For a non-inferiority evaluation, the null hypothesis states that the control intervention is superior to the experimental intervention. The alternative hypothesis is that the experimental intervention is not inferior to the control intervention.

The design of a non-inferiority trial requires specifying the non-inferiority margin, i.e., the extent to which the outcome with the control intervention can exceed that with the experimental intervention and still render the experimental intervention non-inferior to the control intervention. The null hypothesis states that the outcome with the control intervention is at least as large as or exceeds this margin; if the null hypothesis cannot be rejected, then the control intervention is more efficacious than the experimental intervention. Rejection of the null hypothesis is required to establish non-inferiority of the control intervention. It should be noted that, according to the alternative hypothesis, the experimental intervention might perform better than the control intervention, but not to an extent greater than the inferiority margin that has been established.

Because the direction of effect being assessed is one-sided (i.e., the experimental intervention is not inferior to the control intervention), a one-sided hypothesis test is performed. Thus, by not requiring a two-sided hypothesis test, the sample size required will be much lower. However, if the experimental treatment performs better than the control intervention (and the outcome event rate exceeds the non-inferiority margin), one cannot conclude that it is superior, because the trial design was not set up to test this hypothesis.

Before a non-inferiority trial can be undertaken, it is necessary to confirm that the control intervention has been shown to be better than placebo. Furthermore, it is important to select a non-inferiority margin that is small enough to not exceed that which has clinical relevance; choosing a large inferiority margin will risk the generalization of the study findings, because it can be argued that such a large difference is clinically meaningful, suggesting that the control intervention is superior to the experimental intervention. Finally, it has to be assumed that the control intervention is superior to placebo (had such a comparison taken place). To do so requires the inferiority margin to be smaller than the smallest effect size that the experimental intervention would be expected to produce had it been compared with placebo. In this context, for the experimental intervention to be designated as being 'at least as good as' the control intervention, it has to retain at least 50% of the superiority of the control intervention over placebo.[31,32]

ONSET OF TREATMENT (MAXIMIZING MAGNITUDE OF TREATMENT EFFECT)

A major problem in the management of recurrent miscarriage is the assumption that diagnostic tests carried out in the non-pregnant state can identify potential causes of the miscarriages that have already occurred. Treatment is then offered to prevent miscarriage in a subsequent pregnancy. Unfortunately, there is no standardization in many of the treatment protocols regarding the onset of treatment. For example, intravenous immunoglobulin has been administered before conception in some studies, and only after confirmation of the pregnancy

in other studies.[33] Sometimes treatment is instituted only after fetal cardiac activity has been demonstrated, as seen with the use of heparin in women with elevated antiphospholipid levels.[26] In this situation, the likelihood of a successful outcome without treatment once fetal cardiac activity has been demonstrated is relatively high, and will result in efficacy studies failing to accurately quantify the magnitude of the treatment effect with the experimental intervention.

The optimal time of onset of therapy will vary depending on the cause of the recurrent miscarriages, but it makes sense to commence treatment before conception for most causes that can be identified using the current diagnostic protocol. Clearly, consensus on this issue is urgently required so that treatment benefit can be maximized.

CENSORING SUBJECTS WHO FAIL TO CONCEIVE (AVOIDING TREATMENT BIAS)

Another methodological concern in efficacy trials is the practice of restricting the number of cycles of preconceptional treatment patients may undergo. If these women do not conceive, they are withdrawn from the study and are replaced by other women, who take their place in the trial. This strategy violates the principle of randomization and introduces treatment bias by enrolling women with high fecundity rates. It becomes difficult to generalize the results of such trials to the population of women with recurrent miscarriage.

Women with recurrent miscarriage have a longer interpregnancy conception interval compared with those with sporadic miscarriage (i.e., the length of time taken for conception to occur after a previous miscarriage increases with the number of miscarriages).[34,35] The mechanism underlying this observation is not clear. One possible hypothesis is that fear of miscarriage in a subsequent pregnancy induces significant stress that may adversely influence the hypothalamus and result in subtle ovulatory dysfunction.[2] Thus, it is clear that for treatments commenced before conception, a sufficient length of time will be required before pregnancy can be achieved.

For this reason and for the methodological reasons discussed, women enrolled into randomized trials of treatment for recurrent miscarriage should not be withdrawn just because pregnancy has not occurred in a short period of time.

KARYOTYPIC ANALYSIS OF THE ABORTUS (IMPROVING ACCURACY OF TREATMENT EFFECT ESTIMATION)

The risk of aneuploidy arising de novo is present in all pregnancies. Consequently, it is possible that women receiving experimental or control interventions may experience another miscarriage due to a chromosomal aberration, unrelated to the intervention itself (see the debates following Chapter 3). Hence, in efficacy trials, it is prudent to submit all products of conception for karyotypic analysis to exclude the presence of aneuploidy. Without this information, it is impossible to ascertain whether the miscarriage is the result of a failure of the administered intervention or is due to a de novo chromosomal anomaly. The magnitude of the treatment effect will be less accurate without adjusting for the miscarriages that were inevitable because of aneuploidy. However, such adjustments are only reliable if abortus material from all subjects who participated in the trial and had a miscarriage are successfully analyzed.

Improvement in ultrasonographic technology has resulted in images of early pregnancy having higher resolution to permit earlier diagnosis of pregnancy failure – a process that is assisted with serial measurement of serum levels of progesterone and human chorionic gonadotropin. Thus, it is possible to collect fetal and trophoblast tissue electively and prior to the commencement of the miscarriage so that it is in a sterile condition to enable karyotypic analyses to be performed without contamination of the cell culture – a problem that is frequently encountered when tissue is collected in a non-sterile manner after the miscarriage process had commenced. Furthermore, improved techniques in cytogenetics have permitted more accurate and reliable assessments of the products of conception (see Chapter 3).

Given these improvements in diagnostic techniques, it is essential that every effort be made to study the products of conception in every case of miscarriage in therapeutic trials so that a more valid assessment of the efficacy of the experimental treatment can be performed.

SUMMARY

Therapeutic decision-making relies on the availability of good-quality evidence generated from studies of high quality and high internal validity and without bias. In the area of efficacy evaluation of therapy for recurrent miscarriage, the randomized trial is the gold standard and should be designed and executed with attention to the methodological details outlined in this chapter. The starting point requires defining the research objective that is articulated unambiguously as a research question describing the patient population, experimental and control interventions, and outcome of interest. The population should be clearly defined and women with repeated implantation failure should be excluded. The subjects selected for the trial should be randomly allocated to the experimental or control interventions to ensure similarity in the composition of the group. The allocation sequence should be concealed from all investigators and healthcare personnel involved with the trial, so that bias in selecting participants can be avoided.

Whenever possible, attempts should be made to blind subjects, investigators, healthcare personnel providing care, and outcomes assessors so that ascertainment bias can be avoided. Further bias of treatment assessment can be avoided by ensuring that co-intervention does not occur and historical controls are avoided.

Testing the null hypothesis of no difference in outcomes between the experimental and control interventions requires enrolling sufficiently large numbers of participants so that a clinically important treatment effect can be detected. Smaller sample sizes will usually lead to erroneous inferences about treatment efficacy. Wherever possible, stratification should be performed for the number of previous miscarriages. Also stratification, or subgrouping, by female age should be considered.

Treatment should be commenced prior to pregnancy and should be continued for a sufficient length of time to permit pregnancy to occur; postrandomization withdrawals of subjects who fail to conceive after a short period of time should be avoided.

All analyses should be undertaken using an intention-to-treat approach so that postrandomization exclusion of data does not occur. The approach of the study from the perspectives of superiority, equivalence, or non-inferiority should be established before the trial begins, so that the required numbers of participants can be accrued and the hypothesis testing can be directed appropriately. The products of conception should be submitted for karyotypic analysis for all intervention failures, so that more accurate estimates of the effect of treatment can be generated.

Finally, the reporting of the results should follow the guidelines established by the Consolidated Standards of Reporting Trials (CONSORT).[36] This statement consists of a checklist and flow diagram for reporting the results from randomized controlled trials and prompts investigators to ensure that important elements in clinical trial design have been addressed. The issues raised in this chapter are important for creating the basis for using an evidence-based approach to inform therapeutic decisions in the clinical management of recurrent miscarriage.

REFERENCES

1. Jauniaux E, Farquharson RG, Christiansen OB, et al. Evidence-based guidelines for the investigation and medical treatment of recurrent miscarriage. Hum Reprod 2006; 21:2216–22.
2. Daya S. Habitual abortion. In: Copeland LJ, Jarrell JF, eds. Textbook of Gynecology 2nd edn. Philadelphia: WB Saunders, 2000:227–71.
3. WHO recommended definitions, terminology and format for statistical tables related to the perinatal period. Acta Obstet Gynecol Scand 1977; 56:247–53.
4. Tan BK, Vandekerckhove P, Kennedy R, et al. Investigation and current management of recurrent IVF treatment failure in the UK. Br J Obstet Gynaecol 2005; 112:773–80.
5. Nardo LG, Li TC, Edwards RG. Introduction: human embryo implantation failure and recurrent miscarriage: basic science and clinical practice. Reprod Biomed Online 2006; 13:11–12.
6. Laird S, Tuckerman EM, Li TC. Cytokine expression in the endometrium of women with implantation failure and recurrent miscarriage. Reprod Biomed Online 2006; 13:13–23.
7. Stern C, Chamley L. Antiphospholipid antibodies and coagulation defects in women with implantation failure after IVF and recurrent miscarriage. Reprod Biomed Online 2006; 13:29–37.
8. Mardesic T, Ulcova-Gallova Z, Huttelova R, et al, The influence of different types of antibodies on in vitro fertilization results. Am J Reprod Immunol 2000; 43:1–5.
9. Daya S. Immunotherapy for unexplained recurrent spontaneous abortion. Infertil Reprod Med Clinc North Am 1997; 8:65–77.
10. Carp HJA. Investigation and treatment for recurrent pregnancy loss. In: Rainsbury P, Vinniker D, eds. A Practical Guide to Reproductive Medicine. Carnforth, UK. Parthenon, 1997:337–62.
11. Brigham SA, Conlon C, Farquharson RG. A longitudinal study of pregnancy outcome following idiopathic recurring miscarriage. Hum Reprod 1999; 14:2868–71.
12. Carp HJ, Toder V, Torchinsky A, et al. Allogenic leukocyte immunization after five or more miscarriages. Recurrent Miscarriage Immunotherapy Trialists Group. Hum Reprod 1997; 12:250–5.
13. Carp HJA, Toder V, Orgad S, et al. Karyotype of the abortus in recurrent miscarriage. Fertil Steril 2001; 5:678–82.
14. Sullivan AE, Silver RM, LaCoursiere DY, et al. Recurrent fetal aneuploidy and recurrent miscarriage. Obstet Gynecol 2004; 104:784–8.
15. Chalmers TC, Celano P, Sacks HS, et al. Bias in treatment assignment in controlled clinical trials. N Engl J Med 1983; 309:1359–61.
16. Schultz KF, Chalmers I, Hayes RJ, et al. Empirical evidence of bias: dimensions of methodological quality associated with estimates of treatment effects in controlled trials. JAMA 1995; 273:408–12.
17. Khan KS, Daya S, Collins JA, et al. Empirical evidence of bias in infertility research: overestimation of treatment effect in crossover trials using pregnancy as the outcome measure. Fertil Steril 1996; 65:939–45.
18. Daya S. The placebo effect. Evidence-Based Obstet Gynecol 2000; 2:1.
19. Stray Pedersen B, Stray Pedersen S. Etiological factors and subsequent obstetric performance in 195 couples with a prior history of habitual abortion. Am J Obstet Gynecol 1983; 148:140–6.
20. Clifford K, Rai R, Regan L. Future pregnancy outcome in unexplained recurrent first trimester miscarriage. Hum Reprod 1997; 12:387–9.
21. Daya S. Issues in surgical therapy evaluation: the sham operation. Evidence-Based Obstet Gynecol 2000; 2:31–2.
22. Beecher HK. Surgery as placebo. A quantitative study of bias. JAMA 1961; 176:1102–7.
23. Johnson AG. Surgery as a placebo. Lancet 1994; 344:1140–2.
24. American Medical Association. Report of the AMA House of Delegates, 2000 Annual Meeting, Recommendation No. 5. www.ama-assn.org
25. Porter TF, LaCoursiere Y, Scott JR. Immunotherapy for recurrent miscarriage. Cochrane Database Syst Rev 2006; (2):CD000112.
26. Empson M, Lassere M, Craig J, et al. Prevention of recurrent miscarriage for women with antiphospholipid antibody or lupus anticoagulant. Cochrane Database Syst Rev 2005; (2):CD002859.
27. Ioannidis JPA, Haidich A-B, Pappa M, et al. Comparison of evidence of treatment effects in randomized and nonrandomized studies. JAMA 2001; 286:821–30.
28. Glueck CJ, Phillips H, Cameron D, et al. Continuing metformin throughout pregnancy in women with polycystic ovary syndrome appears to safely reduce first-trimester spontaneous abortion: a pilot study. Fertil Steril 2001; 75:46–52.
29. Daya S. Evaluation of treatment efficacy – randomization or observation? Evidence-Based Obstet Gynecol 2001; 3:111–13.
30. Daya S. Issues in assessing therapeutic equivalence. Evidence-Based Obstet Gynecol 2001; 3:167–8.
31. D'Agostino Sr RB, Massaro JM, Sullivan JM. Non-inferiority trials: design concepts and issues – the encounters of academic consultants in statistics. Statist Med 2003; 22:169–86.

32. Jones B, Jarvis P, Lewis JA, et al. Trials to assess equivalence: the importance of rigorous methods. BMJ 1996: 313:36–9.

33. Daya S, Gunby J, Porter E, et al. Critical analysis of intravenous immunoglobulin therapy for recurrent miscarriage. Hum Reprod Update 1999; 5:475–82.

34. Strobino BR, Kline J, Shrout P, et al. Recurrent spontaneous abortion: definition of a syndrome. In: Porter IH, Hook EB, eds Human Embryonic and Fetal Death. New York: Academic Press, 1980: 315.

35. Fitzsimmons J, Jackson D, Wapner R, et al. Subsequent reproductive outcome in couples with repeated pregnancy loss. Am J Med Genet 1983; 16:583–7.

36. Moher D, Schulz KF, Altman D. The CONSORT statement: revised recommendations for improving the quality of reports of parallel-group randomized trials. Lancet 2001; 357:1191–4.

19. Investigation protocol for recurrent pregnancy loss

Howard JA Carp

INTRODUCTION

The patient with recurrent pregnancy loss (RPL) usually seeks a diagnosis of the cause, a prognosis for further pregnancies, and treatment if available. The purpose of an investigation protocol is to assist physicians as to which investigations are worthwhile in order to reach a diagnosis. Various protocols have been published by leading professional organizations such as the Royal College of Obstetricians,[1] the American College of Obstetricians and Gynecologists,[2] the European Society of Human Reproduction and Embryology (ESHRE),[3] and numerous others. However, virtually all protocols tend to classify RPL as one homogeneous condition, and try to suggest a group of investigations or treatment either based on an evidence-based approach or the experience of the particular authors. However, treating RPL as one homogeneous condition takes no account of individual circumstances in different patients. The prognosis is different in different patients. We classify patients into those with a good prognosis and those with a poor prognosis. We have tended to use an approach that differentiates between patients with a good or poor prognosis: primary versus secondary aborters,[4] those with late versus early pregnancy losses (as late losses have a worse prognosis[5]), and recently those losing karyotypically abnormal versus those losing karyotypically normal embryos (as euploid abortions are associated with a worse prognosis than aneuploid abortions[6]). Additionally, treatment is often controversial, as demonstrated by the various debates in this book. We are of the opinion that there may not be one approach to treatment. For example, in antiphospholipid syndrome (APS), low-molecular-weight heparins (LMWH) and aspirin may be the standard treatment, but a different approach is indicated in the patient who continues losing pregnancies despite treatment. In this chapter, some of the standard protocols will be discussed, and some other approaches discussed that may be appropriate in particular patients.

INCLUSION CRITERIA

The standard protocols listed above differ with regard to who should be investigated, and with regard to the criteria for investigation. The ACOG protocol[2] recommends investigation after two or more pregnancy losses, whereas the RCOG[1] and ESHRE[3] protocols only recommend assessment after three or more losses. However, no protocol defines pregnancy loss. A problem arises with preclinical or biochemical pregnancy losses. In these cases, no pregnancy sac can be visualized on ultrasound. No investigation protocol says whether these 'biochemical pregnancies' should be considered pregnancy losses. A positive human chorionic gonadotropin (hCG) level may be due to 'phantom' hCG,[7] an intrauterine pregnancy, or an extrauterine pregnancy. This problem has become especially common since the wide use of in vitro fertilization (IVF), where hCG testing is often performed 12 days after exogenous hCG administration. Although hCG should be cleared from the circulation by 12 days, some may still be present in certain patients, leading to a false-positive result. We have previously defined a biochemical pregnancy as a β-hCG level between 10 and 1000 IU/l in a cycle in which no hCG was administered, no pregnancy sac was demonstrated on ultrasound, and menstruation was delayed by no more than 1 week.[8] This definition has since been accepted by ESHRE.[9] However, we have tended to become more restrictive, and only accept a biochemical pregnancy as such if there are two readings that show a rising level. These pregnancies may be better defined as pregnancies of unknown location (PUL). If they recur three times, the author does consider these events as early pregnancy losses.

Similar confusion surrounds the upper level of pregnancy loss. Traditionally, any pregnancy that has been lost prior to viability was considered as an abortion. The more recent North American definition includes pregnancy losses up to 20 weeks as miscarriages. However, there are many exceptions to this rule. Preston et al,[10] in a leading paper on hereditary thrombophilias, assessed 'miscarriages' as up to 27 weeks. Ober et al, in the paper most often quoted to show that paternal leukocyte immunization is ineffective,[11] included non-consecutive abortions and pregnancies up to 29 weeks (C Ober, personal communication). Laskin et al,[12] in a leading article usually quoted to show that steroids have no place in APS, included patients with pregnancy losses up to 31 weeks. It is difficult to believe that research on patients with two losses at 27, 29, or 31 weeks has relevance to patients with five or more losses of blighted ova. I tend to agree with the conclusions laid out by Farquharson et al,[9] that RPL needs to be much better defined before any relevant investigation or treatment protocols can be determined.

STANDARD PROTOCOLS

The RCOG protocol[1] was originlly published in 1997, and updated in 2003. The protocol attempts to be evidence-based as far as possible. Evidence is classified as in Table 19.1. The recommendations are made for and against various causes of miscarriage, and methods of treatment are graded according to the level of evidence available. Areas lacking evidence are called 'good practice points'. The evidence is mainly taken from the Cochrane Register of Controlled Trials. The guideline recommends

---

Table 19.1 Levels of evidence

Ia. Evidence obtained from meta-analysis of randomized controlled trials

Ib. Evidence obtained from at least one randomized controlled trial

IIa. Evidence obtained from at least one well-designed controlled study without randomization

IIb. Evidence obtained from at least one other type of well-designed quasi-experimental study

III. Evidence obtained from well-designed non-experimental descriptive studies, such as comparative studies, correlation studies, and case studies

IV. Evidence obtained from expert committee reports or opinions and/or clinical experience of respected authorities

---

parental karyotyping, fetal karyotyping, ultrasound, or hydrosonography for uterine anomalies, APS testing and interpretation according to the 'Sapporo' criteria,[13] and treatment with heparin and aspirin. The protocol claims that there is insufficient evidence to assess progesterone and hCG supplementation, bacterial vaginosis, factor V Leiden, or the other hereditary thrombophilias. Assessment of thyroid function, the glucose challenge test, antithyroid antibodies, alloimmune testing and immunotherapy, and assessment of TORCH and other infective agents are not recommended. The RCOG protocol[1] is the generally accepted norm in the UK. The guideline states that a significant proportion of cases of recurrent miscarriage remain unexplained, despite detailed investigation, and that the prognosis for a successful future pregnancy with supportive care alone is in the region of 75%. However, the guideline takes no account of specific types of pregnancy loss, and does not distinguish between different types of patient. There are no suggestions regarding patients who subsequently miscarry despite the reassurance of a 75% prognosis for a live birth. The fact that the guideline states 'The use of empirical treatment in women with unexplained recurrent miscarriage is unnecessary and should be resisted' has denied many British patients with large numbers of miscarriages treatment that may be effective in certain subgroups of patient.

The ACOG guideline[2] is much less dogmatic than the RCOG guideline. Two pregnancy losses are recognized as warranting investigation. The ACOG guideline does not base its recommendations on a strictly evidence-based approach, and does not state that new and controversial etiologies should not be investigated or treated, but that they should be discussed between practitioner and patient. Although the guideline does not take account of different types of patient, or different prognoses, it does state clearly that it should not be construed as dictating an exclusive course of treatment or procedure. The guideline also states that variations in practice may be warranted based on the needs of the individual patient, resources, and limitations unique to the institution or type of practice. Like the RCOG guideline,[1] the ACOG guideline[2] recommends parental karyotyping, and suggests that the couple should be offered prenatal diagnosis if one parent has a chromosomal aberration. The guideline abstains from giving an opinion on karyotyping of the abortus, and reserves judgment on assessment of the uterine cavity. The guideline claims that assessment of the uterine cavity is based on consensus alone, without good evidence. As in the RCOG guideline,[1] there is said to be insufficient evidence to assess luteal phase defect or progesterone or hCG supplements. The ACOG[2] does not recommend assessment of antithyroid antibodies or of infections such as chlamydia, mycoplasma, and bacterial vaginosis. Alloimmune testing, paternal leukocyte immunization and intravenous immunoglobulin (IVIG) are also not recommended.

The ESHRE guideline,[3] like the RCOG guideline,[1] restricts the definition of recurrent miscarriage to three or more consecutive miscarriages. It does take account of different types of patient, as the introduction states 'The number of previous miscarriages and maternal age are the most important covariates and they have to be taken into account when planning therapeutic trials. The ideal trial should have stratification for the number of previous miscarriages and maternal age, with randomization between control and experimental treatments within each stratum'. The protocol discusses investigations of cause and treatment interventions separately, and, unlike the RCOG[1] and ACOG[2] guidelines, does not quote the level of evidence for its recommendations. The protocol

does recommend testing blood sugar levels and thyroid function tests, antiphospholipid antibodies (aPL: lupus anticoagulant (LA) and anticardiolipin antibodies (aCL)), parental karyotyping, and assessment of the uterine cavity by pelvic ultrasound or hysterosalpingography. Hysteroscopy and laparoscopy are reserved as 'advanced investigations', but the protocol does not make clear which patients warrant such 'advanced investigations'. There is a new category of investigations – known as 'investigations that should be used in the framework of a clinical trial'. These include fetal karyotyping, testing of natural killer (NK) cells, luteal phase endometrial biopsy, and homocysteine levels. Treatment is classified separately from investigation in this protocol. Both 'tender loving care' and health advice such as diet and abstention or reduction of coffee intake, smoking, and alcohol are described as established treatments. However, no evidence, results, or references are quoted to justify calling these treatment modalities established treatment. The following are said to require more randomized controlled trials before definite recommendations can be made: aspirin and LMWH or unfractionated heparin for APS, anticoagulants for inherited thrombophilia, progesterone supplementation, IVIG, folic acid in women with hyperhomocysteinemia, and immunization with third-party donor leukocytes. However, immunization with paternal leukocytes is said to be of no proven benefit, nor is multivitamin supplementation. Steroids are said to be associated with more harm than benefit during the first half of pregnancy. Again, no evidence or references are provided.

Table 19.2 contrasts the recommendations for various investigations and treatment modalities in the three protocols. Reliance on these guidelines will leave the physician in a quandary as to which investigations to perform and which treatment to offer.

FACTORS AFFECTING SUBSEQUENT PROGNOSIS

The chance of a third pregnancy loss after two miscarriages is usually quoted to be approximately 20%,

Table 19.2 Comparison of three protocols for the investigation and treatment of recurrent pregnancy loss

Investigation or treatment	RCOG protocol	ACOG protocol	ESHRE protocol
Parental karyotyping	Recommended	Recommended	Recommended
APS assessment (aCL and LA)	Recommended	Recommended	Recommended
Fetal karyotyping	Recommended	Insufficient evidence	Trial required
Uterine cavity assessment	Recommended by ultrasound or hydrosonography	Insufficient evidence	Recommended by ultrasound or hysterosalpingography
Resection of uterine septum	Insufficient evidence	Recommended despite lack of evidence	—
APS assessment (aCL and LA)	Recommended	Recommended	Recommended
Treatment of APS with heparin and aspirin	Recommended	Recommended	Insufficient evidence
Luteal phase investigation	—	Insufficient evidence	Insufficient evidence: trials required
Progesterone or hCG supplementation	Insufficient evidence	Insufficient evidence	Insufficient evidence: more RCTs required
Bacterial vaginosis	Insufficient evidence	Not recommended	—
Hereditary thrombophilias	Insufficient evidence	Insufficient evidence	Recommended as advanced investigation
Anticoagulants for hereditary thrombophilia	Insufficient evidence	Insufficient evidence	Insufficient evidence
Thyroid function	Not recommended	Not recommended	Recommended
Glucose challenge test	Not recommended	Not recommended	Recommended
TORCH testing	Not recommended	Not recommended	Not recommended
Alloimmune testing	Not recommended	Not recommended	Insufficient evidence
Immunotherapy	Not recommended	Not recommended	Insufficient evidence: RCT required for IVIG and third-party leukocytes; PLI no proven effect
'Tender loving care'	Insufficient evidence	—	Recommended
Diet, smoking, alcohol reduction	—	—	Recommended
Folic acid for hyperhomocysteinemia	—	—	Insufficient evidence
Vitamin supplementation	—	—	Not recommended
Steroids	Not recommended	—	Not recommended

APS, antiphospholipid syndrome; aCL, anticardiolipin antibodies; LA, lupus anticoagulant; hCG, human chorionic gonadotrophin; RCT, randomized controlled trial; IVIG, intravenous immunoglobulin; PLI, paternal leukocyte immunization.

and the chance of a fourth miscarriage after three previous miscarriages as approximately 40%. In certain forms of RPL, the recurrence rate is unknown – for example, in recurrent biochemical pregnancies, after IVF, in APS, and in the older woman. However, there are certain factors that help to predict the prognosis:

- number of previous pregnancy losses – as the number of previous losses increases, the chance of a live birth decreases[14,15]
- primary, secondary, or tertiary aborter status – the secondary aborter has a better prognosis than the primary aborter[4]
- karyotype of previous miscarriage – the patient with an aneuploid abortion has a better chance

of a live birth[6] (Figure 3a.1 in Chapter 3a shows prognosis according to fetal karyotype)
- concurrent infertility[14,16]
- maternal age[16,17]
- antipaternal complement-dependent antibodies (APCA) – these have also been reported to be predictive of a successful pregnancy outcome[14,18]
- NK cells[19,20]
- early or late pregnancy losses – patients with late losses tend to have a worse prognosis.[5]

The most important predictive factor is the number of previous miscarriages. Figure 1.1 in Chapter 1 shows the decreasing live birth rate with increasing number of miscarriages. Carp et al[4] have previously published figures for their series.

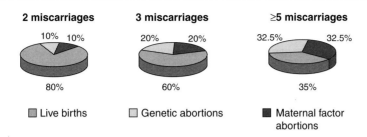

2 miscarriages **3 miscarriages** **≥5 miscarriages**

10% 10%   20% 20%   32.5% 32.5%

80%   60%   35%

☐ Live births   ☐ Genetic abortions   ■ Maternal factor abortions

Figure 19.1 Number of previous abortions and effect of treatment for maternal factors. Patients with two miscarriages have an 80% chance of a live birth if untreated. If 50% of subsequent miscarriages are chromosomally abnormal, any treatment aimed at correcting a maternal cause of miscarriage can only raise the live birth rate from 80% to 90%. A mega-trial is necessary to show a statistical significance between 80% and 90%. Hence, most treatment regimens used on patients with two miscarriages will be ineffective. Treating patients with three miscarriages can only raise the live birth rate by 20%. However, if treatment is used on patients with a poor prognosis, the live birth rate can be raised by 32%, making it relatively easy to show a statistically significant effect of treatment.

After three miscarriages, there was a 55% live birth rate in untreated patients with unexplained RPL (33 of 85 patients). The incidence of live births was 45% after 4 miscarriages (17 of 38 patients), 41% after 5 miscarriages (10 of 24 patients), 13% of patients after 6 miscarriages (2 of 15 patients), and 23% after 7–12 miscarriages (4 of 17 patients).

Figure 19.1 shows the effect of assessing treatment on patients with two miscarriages. If there is a subsequent 80% live birth rate, and 50% of subsequent miscarriages are chromosomally abnormal, any treatment aimed at correcting a maternal cause of miscarriage can only raise the live birth rate from 80% to 90%. In order to show a statistical significance between 80% and 90%, a mega-trial will be required. Hence, any trial that includes patients with two miscarriages will show any treatment to be ineffective. Table 19.3 shows a rough scale of the prognosis according to the various prognostic factors, and should give physicians and patients a rough idea as to the relative prognosis.

'GOOD-PROGNOSIS' PATIENTS

These patients include young patients with two or possibly three first-trimester miscarriages. 'Good-prognosis' patients probably require very little investigation. However, they do require reassurance of their prognosis, and 'tender loving care'.

Ultrasound scans on a regular basis can reassure the patient and their partner that the pregnancy is progressing normally. The early pregnancy centres in the UK are invaluable in this approach, especially if they allow the patient access on a 'walk-in' basis. The patient should be reassured that in the event of another miscarriage, further investigations will be carried out, including karyotyping of the abortus, and possibly embryoscopy. It is doubtful whether 'good-prognosis' patients need pharmacological support on an empirical basis. A question arises regarding patients who have undergone partial investigations. For example, if a patient with

Table 19.3 Relative prognoses according to clinical features

	Good prognosis	Medium prognosis	Poor prognosis
No. of miscarriages	2 3	4	5 6 7 8 9
Age	20s	30s	40s
Karyotype of abortus	Aberrant	Normal	Normal
Primary, secondary, or tertiary aborter	Secondary	Primary or tertiary	Primary or tertiary
Early or late losses	Early	Early	Late
Infertility	Normal fertility		Infertility
APCA	Positive	Negative	Negative
NK cells	Normal		High

APCA, antipaternal complement-dependent antibodies; NK, natural killer.

two blighted ova is found to have a septum, it is questionable whether the septum is the cause, or whether it should be resected. A septum has been described to cause abortions of live fetuses in the second or third trimesters after a 'mini labor'.[21] Therefore, should the septum be left in situ, as there is no evidence that it is the cause, or should it be resected, as it may cause late abortions and preterm labor? These questions should be discussed with the patient and partner. It is important to remember that the patient's views are as valid as those laid down in official guidelines. In any recurrent miscarriage clinic, the majority of patients will have a good prognosis. Their good prognosis should not influence the management of patients with a poor prognosis.

'MEDIUM-PROGNOSIS' PATIENTS

This group of patients will include women with three and possibly four miscarriages. The prognosis for a live birth is approximately 60% after three miscarriages (40% after four miscarriages) (Figure 19.1). If these patients are included in a trial, Figure 19.1 shows that treatment of maternal factors can raise the live birth rate by approximately 25%. Again, a trial of treatment for maternal factors would need large numbers to achieve the power to show a statistically significant benefit from treatment. For example, paternal leukocyte immunization was shown to have a statistically significant benefit in the RMITG trial of 419 patients,[14] but not in the trial by Ober et al[11] with 200 patients. I believe that these patients should be investigated, and the standard protocols assessed above give an indication of the criteria for investigation. In this group of patients, investigation may vary, depending on the clinical presentation. Various clinical presentations and their likely causes are described below. In 'medium-prognosis' patients, treatment should be directed at the cause as far as possible. However, despite extensive investigations, the cause is often not apparent. In these cases, there may be a place for empirical hormone support with progesterone or hCG, as there is evidence[22,23]

(although debatable), that these hormones may improve the prognosis by approximately 25%. This treatment is empirical, as there is no investigation in the interval between pregnancies that can diagnose a hormonal defficiency. A problem may arise when the clinical presentation is at variance with the laboratory investigations. For example, should a patient with aPL and a chromosomally abnormal abortus in a previous pregnancy be treated by anticoagulants? As with 'good-prognosis' patients, skill and experience may be necessary to interpret the results.

If there is a presumptive diagnosis, treatment should be prescribed accordingly. Some examples are given below:

- Opinions are divided as to whether patients with parental chromosomal aberrations have a worse prognosis.[24–26] Additionally, they seem to lose eukaryotypic abortuses.[27] Only a few abortuses inherit the aberration in an unbalanced form (5 of 39 abortuses in the series of Carp et al.[27] However, if the fetus does inherit the chromosomal aberration in an unbalanced form, preimplantation genetic diagnosis (PGD) may be appropriate treatment.
- When fetal karyotypic aberrations are present, there is usually a good prognosis. However, there are a few patients with repeat aneuploidy. This was found in 19% of patients in the series of Carp et al,[27] and 10% of patients in the series of Sullivan et al.[28] PGD is appropriate in cases of repeat aneuploidy.
- aPL are generally accepted as a cause of pregnancy loss. However, no trial has assessed β_2-glycoprotein I (β_2GPI)-dependent antibodies, which might be more relevant than assessing aCL and LA. With our present lack of knowledge, treatment seems to be indicated. However, the 'Sapporo' criteria of two readings at least 6 weeks apart should be observed before a definitive diagnosis.[13] In a questionaire[29] sent to 16 experts in obstetrics, rheumatology, immunology, and internal medicine in the USA, UK, France, Spain, Netherlands, Italy, Israel, Argentina, and Brazil the general opinion was to treat with LMWH

and low-dose aspirin from the moment that pregnancy was diagnosed. However, until now, there has been no evidence that aspirin has a therapeutic effect. On the contrary, a meta-analysis of three trials of aspirin has failed to find any therapeutic effect.[30]

- Hereditary thrombophilias are controversial with regard to their role in pregnancy loss. They seem to be associated with late losses rather than early losses.[10] However, the literature is divided on this issue. We investigate hereditary thrombophilias: protein C and antithrombin activities are measured by chromogenic assays, and free protein S antigen is measured by enzyme-linked immunosorbent assay (ELISA). Patients are diagnosed as having protein C, protein S, or antithrombin deficiency if the value of the corresponding protein is below two standard deviations (SD) of the mean level. Protein C resistance is assessed by clotting techniques. Factor V Leiden, the C677T substitution in the methylenetetrahydrofolate reductase (MTHFR) gene, and the G20210A substitution in the factor II gene are detected by polymerase chain reaction (PCR) amplification. However, these tests are costly. Serum fasting homocysteine levels are possibly better indicators than MTHFR. At present, we treat patients with hereditary thrombophilias with anticoagulants, usually the LWMH enoxaparin. We have found this medication to raise the live birth rate by 25% in a comparative cohort study.[31] Randomized trials are sorely needed in order to determine if this approach is justified.

- There is also a dearth of trials to determine the place of uterine malformations. Classically, hysterosalpingography was used to make the diagnosis of uterine anomalies, but the X-ray is uncomfortable for the patient and can only diagnose the uterine cavity. Hysterosalpingography cannot distinguish between a septate and bicornuate uterus. Recently, hysteroscopy has tended to replace X-ray. Hysteroscopy is associated with much less discomfort, but also cannot distinguish between a septate and bicornuate uterus. However, it is the best procedure for diagnosing

other intrauterine pathology such as polyps, fibroids, etc. Three-dimensional (3D) ultrasound is probably the best procedure for distinguishing between a septate and bicornuate uterus. This distinction is essential if hysteroscopic septotomy is considered. However, 3D ultrasound requires specialized equipment and highly trained staff.

'POOR-PROGNOSIS' PATIENTS

These are the patients with five or more consecutive miscarriages. They have been poorly described in the literature, and have formed the subjects of few trials. We have previously reported that these patients constitute approximately 20% of the patients in the Recurrent Miscarriage Immunotherapy Trialists Group register, and 30% of the patients in our service.[32] The Sheba Medical Center acts as a tertiary referral center for patients with RPL, which may explain the higher number of patients with a poor prognosis in our service. The feature that distinguishes these patients is that they have usually had all the investigations and empirical treatments available. Hormone supplements, anticoagulants, hysteroscopic surgery, and often IVF have been tried. Additionally, there may be APS patients who have failed treatment, patients who continue miscarrying after surgery for uterine anomalies, and, in our service, patients who have been treated with anticoagulants for hereditary thrombophilias without success. However, most of these patients have not had fetal karyotyping performed. After five or more miscarriages, the chance of fetal chromosomal aberrations is less than after three miscarriages. Ogasawara et al[6] have shown clearly that the incidence of chromosomal aberrations decreases with the number of miscarriages. Our approach in these patients is to perform alloimmune testing. This will include a cytotoxic crossmatch between maternal serum and paternal cells to detect APCA. Although the absence of these antibodies may not be relevant after three miscarriages, after five or more miscarriages, APCA are less prevalent than in the parous population.[33] The absence of these antibodies indicates a poorer prognosis,[14] and their presence indicates a better prognosis.[17] The numbers and activity of NK cells can also be helpful. Increased numbers of NK cells have been found in the peripheral blood in RPL,[34] particularly in primary aborters,[35] and in luteal phase endometrial biopsies in RPL.[36] Increased numbers and activity of NK cells have also been associated with a poorer prognosis in the subsequent pregnancy.[37,38]

In 'poor-prognosis' patients in whom other forms of treatment have failed, we do use immunotherapy with either paternal leukocyte immunization or IVIG. Paternal leukocyte immunization has been shown to confer a greater benefit after five or more abortions than after three abortions in two meta-analyses.[15,32] The effect is seen mainly in primary aborters. Other trials and meta-analyses of paternal leukocyte immunization are not appropriate for judging the effect on 'poor-prognosis' patients, as the results have been obscured by the 'good-prognosis' and 'medium-prognosis' patients. IVIG has also not been found to be effective when all patients are judged as a homogeneous group.[39,40] However, when 'poor-prognosis' patients are selected, IVIG has been found to improve the live birth rate.[41–43] Unlike paternal leukocyte immunization, the effect has mainly been seen in secondary aborters.[44] Immunotherapy is probably more appropriate in patients losing karyotypically normal embryos.[45]

As with the 'medium-prognosis' patients, we attempt to karyotype the embryo. If immunotherapy fails, and the embryo is karyotypically normal, surrogacy may offer the only possibility of a live birth. If, however, the pregnancy is karyotypically abnormal, a second pregnancy can be attempted with immunotherapy, as immunotherapy cannot prevent chromosomal aberrations. If, however, the patient loses two karyotypically abnormal embryos, PGD should be offered.

SPECIFIC FORMS OF PREGNANCY LOSS

The majority of RPL are losses of blighted ova, in which no fetal heartbeat, or even a fetal shadow, was ever detected on ultrasound. We tend to assess these patients on the basis of their prognosis, as listed above, and to treat them according to karyotypic findings, and to use immunotherapy if there is a poor prognosis.

RECURRENT SECOND-TRIMESTER FETAL DEATH

This group of patients has a poorer prognosis than that after first-trimester losses.[5] It is therefore justified to investigate and treat after two losses. The chance of a second-trimester loss being due to chromosomal aberrations is less than in first-trimester miscarriages. However, there may be fetal structural anomalies. Hence, detailed ultrasound may assist the diagnosis. Another possibility for diagnosing fetal structural anomalies is embryofetoscopy. Diabetes should be excluded, as it predisposes to fetal anomalies.

Thrombotic mechanisms, due either to APS or to hereditary thrombophilias, are more likely to cause fetal demise than first-trimester miscarriages.[10,46] If either of these is found, in the presence of recurrent second-trimester fetal deaths, treatment by anticoagulants is warranted. New thrombophilias are constantly being identified. Microparticles and protein Z deficiency are two such examples. These thrombophilias are not usually excluded in any investigation protocol. Hence, there may be a place for using anticoagulants on an empirical basis in the absence of APS or hereditary thrombophilia. However, no trial has assessed anticoagulants in unexplained recurrent second-trimester losses.

Drakeley et al[47] have summarized a database analysis of 636 patients attending a UK miscarriage clinic. Second-trimester miscarriages accounted for 25% of miscarriages in their series; 33% tested positive for aPL, there was a 4% prevalence of uterine anomaly, 3% could be explained by infections, and 2% of patients were hypothyroid. In 50% of patients, no diagnosis was apparent. However, hereditary thrombophilias were not investigated in this series.

LOSSES OF LIVE EMBRYOS

Live embryos may be lost in the first or second trimesters. The distinguishing feature of these losses is that the uterus starts to contract, and vaginal bleeding precedes fetal demise. There may be placental separation and retroplacental hematoma formation. These forms of pregnancy loss are relatively rare, comprising approximately 11% of RPL.[48] Losses of live embryos or fetuses are less likely to be due to an embryonic or fetal factor, and more likely to be due to a uterine or other maternal factor. However, patients with this clinical presentation have not been investigated as a separate group. Hence, there is no evidence to support any conclusions about this group. In the first trimester, there is a typical history. Embryonic development is normal. The uterus suddenly starts to contract, and abortion can ensue. Abortion may be fast, within half an hour,[48] or it may take longer. In abortion of live embryos we recommend testing for uterine anomalies and infections. In patients who are pregnant and present with a hematoma, empirical prophylactic antibiotics may have a place in preventing the hematoma from becoming infected. In the case of an infection, uterine contractions follow rapidly, with expulsion of the uterine contents. In the case of second-trimester losses of live fetuses, uterine anomalies, infections, and possibly diabetes (which predisposes to infections) should be investigated. In the presence of contractions in the second trimester, tocolytic agents may be appropriate. Again, the appropriate trials to determine an optimal course of management have not been carried out.

Unfortunately, most patients do not know the character of the miscarriage. They will only know this if ultrasound has previously been performed in order to detect a fetal heartbeat.

MIXED PATTERN OF PREGNANCY LOSSES

In many cases, each pregnancy loss may have a different clinical presentation. For example, there may be a blighted ovum followed by an abortion of a live fetus in the second trimester, followed by a missed abortion. These mixed patterns of pregnancy loss are relatively frequent in patients with three losses, but rare in patients with five or more losses. In patients with a mixed pattern of pregnancy loss, the cause is more likely to be due to chance, and the prognosis is good. Inclusion of these patients in a trial of treatment may well confound the results, and raise the live birth rate of a control group of patients. In our opinion, they probably do not require active treatment. If included in any research protocol, they should be considered as a separate group of patients.

CASE PRESENTATIONS

This section illustrates certain difficult cases in order to show their different presentations and the likely causes and methods of management.

PATIENT 1

This patient, age 22, para 0, presented after six miscarriages between 8 and 9 weeks. No fetal heart had ever been detected, except in the fourth pregnancy, when a fetal heart was said to be present at 6 weeks. However, the pregnancy showed no fetal shadow from 7 weeks onwards until curettage was performed for a blighted ovum at 9 weeks. The fourth pregnancy was found to have a normal 46,XX karyotype. The following features had been investigated and found to be normal. Parental karyotypes were 46,XX and 46,XY. LA, aCL, and hereditary thrombophilias were normal. Hormone levels (luteinizing hormone, follicle-stimulating hormone, and prolactin) were normal. Midluteal progesterone levels were 18 ng/ml. Thyroid function was normal. There was no diabetes. Hysteroscopy showed a normal cavity. APCA were negative. NK-cell testing was not performed at that time. The third pregnancy was treated with progesterone supplements. The fourth and fifth pregnancies were treated with enoxaparin and aspirin on an empirical basis. The sixth pregnancy was untreated. The patient was treated by paternal leukocyte immunization between the sixth and seventh pregnancies. Immunizations were boosted until seroconversion occurred with the development of APCA directed towards paternal HLA antigens. This is our current regimen.[18] The seventh pregnancy was uneventful. No additional medications were administered. The seventh pregnancy terminated in the delivery of a female infant, 3580 g, at 40 weeks. The eighth pregnancy is presently 7 weeks, with a live embryo.

PATIENT 2

This patient, age 24, para 0, presented after three abortions between 12 and 16 weeks. From the history, it was apparent that these were abortions of live fetuses. Hysteroscopy showed a large and thick septum that divided the uterus. The external contour of the uterus was shown to be normal on laparoscopy. The septum was resected hysteroscopically until the fundus of the uterus. The fourth pregnancy terminated as a blighted ovum at 8 weeks. Although a fourth miscarriage may sound like a failure of treatment, this was not so, as the blighted ovum was found to be triploid. The fifth pregnancy terminated as induced labor at 42 weeks, and the sixth pregnancy in spontaneous labor at 40 weeks.

PATIENT 3

This patient, age 30, para 1, a secondary aborter, presented after four midtrimester losses. The first pregnancy terminated as an uncomplicated delivery of a female infant 4050 g. The second pregnancy terminated as a fetal death at 17 weeks, and the third pregnancy as a fetal death at 19 weeks. Parental karyotyping was normal. Glucose challenge tests and thyroid function were normal. Hysteroscopy showed a normal uterine cavity. Thrombophilia testing showed the patient to be homozygous for the MTHFR mutation.[49,50] However, homocysteine levels were normal. The fourth and fifth pregnancies were treated with enoxaparin 40 mg from detection of the fetal heartbeat. However, these pregnancies terminated at 18 and 16 weeks, respectively, with intrauterine fetal deaths. The sixth pregnancy was treated with enoxaparin 80 mg daily. The pregnancy terminated as a cesarean section at 39 weeks. A live male infant of 3240 g was delivered. Although the dose of 40 mg has been compared with 80 mg in a large cohort of patients,[51] and both doses have been found to be equally effective, there may be individual patients in whom the larger doses are required.

PATIENT 4

This patient, age 38, was a secondary aborter with two live births followed by six miscarriages, most of which were missed abortions in which a previous fetal heart was lost between 10 and 12 weeks. Investigation showed APCA to be positive. There was no APS, thrombophilia, or other cause apparent for the miscarriages. The parental karyotypes were 46,XX and 46,XY with a balanced translocation: t(14;13)(p11;q12). The subsequent pregnancy was a missed abortion at 10 weeks. Again, a previously detected fetal heartbeat was lost. This pregnancy was found to be 46,XY, −4, tder(4;13), i.e., monosomy 4. Instead of the second chromosome 4, there was a chromosome with a small section of chromosome 4 and the translocated sections of chromosomes 13 and 14. The patient has been advised to have PGD if she desires another child. PGD will use probes for chromosomes 4, 13, and 14. Meantime, the patient has decided to complete her family with two children.

PATIENT 5

This patient, age 40, para 0, presented after four pregnancy losses. There had been ruptured membranes at 20 weeks, and two intrauterine fetal deaths at 20 weeks, accompanied by hypertension and gestational diabetes. The fourth pregnancy was a missed abortion at 14 weeks. These four pregnancies were achieved from four cycles of zygote intrafallopian transfer (ZIFT). There were no apparent explanations for the pregnancy losses. There was no aPL or hereditary thrombophilia. Hysteroscopy was normal. The parental karyotypes were 46,XX and 46,XY. The fifth pregnancy was achieved by eight cycles of IVF following 22 months of infertility. The fifth pregnancy was treated with aspirin 100 mg. However, the pregnancy was terminated artificially at 22 weeks for severe preeclampsia with HELLP syndrome.

The patient was advised surrogacy. However, she conceived spontaneously while making arrangements for surrogacy. She was treated empirically with enoxaparin 40 mg daily and aspirin 100 mg. At 12 weeks, nuchal translucency screening was normal. A Shirodkar suture was inserted at 13 weeks, due to the previous ruptured membranes at 20 weeks. However, preeclampsia and gestational diabetes developed at 18 weeks, followed by fetal demise. The patient used a surrogate mother who has delivered her a healthy term male infant.

CONCLUSIONS

RPL is not one homogeneous condition. Hence, there is no one protocol that is applicable. The aim of the standard protocols is entirely laudible – to advise physicians with little experience of RPL as to the optimal methods of diagnosis and treatment. Hence, the standard protocols try to guarantee that the patient receives effective treatment, and that ineffective treatment is not used. However, the standard protocols listed above might have done more harm than good, as they treat RPL as one homogeneous group. Hence, their recommendations preclude the treatment of subgroups of patients. The development of an optimal investigation protocol depends on reaching an accurate diagnosis of cause and directing treatment to that diagnosis. Fetal karyotyping and embryoscopy hold out the possibility of more accurately diagnosing embryonic or fetal causes of pregnancy loss. Treatments that have not been shown to be effective when tried on a large cohort of patients may be found to be highly effective when only used on a subgroup of patients with an accurate diagnosis.

REFERENCES

1. Royal College of Obstetricians and Gynaecologists, Guideline No. 17. The Management of Recurrent Miscarriage. London: RCOG, 2003.
2. American College of Obstetricians and Gynecologists. Management of recurrent early pregnancy loss, ACOG Practice Bulletin No. 24, February 2001. Int J Gynecol Obstet 2002; 78:179–90.
3. Jauniaux E, Farquharson RG, Christiansen OB, et al. Evidence-based guidelines for the investigation and medical treatment of recurrent miscarriage. Hum Reprod 2006; 21:2216–22.
4. Carp HJA. Update on recurrent pregnancy loss. In: Ratnam SS, Ng SC, Arulkumaran S, eds. Contributions to Obstetrics and Gynaecology. Singapore: Oxford University Press, 2000.
5. Goldenberg RL, Mayberry SK, Copper RL, et al. Pregnancy outcome following a second-trimester loss. Obstet Gynecol 1993; 81:444–6.
6. Ogasawara M, Aoki K, Okada S, et al. Embryonic karyotype of aborptuses in relation to the number of previous miscarriages. Fertil Steril 2000; 73:300–4.
7. Storring PL, Gaines-Das RE, Bangham DR. International reference preparation of human chorionic gonadotrophin for immunoassay: potency estimates in various bioassay and protein binding assay systems; and international reference preparations of the α and β subunits of human chorionic gonadotrophin for immunoassay. J Endocrinol 1980; 84:295–310.
8. Carp HJA, Toder V, Mashiach S, Rabinovici J. The effect of paternal leukocyte immunization on implantation after recurrent biochemical pregnancies and repeated failure of embryo transfer. Am J Reprod Immunol 1994; 31:112–15.
9. Farquharson RG, Jauniaux E, Exalto N. ESHRE Special Interest Group for Early Pregnancy (SIGEP). Updated and revised nomenclature for description of early pregnancy events. Hum Reprod 2005; 20:3008–11.
10. Preston FE, Rosendaal FR, Walker ID, et al. Increased fetal loss in women with heritable thrombophilia. Lancet 1996; 348:913–16.
11. Ober C, Karrison T, Odem RR, et al. Mononuclear-cell immunisation in prevention of recurrent miscarriages: a randomised trial. Lancet 1999; 354:365–9.
12. Laskin CA, Bombardier C, Hannah ME, et al. Prednisone and aspirin in women with autoantibodies and unexplained recurrent fetal loss. N Engl J Med 1997; 337:148–53.
13. Wilson WA, Gharavi AE, Koike T, et al. International consensus statement on preliminary classification for definite antiphospholipid syndrome. Arthritis Rheum 1999; 42:1309–11.
14. Recurrent Miscarriage Immunotherapy Trialists Group. Worldwide collaborative observational study and metaanalysis on allogenic leukocyte immunotherapy for recurrent spontaneous abortion. Am J Reprod Immunol 1994; 32:55–72.
15. Daya S, Gunby J. The effectiveness of allogeneic leukocyte immunization in unexplained primary recurrent spontaneous abortion. Am J Reprod Immunol 1994; 32:294-302.
16. Cauchi MN, Pepperell R, Kloss M, et al. Predictors of pregnancy success in repeated miscarriages. Am J Reprod Immunol 1991; 26:72–5.
17. Cowchock FS, Smith JB, David S, et al. Paternal mononuclear cell immunization. Therapy for repeated miscarriage: predictive values for pregnancy success. Am J Reprod Immunol 1990; 22:12–17.
18. Orgad S, Gazit E, Lowenthal R, et al. The prognostic value of antipaternal antibodies and leukocyte immunizations on the proportion of live births in couples with consecutive recurrent miscarriages. Hum Reprod 1999; 14:2974–9.
19. Aoki K, Kajiura S, Matsumoto Y, et al. Preconceptional natural-killer-cell activity as a predictor of miscarriage. Lancet 1995; 345:1340–2.
20. Shakhar K, Ben-Eliyahu S, Rosen E, et al. Primary versus secondary recurrent miscarriage: differences in number and activity of peripheral NK cells. Fertil Steril 2003; 80:368–75.
21. Rock JA, Jones HW. The clinical management of the double uterus. Fertil Steril 1977; 28:798–806.
22. Daya S. Efficacy of progesterone support for pregnancy in women with recurrent miscarriage: a meta-analysis of controlled trials. Br J Obstet Gynaecol 1989; 96:275–80.
23. Scott JR, Pattison N. Human chorionic gonadotrophin for recurrent miscarriage. Cochrane Database Syst Rev 2000; (2):CD000101.

24. Carp HJA, Feldman B, Oelsner G, et al. Parental karyotype and subsequent live births in recurrent miscarriage. Fertil Steril 2004; 81:1296–301.

25. Goddijn M, Joosten JH, Knegt AC, et al. Clinical relevance of diagnosing structural chromosome abnormalities in couples with repeated miscarriage. Hum Reprod 2004; 19:1013–17.

26. Sugiura-Ogasawara M, Ozaki Y, Sato T, et al. Poor prognosis of recurrent aborters with either maternal or paternal reciprocal translocations. Fertil Steril 2004; 81:367–73.

27. Carp HJA, Guetta E, Dorf H, et al. Embryonic karyotype in recurrent miscarriage with parental karyotypic aberrations. Fertil Steril 2006; 85:446–50.

28. Sullivan AE, Silver RM, LaCoursiere DY, et al. Recurrent fetal aneuploidy and recurrent miscarriage. Obstet Gynecol 2004; 104:784–8.

29. Tincani A, Branch DW, Levy RA, et al. Treatment of pregnant patients with antiphospholipid syndrome. Lupus 2003; 12:524–9.

30. Empson M, Lassere M, Craig JC, et al. Recurrent pregnancy loss with antiphospholipid antibody: a systematic review of therapeutic trials. Obstet Gynecol 2002; 99:135–44.

31. Carp HJA, Dolitzky M, Inbal A. Thromboprophylaxis improves the live birth rate in women with consecutive recurrent miscarriages and hereditary thrombophilia. J Thromb Haemost 2003; 1:433–8.

32. Carp HJA, Toder V, Torchinsky A, et al. Allogeneic leukocyte immunization in women with five or more recurrent abortions. Hum Reprod 1997; 12:250–5.

33. Carp HJA, Toder V, Mashiach S. Immunotherapy of habitual abortion. Am J Reprod Immunol 1993; 28:281–4.

34. Emmer PM, Nelen WL, Steegers EA, et al. Peripheral natural killer cytotoxicity and CD56+CD16+ cells increase during early pregnancy in women with a history of recurrent spontaneous abortion. Hum Reprod 2000; 15:1163–9.

35. Shakhar K, Ben-Eliyahu S, Loewenthal R, et al. Differences in number and activity of peripheral natural killer cells in primary versus secondary recurrent miscarriage. Fertil Steril 2003; 80:368–75.

36. Clifford K, Flanagan AM, Regan L. Endometrial CD56+ natural killer cells in women with recurrent miscarriage: a histomorphometric study. Hum Reprod 1999; 14:2727–30.

37. Aoki K, Kajiura S, Matsumoto Y, et al. Preconceptional natural-killer-cell activity as a predictor of miscarriage. Lancet 1995; 345:1340–2.

38. Coulam CB, Beaman KD. Reciprocal alteration in circulating TJ6+CD19+ and TJ6+CD56+ leukocytes in early pregnancy predicts success or miscarriage. Am J Reprod Immunol 1995; 34:219–24.

39. Daya S, Gunby J, Clark DA. Intravenous immunoglobulin therapy for recurrent spontaneous abortion: a meta-analysis. Am J Reprod Immunol 1998; 39:69–76.

40. Porter TF, LaCoursiere Y, Scott JR. Immunotherapy for recurrent miscarriage. Cochrane Database Syst Rev 2006; (2):CD000112.

41. Carp HJA, Toder V, Gazit E. Further experience with intravenous immunoglobulin in women with recurrent miscarriage and a poor prognosis. Am J Reprod Immunol 2001; 46:268–73.

42. Yamada H, Kishida T, Kobayashi N, et al. Massive immunoglobulin treatment in women with four or more recurrent spontaneous primary abortions of unexplained aetiology. Hum Reprod 1998; 13:2620–3.

43. Christiansen OB. Intravenous immunoglobulin in the prevention of recurrent spontaneous abortion: the European experience. Am J Reprod Immunol 1998; 39:77–81.

44. Christiansen OB, Pedersen B, Rosgaard A, et al. A randomized, double-blind, placebo-controlled trial of intravenous immunoglobulin in the prevention of recurrent miscarriage: evidence for a therapeutic effect in women with secondary recurrent miscarriage. Hum Reprod 2002; 17:809–16.

45. Clark DA, Daya S, Coulam CB, et al. Implications of abnormal human trophoblast karyotype of the evidence-based approach to the understanding, investigation, and treatment of recurrent spontaneous abortion. Am J Reprod Immunol 1996; 35:495–8.

46. Grandone E, Margaglione M, Colaizzo D, et al. Factor V Leiden is associated with repeated and recurrent unexplained fetal losses. Thromb Haemost 1997; 77:822–4.

47. Drakeley AJ, Quenby S, Farquharson RG. Mid-trimester loss – appraisal of a screening protocol. Hum Reprod 1998; 13:1975–80.

48. Carp HJA, Toder V, Mashiach S, et al. Recurrent miscarriage: a review of current concepts, immune mechanisms, and results of treatment. Obstet Gynecol Surv 1990; 45:657–69.

49. Arruda VR, Von zuben PM, Chiapurini LC, et al. The mutation Ala677-Val in the methylene tetrahydrofolate reductase gene: a risk factor for arterial disease and venous thrombosis. Thromb Haemost 1997; 77:818–21.

50. Nelen WL, Blom HJ, Thomas CM, et al. Methylenetetrahydrofolate reductase polymorphism affects the change in homocysteine and folate concentrations resulting from low dose folic acid supplementation in women with unexplained recurrent miscarriages. J Nutr 1998; 128:1336–41.

51. Brenner B, Hoffman R, Carp HJA, et al. The LIVE-ENOX Investigators. Efficacy and safety of two doses of enoxaparin in women with thrombophilia and recurrent pregnancy loss: the LIVE–ENOX study. J Thromb Haemost 2005; 3:227–9.

20. A patient's perspective

Mindy Gross

I had six miscarriages in less than three years. In retrospect, this seems to be a physical impossibility. Although each miscarriage stands starkly alone in my mind, having six of them in such a short span of time produced a cumulative effect. Each presented me with peculiar challenges and carried its own unique message. On each occasion, I was in a different hospital either in America or in Israel, with different doctors and different walls to witness my misery. It was natural to begin getting that deja vu feeling, 'Haven't I been here before?' Yet, when I looked around, I was forced to admit that – 'No, I had never been *here* before'. Looking back, it seems as if each miscarriage demanded its own identity, its own space in my brain. Each refused to be lumped together with the others.

In retrospect, I had undergone six different and distinct losses. One might think that the loss becomes easier or at least less painful with each successive miscarriage. It doesn't. On the contrary, the physical pain is as fresh and as potent each time. The emotional suffering involved in the loss only increases. It has been said that humans can acclimate themselves to the most horrendous of circumstances; the 'getting used to it' impulse seems to be very strong. This was not the case. I never got used to losing a nascent child.

Although each time I was more prepared on a practical level, I was never prepared on an emotional level. Each miscarriage came as a shock, though the physical symptoms often repeated themselves. The initial trouble always began suddenly; without warning, a stain would appear. Foolishly, I would think 'Could I just wish it away – make believe it didn't exist?' As the sharp pains in my back and cramping increased, I started to ramble, 'Could I have a nervous breakdown simultaneously with a miscarriage?' The hemorrhaging was merciless and, as was now my custom, I grabbed some towels and headed to the car to take me to the hospital.

I had felt pregnant. I had experienced the morning sickness that seemed to last the whole day. Now I wish I hadn't. At least I would have been spared the pain of feeling the symptoms disappear. I was filled to the brim with disappointment. Miscarriage is a death, though perhaps not acknowledged as such by the world outside of the family who have suffered the loss. At the time of my miscarriages, I could not articulate this feeling, but it was very real. I was frightened by the fragility of life. I knew that I had experienced a touch of death, for something had died within me.

The trauma of miscarriage stems from lost hope that was so briefly, and so very vividly, alive. For all of the frustration of infertility, it is one-dimensional, monochromatic – negative, negative, negative, void and nothingness. Miscarriage by contrast is multichromatic. You have hope and a life inside you, and then it is lost – both the child and the hope. Surprisingly, I found that I never became jaded. No matter how many losses, each conception reawakened in me the belief that this time it was going to be different.

The assumption that children will arrive soon or easily, or at least whenever the couple desires them, is a normal assumption, but also a very dangerous one. My family and friends have children. They don't have miscarriages. So, although I may have known intellectually that miscarriages are not that uncommon, my unexpected complications were not part of my everyday consciousness. Infertility and miscarriage are unfortunate things that happen to 'other people'. Since it was too painful to imagine these difficulties in our own lives, when they did occur, I found that I was at a total loss. As the effects of one miscarriage seemed to spill over into the next miscarriage, one truth pervaded my thoughts: I was still barren.

Barren. What a horrible word. It conjures up images of the American southwest, of Arizona and Georgia O'Keeffe's paintings. One of O'Keeffe's favorite motifs is a dry horse's skull sitting on the desert's sand. No signs of life there. Some of the most wretched terrain on earth, incapable of creating and sustaining life. Barren. What a pitiful way to hear oneself described. The label 'fruitless' was so contrary to the way I had perceived myself my whole life. I was always very fruitful, I was a producer. Now I was deficient. I didn't have what it takes to 'produce' in the most valuable of all endeavors – conceiving a child and sustaining a pregnancy.

Bitter. A word I never had an affinity for. Bittersweet chocolate is, to me, a very poor substitute for the real thing: gooey milk chocolate. Bitter implies something unappealing and most certainly not the ideal. Over the span of my years of infertility and often agonizing tests, I asked myself, 'Was I becoming bitter?' I resolved with all my heart that this was one sentiment that would have no place in my vocabulary. Bitterness was a particularly astringent emotion. One whose intensity I felt would be better put to use on other needs and emotions, particularly at such a sensitive time in my life. Bitterness twists one's core personality and corrodes a person's resources and strengths. I was concerned that becoming bitter would have held me back from full participation in and enjoyment of the births of my nieces and nephews as well as countless friends. It would have constricted my own flow of love and giving when that is indeed what I needed to do most.

All I wanted was to have a normal life. After having been married for seven years and wanting children, 'normal' by definition would mean a baby in my arms. Other women I know who have suffered pregnancy losses have also remarked that they too just wanted their lives to be 'normal'. I craved the ordinary, the mundane tasks of motherhood, but they continued to elude me. I also felt confused. I hadn't heard much about miscarriages before, and even if they were relatively commonplace, they were not part of my lexicon. I did read in a book about women suffering from multiple miscarriages the following, which I could strongly relate to. Friedman and Gradstein in their book, *Surviving*

Pregnancy Loss[1] write: 'When you lost your first pregnancy, everyone told you not to worry, it happens to a lot of people. Remember, you are young and healthy and have lots of time to have babies.' But the authors continue, 'Other women have babies so easily; why not you? Lightening is not supposed to strike twice in the same place, and certainly not three or four times.'

My earlier difficulties with conception often left me with a very frightening thought: 'What if I never conceive?' With the miscarriages, I knew my situation was different. Somehow, I believed that in most cases when a woman conceives again and again, the likelihood is that sooner or later a pregnancy should sustain itself. I would periodically remind myself that there were women I knew who never even had the good fortune of having a hope to cling to. Yet, a nagging doubt was lodged in my consciousness and a subtle fear accompanied me wherever I went. My fear was based on the lesson that the miscarriages had taught me. Human existence is very fragile. There are no guarantees.

My body was out of control. First it refused my command to become pregnant and then it refused to hold on to the pregnancy. Since my infertility problems were unexpected, as until now I was a healthy female specimen, this bizarre turn of events caused me to lose my balance. I was young, athletic, never smoked, and only had an occasional glass of wine. Why was my body failing me? I felt that I was twirling in an almost dizzy fashion. Not only was my body out of control, but my life seemed to be spiraling in a direction I could not identify. Once the possibility of childlessness entered my mind, it never departed. It lurked in the shadows of my brain, pushing to the fore at the most unexpected moments. Just when I was enjoying myself, actively engaged in the world around me, the sinking feeling would come rushing back: *I may never, ever give birth to a child. I may never, ever be a natural biological mother.* Paralysis seeped in. It was as if my body froze and my mind locked. Everything was now out of control. I would try to push the ugly thoughts out and concentrate on my life. I focused on my career, my family, my community, and my friends. But the thoughts were still there. The harsh fact of my being a 'habitual aborter' lingered on and on. It aggressively invaded my consciousness and colored my perception of the world. In fact, the cumulative experiences of years of infertility and failed pregnancy had shaken me to my core. My world had suddenly become a whirlwind of intense and mighty emotions. Hope and despair would rage. I found that in the midst of my mundane activities, I was now insecure and frightened. Some of these emotions I felt quite powerfully for the first time in my life. I was distraught and disillusioned. The world had turned bleary.

On a particularly overcast and gloomy day in New York, I entered Brooks Brothers Department Store. Suddenly, I had an overwhelming need to buy a personal diary. The pocket diary I found was maroon and leather and was a present to myself, a consolation prize for bearing circumstances that would crumble many a strong individual. The gold-leafed diary cost more than the budget would normally allow, even if it did bear the distinguished Brooks Brothers insignia. I distinctly remember the day that I bought it. I had been diagnosed with a 'grapefruit-size' ovarian cyst, the latest mishap in my uncontrollable reproductive system. I was nothing less than frenzied, with my cyst surgery looming. With the diary in hand, I hurried to the corner of an enormous Hallmark card store in Manhattan and opened it to the back page. With a burning need, I wrote down the dates, locations and treatments of the miscarriages. I also included the upcoming appointments, the date of my cyst surgery, and all the various treatments I had undergone since the onset of my infertility problems. What if this information would be important some day? How would I remember all the details if I didn't record it somewhere? My response to all my suffering at that time was the emotional equivalent of the diary's blank pages. I was silenced. No words could ever convey the emptiness I felt. But the precise week of each pregnancy loss, each doctor, and each treatment would occupy the gold-leaf pages. Some empty lines would be filled in, in the not too distant future, with the last and most crucial treatment that was yet to come. From time to time, I take out the diary to remember the tears that were shed in that

Hallmark store. Amid the baubles and balloons, the shelves of colorful cards announcing every sort of happy occasion, I was occasionless. I wept and felt my precious lost souls wept with me. I stared in disbelief at the dates and the memories they evoked. I felt weighted down as I held the small maroon diary in my hand. The year 1986 was embossed in gold numbers on the front cover of the book. Could I have imagined what occasion would yet occur during that year?

A well-meaning friend had clipped an article from the local newspaper detailing an experimental treatment for multiple miscarriages. The treatment was initiated in England and was now being offered by a pioneering doctor in Israel. This was actually a rather frequent occurrence; concerned friends would drop by to relay information about some new and innovative medical technology they had learned of from the media. Of course, I very much appreciated their support, but as time passed and no experts had the answers I sought, and all the latest treatments had apparently failed, these suggestions only served as a constant reminder of my childlessness. I truly felt loved by all those who called and cared enough to keep me in their thoughts and prayers. No doubt it was my pain and my insecurity about the future that made each suggestion so difficult. I was tired of being disappointed, sick of hanging my hope of becoming a mother on some new innovative medical treatment. Looking back, I think I was also tired of disappointing everyone around me. This particular newspaper article was especially ill-timed; it arrived as the hemorrhaging of my sixth consecutive miscarriage worsened. As I lay on my bed, the only thing I could be sure of was that I didn't want to look at, much less consider, any new 'treatments'. I certainly could not face another doctor. Each new doctor would need my medical history, and with each retelling I found myself reliving. Six miscarriages, six different doctors, six different hospitals. Could I tell this sorrowful tale one more time? I crumpled the article and placed it in the wastepaper basket next to my bed amongst all of the tear-filled tissues. The cramping continued and I knew with certainty that I couldn't and wouldn't ever have the energy to face another treatment protocol. In fact, the only thing I wanted was to survive this most recent hardship and sit very still, by myself, for a long, long time.

As the bleeding intensified, I could fool myself no longer. I needed a doctor. I turned to the wastepaper basket. The discarded ball of newspaper stared up at me. I felt it was actually challenging me – daring me to try once again. Suddenly, that rejected article became the focus of my anger, frustration, and all my hope. My decision to take an experimental treatment was not an easy one. I was concerned with the unclear repercussions, but the confidence and sincere concern of my doctor helped me move forward. Treatments in general are not just the filling of prescriptions, scheduling doctors' appointments, and undergoing procedures. The word 'treatment' equals the word 'hope'. It was therefore very difficult for me to see any treatment as routine.

Infertility and pregnancy loss presented me with challenges and choices that were often painful and difficult to make. My personal suffering had been well hidden behind the guise of a 'normal life'. As a result, the life crisis that evolved with my pregnancy losses was often misunderstood. Pregnancy loss creates isolation, an overwhelming feeling of sadness. I felt vulnerable and out of control. These are intense and powerful emotions, which need to be recognized, identified, and dealt with. My own personal experience was that my spirit could be crushed or elated by the result of a blood test, because its results meant the difference between life and death in pregnancy, or between a healthy organ and a diseased one. Each doctor's visit became a focal point, a touchstone, a painful reality check as to how realistic it was to believe that motherhood was still within my grasp. Now nearly twenty years later from the birth of the first of my three children, writing this chapter still evokes such powerful emotions that it is as if it is in 'real time'. Tears flow freely. Painful memories are now intertwined with joy that soars and knows no bounds. The years of infertility and multiple pregnancy loss will always be an integral part of my most essential self. That self came to motherhood with profound blessings from G-d and the pioneering and brave efforts of dedicated doctors and hospital staff, all to whom I am forever grateful.

REFERENCE

1. Friedman R, Gradstein B. Surviving Pregnancy Loss: A Complete Sourcebook for Women and Their Families. Boston: Little, Brown, 1992.

Index

N.B. Page numbers in *italic* denote figures and tables.